ONE WEEK LOAN

Renew Books on PHONE-it: 01443 654456

Books are to be returned on or before the last date below

Better Than Conscious?

Strüngmann Forum Reports

The Ernst Strüngmann Forum is made possible through the generous support of the Ernst Strüngmann Foundation, inaugurated by Dr. Andreas and Dr. Thomas Strüngmann.

Additional support for this Forum was received from:
Deutsche Forschungsgemeinschaft (German Science Foundation),
the Dresdner Bank, and the city of Frankfurt.

Better Than Conscious?

Decision Making, the Human Mind, and Implications for Institutions

Edited by

Christoph Engel and Wolf Singer

Program Advisory Committee:

Christoph Engel, Paul Glimcher, Kevin McCabe,
Peter J. Richerson, Lael Schooler, and Wolf Singer

The MIT Press

Cambridge, Massachusetts
London, England

© 2008 Massachusetts Institute of Technology and
the Frankfurt Institute for Advanced Studies

Series Editor: J. Lupp
Assistant Editor: M. Turner
Photographs: U. Dettmar
Typeset by BerlinScienceWorks

MIT Press books may be purchased at special quantity discounts
for business or sales promotional use. For information, please email
special_sales@mitpress.mit.edu or write to Special Sales Department,
The MIT Press, 55 Hayward Street, Cambridge, MA 02142.

The book was set in TimesNewRoman and Arial.
Printed and bound in China.

Library Congress Cataloging-in-Publication Data

Ernst Strüngmann Forum (2007 : Frankfurt, Germany)
  Better than conscious? : decision making, the human mind, and implications
for institutions / edited by Christoph Engel and Wolf Singer.
     p. ; cm. — (Strüngmann Forum reports)
  Forum held June 10–15, 2007 in Frankfurt, Germany.
  Includes bibliographical references and index.
  ISBN 978-0-262-19580-5 (hardcover : alk. paper)
  1. Decision making—Physiological aspects—Congresses. 2. Decision
making—Social aspects—Congresses. 3. Cognitive neuroscience—
Congresses. I. Engel, Christoph, 1956– II. Singer, W. (Wolf) III. Title. IV.
Series.
  [DNLM: 1. Brain—physiology—Congresses. 2. Cognitive Science—
Congresses. 3. Decision Making—Congresses. 4. Mental Processes—
Congresses. WL 300 E727b 2008]
  QP395.E76 2007
  612.8—dc22
                        2008000030

Contents

The Ernst Strüngmann Forum   vii

List of Contributors   ix

Preface   xiii

1   **Better Than Conscious?**
The Brain, the Psyche, Behavior, and Institutions   1
Christoph Engel and Wolf Singer

2   **Conscious and Nonconscious Processes:**
Distinct Forms of Evidence Accumulation?   21
Stanislas Dehaene

3   **The Role of Value Systems in Decision Making**   51
Peter Dayan

4   **Neurobiology of Decision Making: An Intentional Framework**   71
Michael N. Shadlen, Roozbeh Kiani, Timothy D. Hanks,
and Anne K. Churchland

5   **Brain Signatures of Social Decision Making**   103
Kevin McCabe and Tania Singer

6   **Neuronal Correlates of Decision Making**   125
Michael Platt, Rapporteur
Peter Dayan, Stanislas Dehaene, Kevin McCabe,
Randolf Menzel, Elizabeth Phelps, Hilke Plassmann,
Roger Ratcliff, Michael Shadlen, and Wolf Singer

7   **The Evolution of Implicit and Explicit Decision Making**   155
Robert Kurzban

8   **Passive Parallel Automatic Minimalist Processing**   173
Roger Ratcliff and Gail McKoon

9   **How Culture and Brain Mechanisms**
Interact in Decision Making   191
Merlin Donald

10   **Marr, Memory, and Heuristics**   207
Lael J. Schooler

11   **Explicit and Implicit Strategies in Decision Making**   225
Christian Keysers, Rapporteur
Robert Boyd, Jonathan Cohen, Merlin Donald, Werner Güth,
Eric Johnson, Robert Kurzban, Lael J. Schooler, Jonathan Schooler,
Elizabeth Spelke, and Julia Trommershäuser

12   **How Evolution Outwits Bounded Rationality:**
     The Efficient Interaction of Automatic and
     Deliberate Processes in Decision Making
     and Implications for Institutions   259
     Andreas Glöckner

13   **The Evolutionary Biology of Decision Making**   285
     Jeffrey R. Stevens

14   **Gene–Culture Coevolution and the**
     Evolution of Social Institutions   305
     Robert Boyd and Peter J. Richerson

15   **Individual Decision Making and the**
     Evolutionary Roots of Institutions   325
     Richard McElreath, Rapporteur
     Robert Boyd, Gerd Gigerenzer, Andreas Glöckner,
     Peter Hammerstein, Robert Kurzban, Stefan Magen,
     Peter J. Richerson, Arthur Robson, and Jeffrey R. Stevens

16   **The Neurobiology of Individual Decision Making,**
     Dualism, and Legal Accountability   343
     Paul W. Glimcher

17   **Conscious and Nonconscious Cognitive**
     Processes in Jurors' Decisions   371
     Reid Hastie

18   **Institutions for Intuitive Man**   391
     Christoph Engel

19   **Institutional Design Capitalizing on the**
     Intuitive Nature of Decision Making   413
     Mark Lubell, Rapporteur
     Christoph Engel, Paul W. Glimcher, Reid Hastie,
     Jeffrey J. Rachlinski, Bettina Rockenbach, Reinhard Selten,
     Tania Singer, and Elke U. Weber

Name Index   433

Subject Index   443

The Ernst Strüngmann Forum

The Ernst Strüngmann Forum is founded on the tenets of scientific independence and the inquisitive nature of the human mind. Through its innovative
communication process, the Ernst Strüngmann Forum facilitates the continual
expansion of knowledge by providing a creative environment within which
experts can scrutinize high-priority issues from multiple vantage points.

The themes that are selected transcend classic disciplinary boundaries; they
address topics that are problem-oriented and of high-priority interest. Proposals are submitted by leading scientists active in their field and are selected by a
scientific advisory board, comprised of internationally recognized members.

This particular theme began when Christoph Engel and Wolf Singer submitted a proposal entitled, "Better than Conscious? Exploiting the Capacity of
Humans to Reach Decisions by Both Serial and Parallel Processing of Information." Their intent was to explore, with their colleagues, the human ability
to reach decisions consciously as well as without conscious control; deliberate and intuitive; explicit and implicit; through the processing of information serially as well as in parallel; with a general-purpose apparatus or with
task-specific neural subsystems. They envisioned the analysis to take place
on four levels—neural, psychological, evolutionary, and institutional—and
hoped that the resulting discussion could be beneficial in the design of better
institutional interventions.

Paul Glimcher, Kevin McCabe, Peter J. Richerson, and Lael Schooler joined
them as members of the steering committee. Together they invited colleagues
from the areas of anthropology, neuroscience, law, evolutionary biology, behavioral science and economics to join them in Frankfurt for a focal meeting.
Held on June 10–15, 2007, a lively week of discussions ensued within a most
stimulating setting.

The results of the entire process have been set down in this Strüngmann
Forum Report. It is not meant to be a consensus document. The individual
chapters give a sense of the scope of the topics considered, and the group
reports (Chapters, 6, 11, 15, and 19) distill the intense dialogue that evolved.
In this regard, Michael Platt, Christian Keysers, Richard McElreath and Mark
Lubell deserve special mention. As rapporteurs of the discussion groups, their
task was certainly not easy. Neither was the job of the moderators, so ably assumed by Wolf Singer, Eric Johnson, Peter Richerson, and Jeffrey Rachlinksi.
We are grateful to them for assuming these responsibilities.

Everyone—the chairpersons, steering committee, authors and coauthors—
brought to the process not only their congenial personalities but a willingness to

question and go beyond that which is already known. The intellectual challenge was complex, and we do not purport to have discovered a magic formula. Our hope is that this volume will stimulate further dialogue and broaden the lines of enquiry, so that answers to the many pressing issues may eventually be found.

A communication process of this nature requires, first and foremost, institutional stability as well as an environment that promotes and guarantees free thought. On behalf of everyone involved, I wish to express our deepest gratitude to Dr. Andreas and Dr. Thomas Strüngmann. As the founders of the Ernst Strüngmann Foundation, named in honor of their father, their generous support and belief in this process has enabled the Ernst Strüngmann Forum to conduct its work in the service of science.

Julia Lupp, Program Director, Ernst Strüngmann Forum
Frankfurt Institute for Advanced Studies (FIAS)
Ruth-Moufang-Str. 1, 60438 Frankfurt am Main, Germany
http://fias.uni-frankfurt.de/esforum/

List of Contributors

Robert Boyd   UCLA Department of Anthropology and Center for Behavior Evolution and Culture, 341 Haines Hall, Box 951553, Los Angeles, CA 90095–1553, U.S.A.

Anne K. Churchland   Howard Hughes Medical Institute, Department of Physiology and Biophysics, University of Washington, Box 357290, Seattle, WA 98195–7290, U.S.A.

Jonathan D. Cohen   Department of Psychology, Princeton University, Green Hall, Princeton, NJ 08544, U.S.A.

Peter Dayan   Gatsby Computational Neuroscience Unit, UCL, Alexandra House, 17 Queen Square, London WC1N 3AR, U.K.

Stanislas Dehaene   Inserm-CEA Cognitive Neuroimaging Unit, CEA/SAC/DSV/DRM/NeuroSpin, Bâtiment 145, Point Courrier 156, 91191 Gif/Yvette, France

Merlin Donald   Department of Cognitive Science, Case Western Reserve University, Crawford Hall, 612C, 10900 Euclid Ave., Cleveland, OH 44106–7068, U.S.A.

Christoph Engel   Max Planck Institute for Research on Collective Goods, Kurt-Schumacher-Str. 10, 53113 Bonn, Germany

Gerd Gigerenzer   Center for Adaptive Behavior and Cognition, Max Planck Institute for Human Development, Lentzeallee 94, 14195 Berlin, Germany

Paul W. Glimcher   Center for Neuroeconomics, New York University, 4 Washington Place, New York, NY 10003, U.S.A.

Andreas Glöckner   Max Planck Institute for Research on Collective Goods, Kurt-Schumacher-Str. 10, 53113 Bonn, Germany

Werner Güth   Max Planck Institute of Economics, Strategic Interaction Group, Kahlaische Str. 10, 07745 Jena, Germany

Peter Hammerstein   Institute for Theoretical Biology, Humboldt University Berlin, Invalidenstr. 43, 10115 Berlin, Germany

Timothy D. Hanks   Howard Hughes Medical Institute, Department of Physiology and Biophysics, University of Washington, Box 357290, Seattle, WA 98195–7290, U.S.A.

Reid Hastie   Graduate School of Business, Center for Decision Research, University of Chicago, 5807 S. Woodlawn Avenue, Chicago, IL 60637, U.S.A.

Eric J. Johnson   Columbia Business School, Center for Decision Sciences, Columbia University, 3022 Broadway, New York, NY 10027, U.S.A.

Christian Keysers   BCN Neuro-Imaging Center, University Medical Center Groningen, A. Deusinglaan 2, 9713 AW Groningen, The Netherlands

Roozbeh Kiani   Howard Hughes Medical Institute, Department of Physiology and Biophysics, University of Washington, Box 357290, Seattle, WA 98195–7290, U.S.A.

Robert Kurzban   Department of Psychology, University of Pennsylvania, 3720 Walnut St., Philadelphia, PA 19104, U.S.A.

Mark Lubell   Department of Environmental Science and Policy, University of California, Davis, One Shields Avenue, Davis, CA 95616, U.S.A.

Stefan Magen   Max Planck Institute for Research on Collective Goods, Kurt-Schumacher-Str. 10, 53113 Bonn, Germany

Kevin McCabe   Center for the Study of Neuroeconomics, George Mason University, 4400 University Drive, Fairfax, VA 22030, U.S.A.

Richard M. McElreath   Department of Anthropology, University of California–Davis, One Shields Ave, Davis, CA 95616–8522, U.S.A.

Gail McKoon   Department of Psychology, Ohio State University, 1835 Neil Avenue, Columbus, OH 43210, U.S.A.

Randolf Menzel   Institute for Biology, Freie Universität Berlin, Königin-Luise-Str. 28–30, 14195 Berlin, Germany

Elizabeth Phelps   Department of Psychology, New York University, 6 Washington Place, New York, NY 10003, U.S.A

Hilke Plassmann   Division of the Humanities and Social Sciences, California Institute of Technology, 1200 E. California Blvd., Pasadena, CA 91125, U.S.A.

Michael Platt   Department of Neurobiology, Duke University Medical Center, Bryan Research Building, Durham, NC 27710, U.S.A.

Jeffrey J. Rachlinski   Cornell Law School, Cornell University, Myron Taylor Hall, Ithaca, NY 14853-4401, U.S.A.

Roger Ratcliff   Department of Psychology, Ohio State University, 1835 Neil Avenue, Columbus, OH 43210, U.S.A.

Peter J. Richerson   Dept. of Environmental Science and Policy, University of California, Davis, One Shields Avenue, Davis, CA 95616, U.S.A.

Arthur Robson   Department of Economics, Simon Fraser University, 8888 University Drive, Burnaby, British Columbia V5A 1S6, Canada

Bettina Rockenbach   Center for Empirical Research in Economics and, Behavioral Sciences, University of Erfurt, Nordhäuser Str. 63, 99089 Erfurt, Germany

Jonathan W. Schooler   Department of Psychology, University of British Columbia, 2136 West Mall Avenue, Vancouver, British Columbia V6T 1Z4, Canada

Lael J. Schooler   Center for Adaptive Behavior, Max Planck Institute of Human Development, Lentzeallee 94, 14195 Berlin, Germany

Reinhard Selten   Juridicum, University of Bonn, Adenauerallee 24–42, 53113 Bonn, Germany

Michael N. Shadlen   Howard Hughes Medical Institute, Department of Physiology and Biophysics, University of Washington, Box 357290, Seattle, WA 98195–7290, U.S.A.

Tania Singer   Institute for Empirical Research in Economics, University of Zurich, Blümlisalpstr. 10, 8006 Zurich, Switzerland

Wolf Singer   Max Planck Institute for Brain Research, Deutschordenstr. 46, Frankfurt am Main, Germany

Elizabeth Spelke   Department of Psychology, Harvard University, 33 Kirkland St., Cambridge, MA 02138, U.S.A.

Jeffrey R. Stevens   Center for Adaptive Behavior and Cognition, Max Planck Institute for Human Development, Lentzeallee 94, 14195 Berlin, Germany

Julia Trommershäuser   Department of Psychology, Giessen University, Otto-Behaghel-Str. 10F, 35394 Giessen, Germany

Elke U. Weber   Graduate School of Business, Columbia University, 716 Uris Hall, 3022 Broadway, New York, NY 10027, U.S.A.

Preface

Scientific disciplines are like children. This may seem to be an awkward metaphor, but in one important respect there is a parallel. Jean Piaget taught us that human development advances in stages. Children cannot but stumble into situations "when they no longer understand the world." Assimilating the new experiences to their previous body of knowledge no longer works. They are taken by surprise. They are forced to reconstruct their world by way of accommodation.

An experience akin to this occurred at the outset of this collective endeavor. For one of the editors of this volume, it was an established piece of truth that, in all but the most trivial situations, rational choice models do not describe the mental process. Cognitive resources are way too limited. Radically simple search and decision rules are the obvious way out. Actually this academic was so convinced that he organized a meeting entitled "Heuristics and the Law" in 2004 to flesh out normative implications, together with the leading figure in heuristics research, Gerd Gigerenzer. Then he stumbled into another contributor to this volume, Paul Glimcher. Paul showed that even monkeys use one of the most taxing tools of rational choice analysis, Bayesian updating. Are monkeys really superior to humans? This vexing question triggered the present collaboration between the two editors of this volume.

Of course they are not, was the obvious answer. To perform information-rich mental operations, humans do not engage in consciously controlled deliberation. They rely on consciously not accessible, automatic, parallel processing. At most, the end result is propelled back to consciousness as an intuition.

What can we say about the underlying neural processes? How does the brain know that it has reached a decision? How can we tell the many possible conceptualizations of the psychological divide from each other? If the consciously not controlled mental apparatus is so powerful, why did conscious, deliberate, serial control evolve at all? What does all of this mean for the analysis and the design of institutions?

This inaugural Ernst Strüngmann Forum provided a perfect framework for posing these bold questions, and for making quite a bit of progress: in asking yet sharper questions; in identifying bones of contest and lacunae; in sketching promising avenues for further research; and in offering some first answers. Our deep gratitude is with the Ernst Strüngmann Forum. The Forum has done everything to express its trust in our ability to turn daring questions into a thought-provoking product. Julia Lupp and her collaborators have brought all their expertise and inventiveness to bear, so that we could experience a unique environment of true academic freedom. We all will be keeping the warmest recollections of a fascinating week in Frankfurt and of a most productive process in the preparation of this culminating point, and in our attempts to harvest after the event.

Science is a collective endeavor by definition. However, joint work hardly ever becomes as productive and as engaging.

The Editors

1

Better Than Conscious?

The Brain, the Psyche, Behavior, and Institutions

Christoph Engel[1] and Wolf Singer[2]

[1]Max Planck Institute for Research on Collective Goods, 53113 Bonn, Germany
[2]Max Planck Institute for Brain Research, 60528 Frankfurt am Main, Germany

Abstract

The title of this chapter is deliberately provocative. Intuitively, many will be inclined to see conscious control of mental process as a good thing. Yet control comes at a high price. The consciously not directly controlled, automatic, parallel processing of information is not only much faster, it also handles much more information, and it does so in a qualitatively different manner. This different mental machinery is not adequate for all tasks. The human ability to deliberate consciously has evolved for good reason. However, on many more tasks than one might think at first sight, intuitive decision making, or at least an intuitive component in a more complex mental process, does indeed improve performance. This chapter presents the issue, offers concepts to understand it, discusses the effects in terms of problem-solving capacity, contrasts norms for saying when this is a good thing, and points to scientific and real-world audiences for this work.

Illustrations

Combining Quantities

$2 + 2 = ?$ What a stupid question! As of the first grade, most everyone can easily answer this. If you do not believe it, let us prove it. Assume the answer was 4. One of the axioms of arithmetic posits that addition is revertible:

$$a + b = c \Leftrightarrow c - b = a. \tag{1}$$

Thus, from the original question we have $a = 2$ and $b = 2$. Then according to the right-hand side of Equation 1, we must have:

$$c - 2 = 2 \Rightarrow c = 2 + 2 = 4. \tag{2}$$

You are not convinced by the proof? Well, since you are still not content, here is an apple. Here is another apple. How many apples are on the table? Let's count them: one apple, two apples, period. Now let's do the same operation with two more apples, on the desk. Now we have two apples on the table, and two on the desk, right? What if we put all apples on the table? Well, let's count again: 1, 2, 3, 4. Convincing?

Yes, but a category error. Our proof was axiomatic. We exploited the axiom that addition and subtraction are perfectly revertible. However, by definition, an axiom cannot be proven. One can only design proofs built upon axioms that are accepted by the community to which one is speaking. Our second argument, by contrast, utilized the counting routine. It relied on (a) a social practice that all of us have been taught in childhood, (b) a piece of language, and (c) the concept of natural numbers situated behind this language. You probably had no difficulty following the second example since you share this social practice, the meaning of the names for natural numbers, and the experience that there is a reliable mapping between the two of these and simple arithmetic. Ultimately, however, the second example does not constitute a proof; instead it is simply an appeal to shared cultural practice.

Of course, both this practice and the axiomatic system are very useful. What if we put two oranges on the table and two oranges on the desk? Dead easy: $2 + 2 = 4$. And what if we put two apples on the table and two oranges on the desk? How many pieces of fruit do we have on the table if we move the oranges from the desk to the table? Dead easy again: $2 + 2 = 4$. Try this task on a two-year-old and be prepared for a number of surprises. Which of the two tasks would you, as an adult, expect to be more difficult? You would probably guess the second, since it implies abstraction. Yet it has been shown that most two- to three-year-olds fully understand the abstract concept of numerosity (Wynn 1992). Once they know the numbers up to 20, it is even easy for them to extend their mathematical ability beyond that frontier, simply by asking them to repeat the operations of addition and subtraction (Lipton and Spelke 2005).

It is, however, much more difficult for children to map the counting routine and the names of numbers they associate with the abstract concept (Wynn 1992). Only by age four do children understand that the words of the counting routine refer to numerosity and that the routine itself functions to enumerate the items (Hauser and Spelke 2005). If children apply the counting routine to a novel set of objects, they perform well, up to the limit to which they have learned numbers. However, if you then ask them—How many of these objects are there?—only 16% of the 2½-year-olds are able to give the correct answer, as are only 55% of the 3½-year-olds (Wynn 1990). If a child at age 2½ is told that a pile contains "four fish," and then two fish are removed, the child will insist that the pile still contains four fish (Condry et al. 2003). Although the child uses the counting words correctly in the counting routine, she evidently interprets each word above one as simply meaning "more than one" (Hauser and Spelke 2005).

How do other primates perform on the same tasks? Consider "Ai," a chimpanzee from the Primate Research Center in Kyoto, who for over twenty years has been involved in experiments that test her cognitive abilities (Matsuzawa et al. 2006). Initially, Ai interpreted "1" as "one" and "2" as "more than one." With further training, Ai learned to apply "2" and "3" correctly, but the amount of training needed to make this incremental move was no different from the amount of training needed for the first two integers. When the symbol "4" was introduced, Ai's performance fell to chance on "3"; she evidently interpreted "3" as "more than two." Ai has not progressed beyond the symbol "9" after twenty years of training. Chimpanzees learn the integer list through brute association, mapping each symbol to a discrete quantity. Human children, however, learn by making an induction from a limited body of evidence (Hauser and Spelke 2005).

Is solving the task $2 + 2 = ?$ on two apples and two oranges lying on a table a conscious activity? Before reading the above paragraphs, you may have again thought: What a stupid question! Yet defining consciousness is tricky business. For the moment let us agree that mental activity can be considered "conscious" if a person is aware of the activity. One is even more on the safe side if the individual is able to report this mental activity. That said, we would bet that not only is a toddler unable to report how she maps the names of natural numbers to the abstract concept of numerosity but, most likely, if you are not a cognitive scientist, you have also not been aware of the need to do that mapping before you perform the simple task of saying how many pieces of fruit are on the table. What patently appears to be a conscious activity capitalizes heavily on nonconscious mental processes.

$2 + 3 = ?$ Is the mental process for solving this problem, say again in apples, any different from solving $2 + 2 = ?$ Heavens no, you may think: this is again primitive arithmetics. Yet if one measures reaction times, there is a huge difference, although the example is a bit tricky in that it is on the borderline. To make the difference net, let us compare $2 + 1$ with $2 + 3$. The reaction time on $2 + 1$ is on the order of 40–100 ms above the baseline per item. For $2 + 3$, it goes up to 250–350 ms above the baseline per item. Thus, to complete the second task, subjects need at least four times the time required to finish the first computation. This suggests that different mental mechanisms are involved. The process of counting fewer than (and sometimes up to) four items is an automatic, preattentive activity related to vision (Trick and Pylyshyn 1994). Humans are thus able to perform the first task $(2 + 1)$ in a totally nonconscious way.

For a final example, consider the following: On the table as well as on the desk, there stands a bowl containing dried beans. You are asked to estimate whether the total amount of beans from the bowls on the table and desk is enough to fill an empty bucket on the floor. Now, if a computer were to solve this problem, you would have to specify the following: how many beans of average size are necessary to fill the bucket? How many beans are, at the minimum, in either bowl? The computer would then add up these two numbers and compare them to the threshold of the bucket. Without these numbers, the computer would be helpless. Not so for human subjects, for along with the mental machinery for exact counting, humans possess a second mechanism that enables an approximate assessment of large numbers to be made. This mechanism is even able to perform simple arithmetic operations, such as addition or subtraction. The key feature, the tool for approximating quantity without counting, relies on an automatic process (Dehaene 1997).

Determination of Guilt

As long as a country is not at war, no other governmental activity interferes as severely in its citizens' lives as the criminal justice system. In some countries, a citizen accused of a crime risks being sentenced to death. In all countries, prison terms are possible. A precondition for sentencing an accused citizen (the defendant) is to prove to the requisite standard that she has indeed committed the crime to which she is accused. Defining this standard presents the legal order with a serious dilemma: unless the defendant pleads guilty, past events must be reconstructed to arrive at a decision. Reconstructing past events, however, is prone to errors. The risk of incorrect decisions is further aggravated by the adversarial nature of courtroom procedure. In their attempts to exact a decision in their favor, both the attorney general and the counsel for the defense deliberately try to influence the court; neither is likely to present a fair account of the events. The legal order has to satisfy two goals:

1. Materially wrong decisions should be avoided. (Of course, convicting an innocent is worse than acquitting a guilty defendant. In the parlance of signal-detection theory: false alarms matter more than false misses. Still, both lead to suboptimal decisions.)
2. The supreme exercise of sovereign powers should be ostensibly as correct as possible; the rules of law and principles of democracy demand this.

These two goals are often in conflict, because nonconsciously controlled or reportable decisions or elements that contribute to the decision are often more reliable.

Consider the process by which the legal system determines whether a witness has actually observed the defendant at the crime scene: A lineup is organized, where the accused is interspersed with a sufficient number of similar-looking individuals. If the witness is able to single out the defendant, a first level of proof has been established. Of course, the legal system understands that this method is subject to error (Sporer et al. 1996), and thus it is also standard practice to ask the witness how confident she is, as well as to observe signals such as body language or the nuances of utterances. During this process, both the witness and the legal system rely on intuitive judgment, which, by its very nature, is not controllable or reportable. Only the results of this process can be reported.

Recent research by Sauerland and Sporer (2007) has analyzed this more thoroughly. In a mock lineup, the reaction times of witnesses were measured and post-experiment reports matched to the results. When witnesses made an intuitive, holistic judgment, they did so at a much faster speed, and the outcome was much more reliable than if they had looked for certain criteria (e.g., hair color, shape of the nose, or thickness of the eyebrows). Thus, intuition beats deliberation.

In most criminal cases, though, conflict is not confined to an isolated aspect of the case. A whole series of events may be in dispute. To address these, the attorney general typically tells a story to explain the events and establish guilt. Tactically, the defendant and her counsel must decide whether they are better off telling a competing story or contradicting key features of the attorney general's story. Moreover, under criminal procedure, any feature of the story that is disputed must be formally proven. It is again a tactical issue for both parties to determine the order for the presentation of the evidence and counterevidence. Typically, the judge and/or the jury listen to evidence in a scrambled order, and it remains incomplete until the end. Experimental work with mock juries has shown that provisional stories are worked out as the evidence is presented. Jurors are content to convict if, after hearing all the evidence, there is a convincing story, with no conspicuous holes, and with no striking pieces of counterevidence (Hastie et al. 1983; Hastie 1993). In other words, juries and judges ultimately rely on a consciously uncontrolled mental process, namely intuition.

Subsequent research has deciphered the underlying mental mechanism. It has been found that a person determines whether a story is "convincing" once coherence is generated among the pieces of evidence. In this process, world knowledge defines base rates, and these rates are updated in light of the evidence. Subjects give progressively more weight to evidence that supports their preferred story while progressively underrating conflicting evidence. The process of re-weighting continues until the requisite mental standard for being convinced is reached, or until the process is stopped because the evidence is patently conflicting (Simon 1998; Simon et al. 2001).

This is troubling news for the legal order. A typical crime has far too many degrees of freedom to lend itself to any form of rigorous scientific fact-finding. Typically, until the end of a court case, there remains a certain degree of uncertainty. The legal order cannot exclude the possibility that judges and juries engage in sense-making. Actually, continental legal orders do so quite openly: They do not exclusively define the standard of proof in objective terms. They do not ask for a 95% or 99% probability that the defendant has committed the crime. Rather they ask a judge to rely on her *conviction intime*. A judge must be able to overcome her doubts or she must acquit the defendant (Schulz 1992). Psychological work on consistency maximization via parallel constraint satisfaction explains why this doctrinal requirement is meaningful (Glöckner, this volume). However, work on coherence-based reasoning demonstrates that the mechanism is not free of errors.

Playing against an Opponent

Workable competition is a beautiful institution; it forces actors on both sides of the market to reveal their preferences. Competition is a direct mechanism (Bolton and Dewatripont 2005). A seller has nothing to gain from withholding quantity or from demanding a price above marginal cost. A buyer has nothing to gain from refusing to deal, as other sellers or other buyers would make the profit. In game theoretic terms, workable competition forces all actors to play a game against Nature (Straffin 1993). It does not make sense for them to treat the other market side as a strategic actor.

The world looks very different if the other market side is small, or if the entry of new buyers or sellers into the market is unlikely (Baumol 1982). Here a seller is best off if she sets a high price or keeps the quantity sold low. Likewise a buyer is best off if she refuses to buy an expensive item, although the price for this one unit is below its marginal revenue. If she does, some units will not sell, but the units that are traded are sold cheaper. Thus, she cashes in on a distributional gain.

Game theory offers a highly elegant technology for solving the resulting conflicts of strategic interaction. Its mainstay is the Nash equilibrium (Nash 1951). Either player plays a best response, given that the other player also plays a best response. Most experimental economics is about testing the predictions of game theory in the lab. Not surprisingly, experimental subjects systematically deviate from these predictions in a host of games (i.e., strategic situations). Typically, this is taken as evidence for cognitive biases (Kahneman and Tversky 2000), as well as for motivational dispositions that deviate from utility maximization (Kagel and Roth 1995). Less attention has been given to the fact that experimental evidence also speaks to the conscious/nonconscious divide.

A pertinent piece of evidence for this is provided by Ariel Rubinstein, one of the leading game theorists. Rubinstein has set up a web site designed to help his colleagues teach game theory. A set of rather tricky games is presented, and teachers are invited to have their class play these games online in private the day before the respective topic is taught in class. The teacher then receives statistical information back from Rubinstein's site as to how the pupils performed on these games. As a by-product, Rubinstein records reaction times. In most of these games, a characteristic picture is seen. Although in theory there should be plenty of strategies taken, students utilized only a very few. More interestingly, for some of these strategies, reaction times are much shorter than for others. Apparently, only a few strategies are highly intuitive (Rubinstein 2007).

Consider the following, relatively simple example: Subjects were asked to be the row player against an anonymous opponent (the column player) in the

	L	R
T	2, –2	0, 0
B	0, 0	1, –1

Figure 1.1 Ariel Rubinstein's game.

game depicted in Figure 1.1. Read this matrix the following way: the row player has the choice of selecting either the top (T) or the bottom (B); the column player chooses between left (L) and right (R). There are four possible combinations of actions: TL, TR, BL, BR. In each of the four cells, the left number represents the row player's payoff; the right number is the payoff for the column player. If both players are fully rational, they would attempt to select the best response: What would the row player want to do if she knew that the column player would play left? Since 2 is more than 0, the row player would want to play top. Similarly, you can make the comparisons for all four cells, and for both players. In the matrix, the resulting best responses are underlined. Note that in no cell are two payoffs underlined. Whatever the other player does, the first player would want to do something different. In game theoretic parlance: the game has no Nash equilibrium in pure strategies. The only equilibrium of this game is in mixed strategies. The row player has to randomize between her two actions, anticipating that the column player will do the same. In this equilibrium, the row player would play top with probability 1/3, and bottom with the corresponding probability 2/3. Likewise, the column player would play left with probability 1/3, and right with probability 2/3.

If you have never been exposed to game theory, you will certainly not find this solution intuitive. In experiments, subjects find it pretty hard to randomize, if the possibility of an equilibrium in mixed strategies dawns on them at all. Moreover, Rubinstein has assigned you the role of the row player. This is a comfortable position. In the worst of all cases, you come out even. In the *TR* and *BL* cells, you make zero profit. However in both the *TL* and the *BR* cells, you expect a positive profit. Admittedly, it goes at the expense of your opponent. The game is a zero sum game. All you win is taken away from your opponent. Therefore, if you believe deeply in altruism, you would rather play bottom. That way you will make sure that your opponent cannot suffer a big loss. However, most of us are probably not that altruistic. We are rather attracted by the chance to make a big gain in the *TL* cell. That is at any rate what 67% of Ariel Rubinstein's subjects did, and those who did took less time to make up their minds. The median reaction time for those who choose top was 37 seconds, while the median for those who choose bottom was 50 seconds. Admittedly, 37 seconds is still quite a bit of time, and we must be careful in interpreting the difference. It seems safe to say that subjects found playing top more intuitive, even if they have not reached that conclusion exclusively with their automatic system. In other games the differences in reaction times were even more impressive. Since, however, most of these games require more game theoretic knowledge, they are not reported here.

For the purposes of this book, there are two implications: even at the very heart of rational choice theory, in strategic interaction, we should be prepared for actions that are influenced by nonconscious mental operations. Whether this is good news or not depends crucially on the structure of the game. In the concrete case, if the opponent anticipates you to be greedy, she will play right, which makes her best off, and you go home with nothing. She might discover this since she is smart, or she might counter your intuition with her intuition, saying that there are more egoists than altruists in the population. Now if you (intuitively) anticipate this, it is better to play bottom. A bird in the hand is worth two in the bush. Yet if your opponent is really clever, she will outwit this move, and play left, which again leaves you with nothing. Of course you could counter this by playing top and would be in the best of all worlds, ad infinitum. In this class of games, intuition does not offer an easy way out. In many others, however, it does.

Concepts

How Many Agents Are Involved?

Actually, the presentation of the issue in the examples already makes an assumption that need not be uncontroversial. Conscious decision making and nonconscious decision making are seen as two distinguishable processes. Humans possess (at least) two different mental apparatuses that make decisions: one operates under conscious control; the other does not. This view does not exclude the possibility that both machineries interact, nor does it mean that either machinery has an exclusive domain, to which the other has no or only rare access. Both machineries need not be in competition at all times. Nonetheless, this perspective treats human decision makers as multiple agents.

Once one allows for this possibility, there is no need to limit the number of agents to just two. There might be an emotional agent, distinct from a more cold-blooded one. There might be a general-purpose agent, distinct from a more task- or context-specific agent. There might be an agent for a decision taken by the individual alone, distinct from an agent for participating in group decision making.

If there is more than one agent, the interaction between them becomes the issue. Do the agents simultaneously work on the same task? If so, how are conflicts resolved? Is there something like a master and slave mode that gives one of the agents control over what the other does? Is it possible to split a decision task such that several agents provide well-defined inputs? If so, how are these inputs integrated, and by which agent? Is there something like a meta-decision that assigns a new task to one of the agents? If so, is this meta-decision taken by just one (superior?) agent, or by some form of competition between the potentially pertinent agents? Is the meta-decision taken centrally or decentrally? In metaphorical terms: Is the interaction of multiple mental agents better captured by a firm or by a market model?

Definitions

Defining consciousness is as unpleasant as nailing a pudding to the wall. In our experience, we do not take all decisions the same way. Not so rarely, we feel driven by forces that we do not understand, we do not control, we do not predict. From these we feel we can distinguish other decisions. Colloquially we call them conscious. All attempts to draw an exact line between conscious and the nonconscious, however, meet with objections. For example:

1. A decision may be considered to have been consciously made if a person is able to report the information taken into consideration as well as the way in which it was processed. Such a definition could very well be too narrow, for the person could merely lack language or suffer from deception, as shown with the arithmetic example.
2. A decision may be considered to be conscious if a person is aware of the mental process leading to it. This definition may be too broad. If I ponder over a difficult problem, and all of a sudden I see the solution, I know it when I see it, but I have at best guessed where it came from.
3. A decision may be considered to have been consciously made when the prefrontal cortex has been engaged. Again, this explanation may be too narrow, as neuroimaging demonstrates that there is a gradual shift between almost no and very far-reaching activation. Intermediate states like "preconsciousness" can be identified (Dehaene et al. 2006).

Clusters

Even if we can agree on one definition for consciousness, how do we describe the borderline area between related concepts: deliberate versus intuitive; explicit versus implicit; controlled versus automatic; serial versus parallel; analytic versus holistic; slow versus rapid; ad hoc versus learned; plastic versus patterned? One can certainly come up with examples that fall into the first category on pretty much all of these dimensions. For example, if I am a game theorist, and a friend approaches me with a serious problem of strategic interaction, I can sit down and work out a formal model exploiting all the many degrees of freedom game theory gives me, even though it will take me considerable time to do so. Likewise there are examples that fall into the second category on almost all of these dimensions: When I drive to work in the morning, almost all of the many decisions I make en route will be fast and automatic; I will process information in parallel, will rely heavily on prepackaged routines learned in driving school and improved in my later driving experience.

However it is not difficult to identify examples that fall into one side of some dimensions and to another side in others. The three illustrations given at the beginning of this chapter demonstrate this:

1. To do arithmetic, we must combine our understanding of numerosity with our knowledge of names for numbers. For most of us, neither mental process is consciously accessible. Thus, we build our conscious ability to perform mathematical operations on these nonconscious foundations.

2. When deciding whether a defendant has committed the crime, a jury certainly makes an effort to discuss the explicit relevance of the pieces of evidence heard in court. Ultimately, however, jury members cannot avoid, and should not try to avoid, making sense out of the evidence. They become aware of the result, but not of the mental machinery that generates coherence to produce the result.

3. When we decide how to act in the presence of an opponent, we may wish to exploit our knowledge of game theory. However, all of our training does not help if we fail to combine it with a sense of how this specific opponent is going to act. Only in the closed world of game theory can we take it for granted that our opponent is a rational utility maximizer. If our opponent deviates from these assumptions, and experimental economics has shown that many do, we are best off to optimize using a best guess about the type of behavior that our opponent will choose.

These illustrations raise questions; they unfortunately do not point to the answers. Behavior can be clustered along the dimensions listed above. Fine. Behavior need not be clustered along the dimensions listed above. Also fine. When, however, is it clustered? Along which dimensions are clusters more likely than along others? Are there systematic correlations between tasks or environments and certain clusters? Are there other systematic correlations between personality and certain clusters? Is clustering a matter of learning and training? Are interaction partners able to predict or influence these clusters?

Effects

Is Rational Choice Descriptively Correct?

Mental mechanism matters. Human subjects react differently to changes in their environment, depending on how they process information. Since the cognitive revolution in psychology, this view has been widely held (Chomsky 1959). Ultimately, to define the effects on performance, one needs to map the distinctions listed in the previous section to modes of decision making or problem solving. This raises the issue of clusters: Which combinations of features are at all feasible? How permanent are these combinations? Are the combinations human universals, or are they distributed in the population? How do individuals acquire problem-solving modes? How do they map onto perceived features of problems? What is the role of institutions in triggering, or in even generating, specific clusters?

Some of these questions have been addressed elsewhere (Engel and Weber 2006). For our purposes here, we will slight the clustering problem and ask a simplified question: Provided that an adequate cluster of features has formed, what is the effect of foregoing conscious control?

Since the time of the grand Roman orators, the *argumentum ad absurdum* has been a powerful rhetorical weapon. In the crusade against the rational choice model, an *argumentum ad absurdum* is frequently proffered . The power of this model rests on the ability to reduce social interaction to an exercise in arithmetic: Define the utility function for each individual who is part of the conflict. Create a common currency (e.g., money). Use this currency to quantify the initial endowments of all individuals. Translate all features of the environment into cost, again quantified by means of the common currency. Say exactly who knows what. If individuals move sequentially, define the timeline. Assume that all individuals have exclusively one goal, and that everyone realizes that all others have this goal: the maximization of their utility, given all constraints. Then, with this setup, you can calculate the equilibrium. Granted, the mathematical skills required for this were not taught in most secondary schools. However, after a few weeks of practice, a person should be able to derive the correct solution to standard optimization problems.

All of us solve problems throughout the day, don't we? Yet the percentage of humans able to solve even a simple optimization problem is far below 1%. Even to the most enthusiastic defenders of the rational choice model, it seemed obvious, therefore, that the model does not describe the underlying mental mechanism. Economists tend to say: it is only an "as-if" model (Friedman 1953). Psychologists would use different terms for the same statement. The rational choice model is at best paramorphic, not isomorphic (Fischhoff et al. 1981). Standard reasoning has it that, in the black box of the human mind, some process is going on that one would not really want to understand, but that ultimately converges to yield the predictions of the rational choice model. Specifically, the defenders of the rational choice model claim that individuals ultimately adapt to restrictions, and to the forces of competition, in particular (Friedman 1953).

So goes the *argumentum ad absurdum*. The argument is powerful since it resonates with our experience. Most of us just cannot reach the answer via mathematics. Even those who have the prerequisite skills would agree that it takes more effort than a person can afford in daily activities. In our experience, cognitive resources are severely limited. Actually, the limitations begin even before a person learns mathematics. Most individuals have a memory span of seven plus/minus one item (Wechsler 1945). Even in simple problems of strategic interaction, this is not enough. Think back to Ariel Rubinstein's game: Before you realize that the game does not have a solution in terms of pure strategy, you must have tried out all combinations for both players and memorized the results. To calculate each best response, you must compare two payoffs. Even if we ignore the information about structure, we need to compare the correct payoffs, or 2 × 8 items. We are only less aware of this second limitation since we are so dependent on external aids. We realize that this is going to be tricky business, and thus reach for paper and a pencil.

What if we have fallen prey to an illusion? Until Galileo, it seemed clear that the Earth was flat, and that the Sun and the Moon circled around it. Subsequently, science has convinced us that the Earth is a sphere that circles around the Sun. Will science also be able to convince us that the rational choice model pretty much captures what happens in our mind when we solve a problem of strategic interaction? Science is not there yet, and it is difficult to know whether it will arrive at exactly the mechanism assumed by the model. Still, it is much closer than most of us would find intuitive.

The main barrier to the formation of descriptively adequate intuitions about mental mechanisms is consciousness. We possess the ability to handle information consciously and to derive from this a plan for action. We are, however, misled to believe that this fully describes the underlying mental mechanism. Psychology has demonstrated that we are able to handle vast amounts of information in almost no time, nonconsciously (Glöckner 2007). Neuroscience has demonstrated that we are able to record fine-grained information about positive and negative utility, and that we update this information in light of every single new experience, nonconsciously (Glimcher 2003). With these ingredients, a mechanism pretty close to the assumptions of rational choice theory could be implemented.

Decisions on Incomplete Factual Basis

Even the most faithful believers in the rational choice model do not claim that it describes the underlying mental mechanisms of a chess player (de Groot 1965). Chess is a deterministic problem: the chessboard is exactly defined, as is the composition of the chessmen, their moves, and the rules of conflict that govern two chess pieces on the same field. In a world without resource limitations, one could thus calculate the optimal way to play a game of chess. More interestingly, one could calculate the optimal sequence of future moves, given that the opponent has moved in some known way in the past. For quite a few years, computers have succeeded in beating the world champion in chess. How do they accomplish this? Do they achieve success through brute force, making innumerable calculations? To the contrary, the computers employed heuristics, and the reason is straightforward. In a game of chess, there are so many degrees of freedom that combinatorics explode. Likewise even the stupendously powerful, nonconscious, parallel-processing mechanism in the human mind is overwhelmed (Gigerenzer et al. 1999).

Many real-life problems are even worse. Often we have to decide on an issue when we do not have access to complete information. For example, in competition, we know that our competitor is working on a process innovation, but we do not know how likely she is to succeed. We also do not know how much this innovation would reduce her production costs, if she were to succeed. Should we also spend money to find a cheaper way of manufacturing the product? Would we still make enough profit once our competitor has reduced her price (e.g., since her capacity remains limited)? In principle, there are three reasons why information may be incomplete: (a) we may be attempting to know something that no one else knows, or that cannot be communicated in a credible way; (b) the price of generating or acquiring the information is prohibitive; (c) some overriding legal or social norm prevents us from gaining access to the information.

When the factual basis is incomplete, we must decide under uncertainty. Some forms of uncertainty lend themselves to rational choice analysis, and hence to the calculation of optimal responses. For example, if uncertainty is stochastic, and we know the probability distribution, we can calculate expected values. If we do not know the probability distribution, we can replace it by our beliefs (Savage 1954). If uncertainty is strategic in nature, and we have reason to believe that our opponents maximize utility, we can use game theory to base our decision. If the problem space is well defined, but we do not know the combination of features, we can introduce an artificial move of Nature and again use game theory (Harsanyi 1967–1968). However, many real-life problems are plagued by an element of pure ignorance (Kirzner 1994). The problem space is at least partly not defined. We are down to guesswork.

Interestingly, the nonconscious mental machinery is pretty good at that as well. It is prepared to produce decent responses to problems that are only partly defined. It is permanently engaged in making sense out of the available information and in creating meaning (Glöckner, this volume). To that end, it relies on deliberately fuzzy tools like exemplars and schemas. In an exemplar, the individual happens to know a good response to a graphically described problem. This may be an earlier good or bad experience, a good story about someone else's experiences, or a colorful counterfactual. The individual transposes the solution by way of analogy (Smith and Zárate 1992; Juslin et al. 2003). A schema is less tightly linked to a full story. In memory, the individual has stored a more or less rich description of a concept and matches the available information to this concept. In so doing, more weight is given to the presence, or the absence, of what the person sees to be the key factors (Bartlett 1932). All of this happens rapidly, and only the result is perceived consciously.

Insight

Every scientist has experienced insight: after struggling with a problem for hours, days, or even years, out of the blue, the way forward suddenly appears—fully convincing and often far simpler than expected. Lawyers are trained to achieve similar results through a method known as hermeneutics. Given an overly rich set of potentially relevant facts of the case as well as an overly rich set of legal rules, doctrinal lawyers progressively narrow down, through an iterative process, the interpretations of code as well as the interpretations of the facts, until they match. In legal jargon, this end result is called syllogism. In all but the most simple cases, there is a dose of creativity, or insight, in this hermeneutical exercise. All of a sudden, a doctrinal lawyer sees an appropriate selection of facts and an appropriate doctrinal twist, which results in a match. Afterwards, she is able, and obliged for that matter, to tell an explicit, fully consistent story. This, however, is only a technology for the representation of a decision that has been found otherwise. Specifically, the doctrinal lawyer is able to construct an explicit representation of a decision, but she does not have access to the mental process that has led her to find this result (Engel 2007).

Both scientists and doctrinal lawyers capitalize on insight (Bullbrook 1932). There is reason to believe that the mental process behind insight is closely related to the parallel constraint satisfaction mechanism that has already been presented in explaining how judges and juries assess the evidence. The key feature in the model, which also helps us understand insight, is attractor dynamics. The mind strives for generating meaning out of what initially looks like inconsistent evidence. It does so in deflating some while inflating other elements, until a qualitatively new, coherent picture emerges. The same holds when we search for a solution to what initially looks like an intractable problem. Not only is this process consciously not accessible; when subjects are induced to verbalize, their ability to find the solution deteriorates (Schooler 1993).

Norms

Performance

When is a decision "better than conscious"? The answer depends on the norm. The primary goal must be performance. Is the individual likely to perform better on the task at hand if she forgoes conscious deliberation and lets the nonconscious mental apparatus do all the work, or at least part of it (Hammond et al. 1987)? In deterministic problems, at least after the fact, performance can be assessed in an unequivocal way. If the problem is aggregating two apples and two oranges into four pieces of fruit, every answer that is not "four" is materially wrong. We may dispute whether this assessment follows from a violation of the axioms, or from a violation of social practice. However we have no doubt that being materially correct is the norm.

For the other two illustrations (i.e., guilt determination and competition), defining the norm is not so easy. Is the decision "guilty" below standard if, a few years later, DNA evidence proves that the defendant was not at the crime scene? The decision is certainly materially wrong, but is "truth" the appropriate standard? Ultimately, the legal order leaves this unanswered. In most legal orders, later DNA evidence on personal identity is sufficient to re-open proceedings. Yet as long as the new procedure is pending, the old judgment is still valid and, for example, it is possible to keep the defendant in prison until the former judgment has been formally repealed. Why is that? A radical improvement in the evidence, after the final ruling has been given, is a rare event. New, but less compelling evidence, however happens quite frequently. If this type of evidence sufficed to call earlier judgments into question, many judgments would be provisional, at best. To avoid this situation, the legal order is content with judgments that are "good enough," and procedural codes exist to define the necessary criteria. Typically, the standard has two elements. First, a final judgment must be based on evidence that, at least at face value, looks conclusive. Second, the requisite procedural safeguards for making the decision may not have been grossly violated.

Legal safety, the reliability of judgments, respect for the courts: these are all secondary goals. Yet behind each of them is the problem of defining the primary goal. Rare instances notwithstanding, for which DNA evidence is the best approximation, the legal system has no chance of ever fully establishing the truth. Instead, it must reach a decision based on an incomplete set of information. The legal system must face the very real chance of making materially wrong decisions. All it can attempt to do is to avoid patently wrong decisions. In reality, the problem goes deeper. In almost all legal cases, even after the fact, nobody will ever be able to say with certainty whether the decision has been materially right or wrong. The legal order has reacted by defining standards of proof. In criminal justice, the American legal order requires guilt to be established "beyond reasonable doubt." This obviously does not constitute certainty. It is sufficient if the judgment is based on evidence that makes guilt so highly probable that a reasonable person would exclude alternative explanations. Note the implication: if this standard was met in the original judgment, the conviction met the standard although the defendant was innocent.

Seemingly, with Ariel Rubinstein's game, one is back to determinism. Remember the game has a unique equilibrium, in mixed strategies, where the row player plays top with probability 1/3, and the column player plays left with probability 1/3. Yet this is a best response for the row player only if she believes the column player to maximize expected utility. This need not be true. The column player might be risk averse. In the interest of making sure that she is not left with her worst payoff, –2, she might always play right. From Figure 1.1 we already know that, if this is what the row player believes, she should play bottom, to secure her second best outcome, 1. Or the column player might be puzzled by the game and flip a coin. If the coin is fair, this gives probability 1/2 to both left and right. If this is what the row player believes, her best response is not matching this, but playing top with certainty. In expected values, this gives her:

$$\frac{1}{2}(TL)+\frac{1}{2}(TR)=\frac{1}{2}(2)+\frac{1}{2}(0)=1. \qquad (3)$$

Were she to match, she would only have:

$$\frac{1}{4}(TL)+\frac{1}{4}(TR)+\frac{1}{4}(BL)+\frac{1}{4}(BR)=\frac{1}{4}(2)+\frac{1}{4}(0)\frac{1}{4}(0)+\frac{1}{4}(1)=\frac{3}{4}. \qquad (4)$$

From this, one learns that only the calculation of the best response is fully determined, but that there is uncertainty about the behavior of the opponent. If the game is played only one time, and if the opponent is anonymous, the row player can at most rely on her world knowledge to base her selection. If she has read Ariel Rubinstein's paper, she might surmise that column players have the opposite propensity of row players. Since they are hit rather badly in the top left cell, they might, on average, be more inclined to play right. In that case, the row player is in a difficult situation. Let us indicate the subjective probability of the column player playing right by a, which we assume to be larger than 1/2. This implies the belief that she plays left with corresponding probability $(1 - a)$. If the row player plays bottom, she expects to earn $a \times 1 = a$. If she plays top, she expects $(1 - a)2$. She is indifferent between playing top and bottom if $a = (1 - a)2 \Rightarrow a = 2/3$.

Actually, this is exactly the probability distribution if the column player plays her best response. Making the other player indifferent is how a rational player determines probabilities in the mixed equilibrium. Consequently, if the row player maximizes utility, it is not enough for her to hypothesize that the column player would privilege right. She must believe her to privilege this action very strongly.

Rare events like frequency auctions notwithstanding, in reality people do not look up the literature on experimental games before they decide on strategic action. Instead the row player might rely on common sense to come up with the same hypothesis. Common sense basically works through the construction of a simple counterfactual: were I the column player, what would I do? Are others likely to be similar to me? To come up with these assessments, the row player would have to rely heavily on her intuition.

Secondary Goals

Until now, our analysis has ignored decision cost, which may be prohibitive. Imagine a two-person, simultaneous game where each player has to choose between four different actions. In reality, this is not a very rich setting; however, it means that a player must calculate best responses for 16 cells. Since a player must also know the best responses of the opponent, 32 results are needed. Now imagine that the game has no equilibrium in pure strategies. If a player starts calculating the mixed equilibrium over four strategies, she must solve a system of four equations in three unknowns. This will take some time and could potentially introduce a calculation error. The player may not have time or may not trust the calculations. Such a game is, of course, still manageable; however, if complexity is introduced, calculation becomes overwhelming. Recall chess. In statistical jargon, the game is NP-hard. No one could just calculate best responses.

The legal example of guilt determination epitomizes secondary goals which are, metaphorically speaking, measured in a different normative currency. Society is not content with judges merely reaching materially acceptable decisions. We want them to give reasons that the defendant can understand. We want them to demonstrate to the public at large that the legal system works properly. We want them to expose themselves to peer review by the upper courts and the wider legal community. We want them, as a side benefit of deciding the concrete case, to contribute to the evolution of the legal order (Engel 2001).

Audiences

Who should be interested in better understanding the power of nonconscious (elements in) decision making and problem solving? Psychologists, of course, since decision making and problem solving are their business. Neuroscientists as well, since searching for the neural correlates of nonconscious decision making provides them with a stimulating set of challenging research questions. But equally so, economists. Although economics has experienced a powerful behavioral revolution, this has only very tentatively evolved into a cognitive revolution. Economics, as a discipline, is not very attentive to mental mechanisms. The ideas expressed throughout this volume, however, demonstrate that taking nonconscious decision making seriously would be very productive for the field.

Last, but certainly not least, nonconscious decision making and problem solving are issues of great importance for institutional analysis and design. The illustration given of guilt determination has served as one example. Relevance, however, is not confined to understanding the workings of the legal system. We must also gain a more adequate sense of those individual and social problems that institutions set out to address. To date, most institutional analysis and, in particular, most new institutional economics build on the assumption that institutional addressees decide deliberately. In many practically, and for that matter, legally relevant contexts, this is factually wrong. If the power of the nonconscious were properly taken into account, institutional designers would come up with different, more adequate interventions.

Acknowledgments

Helpful comments on an earlier version by Andreas Glöckner and Julia Lupp are gratefully acknowledged.

References

Bartlett, F. C. 1932. Remembering. A Study in Experimental and Social Psychology. Cambridge: Cambridge Univ. Press.

Baumol, W. J. 1982. Contestable markets. An uprising in the theory of industry structure. *Am. Econ. Rev.* **72**:1–15.

Bolton, P., and M. Dewatripont. 2005. Contract Theory. Cambridge, MA: MIT Press.

Bullbrook, M. E. 1932. An experimental inquiry into the existence and nature of "insight." *Am. J. Psychol.* **44**:409–453.

Chomsky, N. 1959. A review of B.F. Skinner's verbal behavior. *Language* **35**:26–58.

Condry, K. F., E. Gramzow, and G. A. Cayton. 2003. Toddler counting. Three-year-olds' inferences about addition and subtraction. Poster presented at the 70th Biennial Meeting of the Society for Research in Child Development, Tampa, FL.

de Groot, A. D. 1965. Thought and Choice in Chess. The Hague: Mouton.

Dehaene, S. 1997. The Number Sense. How the Mind Creates Mathematics. New York: Oxford Univ. Press.

Dehaene, S., J.-P. Changeux, L. Naccache, J. Sackur, and C. Sergent. 2006. Conscious, preconscious, and subliminal processing. A testable taxonomy. *Trends Cogn. Sci.* **10**:204–211.

Engel, C. 2001. Die Grammatik des Rechts. In: Instrumente des Umweltschutzes im Wirkungsverbund, ed. H.-W. Rengeling and H. Hof, pp. 17–49. Baden-Baden: Nomos.

Engel, C. 2007. The psychological case for obliging judges to write reasons. In: The Impact of Court Procedure on the Psychology of Judical Decision Making, ed. C. Engel and F. Strack, pp. 71–109. Baden-Baden: Nomos.

Engel, C., and E. U. Weber. 2006. The impact of institutions on the decision how to decide. MPI Collective Goods Preprint No. 2006/19. http://ssrn.com/abstract=935024.

Fischhoff, B., B. Goitein, and Z. Shapira. 1981. Subjected expected utility. A model of decision-making. *J. Am. Soc. Info. Sci.* **32**:391–399.

Friedman, M. 1953. Essays in Positive Economics. Chicago: Univ. of Chicago Press.

Gigerenzer, G., P. M. Todd, and ABC Research Group. 1999. Simple Heuristics that Make Us Smart. New York: Oxford Univ. Press.

Glimcher, P. W. 2003. Decisions, Uncertainty, and the Brain: The Science of Neuroeconomics. Cambridge, MA: MIT Press.

Glöckner, A. 2007. Does intuition beat fast and frugal heuristics? A systematic empirical analysis. In: Intuition in Judgment and Decision Making, ed. H. Plessner, C. Betsch, and T. Betsch. Mahway, NJ: Lawrence Erlbaum, in press.

Hammond, K. R., R. M. Hamm, J. Grassia, and T. Pearson. 1987. Direct comparison of the efficacy of intuitive and analytical cognition in expert judgment. IEEE Transactions. *Systems, Man, & Cybernetics* **17(5)**:753–770.

Harsanyi, J. 1967–1968. Games with incomplete information played by "Bayesian" players. *Management Sci.* **14**:159–182, 320–224, 486–502.

Hastie, R. 1993. Inside the Juror. The Psychology of Juror Decision Making. Cambridge: Cambridge Univ. Press.

Hastie, R., S. Penrod, and N. Pennington. 1983. Inside the Jury. Cambridge, MA: Harvard Univ. Press.

Hauser, M. D., and E. S. Spelke. 2005. Evolutionary and developmental foundations of human knowledge: A case study of mathematics. In: The Cognitive Neurosciences III, ed. M. S. Gazzaniga, pp. 853–864. Cambridge, MA: MIT Press.

Juslin, P., H. Olsson, and A.-C. Olsson. 2003. Exemplar effects in categorization and multiple-cue judgment. *J. Exp. Psychol.: Gen.* **132**:133–156.

Kagel, J. H., and A. E. Roth, eds. 1995. The Handbook of Experimental Economics. Princeton, NJ: Princeton Univ. Press.

Kahneman, D., and A. Tversky. 2000. Choices, Values, and Frames. Russell Sage Foundation. Cambridge: Cambridge Univ. Press.

Kirzner, I. 1994. On the economics of time and ignorance. The market process. In: Essays in Contemporary Austrian Economics, ed. P. J. Boettke und D. L. Prychitko, pp. 38–44. Brookfield: Elgar.

Lipton, J. S., and E. S. Spelke. 2005. Preschool children master the logic of number word meanings. *Cognition* **98**:57–66.

Matsuzawa, T., M. Tomonaga, and M. Tanaka, M., eds. 2006. Cognitive development in chimpanzees. *Intl. J. Primatology* **28(4)**:965–967.

Nash, J. 1951. Non-cooperative games. *Annals Math.* **54**:286–295.

Rubinstein, A. 2007. Instinctive and Cognitive Reasoning: A Study of Response Times. *Econ. J.*, in press.

Sauerland, M., and S. L. Sporer. 2007. Post-decision confidence, decision time, and self-reported decision processes as postdictors of identification accuracy. *Psychol. Crime Law*, in press.

Savage, L. J. 1954. The Foundations of Statistics. New York: Wiley.

Schooler, J. W. 1993. Thoughts beyond words: When language overshadows insight. *J. Exp. Psychol.: Gen.* **122**:166–183.

Schulz, J. 1992. Sachverhaltsfeststellung und Beweistheorie: Elemente einer Theorie strafprozessualer Sachverhaltsfeststellung. Köln: Heymanns.

Simon, D. 1998. A psychological model of judicial decision making. *Rutgers Law J.* **30**:1–142.

Simon, D., L. B. Pham, Q. A. Le, and K. J. Holyoak. 2001. The emergence of coherence over the course of decision making. *J. Exp. Psychol.: Learn. Mem. Cogn.* **27**:1250–1260.

Smith, E. R., and M. A. Zárate. 1992. Exemplar-based model of social judgement. *Psychol. Rev.* **99**:3–21.

Sporer, S. L., R. S. Malpass, and G. Köhnken. 1996. Psychological Issues in Eyewitness Identification. Mahwah, NJ: Lawrence Erlbaum.

Straffin, P. D. 1993. Game Theory and Strategy. Washington, D.C.: Mathematical Assoc. of America.

Trick, L. M. and Z. W. Pylyshyn. 1994. Why are small and large numbers enumerated differently? A limited-capacity preattentive stage in vision. *Psychol. Rev.* **101**:80–102.

Wechsler, D. 1945. A standardized memory test for clinical use. *J. Psychol.* **19**:87–95.

Wynn, K. 1990. Children's understanding of counting. *Cognition* **36**:155–193.

Wynn, K. 1992. Children's acquisition of the number words and the counting system. *Cogn. Psychol.* **24**:220–251.

2

Conscious and Nonconscious Processes

Distinct Forms of Evidence Accumulation?

Stanislas Dehaene[1,2,3,4]

[1] INSERM, U562, Cognitive Neuroimaging Unit, 91191 Gif/Yvette, France
[2] CEA, DSV/I2BM, NeuroSpin Center, 91191 Gif/Yvette, France
[3] Univ Paris-Sud, IFR49, 91191 Gif/Yvette, France
[4] Collège de France, 75005 Paris, France

Abstract

Among the many brain events evoked by a visual stimulus, which ones are associated specifically with conscious perception, and which merely reflect nonconscious processing? Understanding the neuronal mechanisms of consciousness is a major challenge for cognitive neuroscience. Recently, progress has been achieved by contrasting behavior and brain activation in minimally different experimental conditions, one of which leads to conscious perception whereas the other does not. This chapter reviews briefly this line of research and speculates on its theoretical interpretation. I propose to draw links between evidence accumulation models, which are highly successful in capturing elementary psychophysical decisions, and the conscious/nonconscious dichotomy. In this framework, conscious access would correspond to the crossing of a threshold in evidence accumulation within a distributed "global workspace," a set of recurrently connected neurons with long axons that is able to integrate and broadcast back evidence from multiple brain processors. During nonconscious processing, evidence would be accumulated locally within specialized subcircuits, but would fail to reach the threshold needed for global ignition and, therefore, conscious reportability.

An Experimental Strategy for Exploring Consciousness

Although the nature of consciousness remains a formidable problem, Lionel Naccache and I argue that it can be approached through behavioral and brain-imaging methods:

> The cognitive neuroscience of consciousness aims at determining whether there
> is a systematic form of information processing and a reproducible class of neuro-
> nal activation patterns that systematically distinguish mental states that subjects
> label as "conscious" from other states (Dehaene and Naccache 2001).

In that respect, identifying the neural bases of consciousness need not be any
more difficult than, say, identifying that of other states of mind (e.g., face perception or anger). Bernard Baars (1989) outlined a simple *contrastive method* which, in his own terms, consists simply in contrasting pairs of similar
events, where one is conscious but the other is not. Baars noted that in the
last forty years, experimental psychology and neuropsychology have identified
dozens of contrasts relevant to consciousness. Examples include normal vision versus blindsight; extinguished versus seen stimuli in patients with hemi-
neglect; masked versus nonmasked visual stimuli; habituated versus novel
stimuli; accessed versus nonaccessed meanings of ambiguous stimuli; distinctions within states of consciousness (sleep, coma, wakefulness, arousal);
voluntary versus involuntary actions; or even explicit problem solving versus
implicit "incubation."

   In this chapter, I focus on the masking paradigm, perhaps the simplest and
most productive situation in which to study conscious access in normal subjects. During masking, a target visual stimulus is flashed briefly on a computer
screen. It can be followed or preceded by a "mask": another visual stimulus
presented at the same screen location or just nearby. Under the right conditions, presentation of the mask erases the perception of the target stimulus, and
subjects report that they are no longer able to see it. Yet the target stimulus still
induces behavioral priming effects and brain activation patterns which correspond to nonconscious or "subliminal" (below threshold) processing. Focusing
on what types of processing can occur under subliminal masking conditions,
and what additional processes unfold once the stimulus is unmasked, can thus
shed considerable light on the nature of conscious access.

How Do We Measure Whether Conscious Access Occurred?

As mentioned above, once an appropriate paradigm such as masking is available, studying the cerebral correlates of conscious access need not be more
difficult than, say, studying face perception. In both cases, one correlates brain
activity with the presence or absence of the relevant aspect of the stimulus
(face vs. nonface stimulus, or conscious vs. nonconscious perception). What is
special about conscious access, however, is that it is defined solely in subjective terms. Thus, Lionel Naccache and I have argued:

> The first crucial step is *to take seriously introspective phenomenological reports.*
> Subjective reports are the key phenomena that a cognitive neuroscience of con-
> sciousness purports to study. As such, they constitute primary data that need to

be measured and recorded along with other psychophysiological observations (Dehaene and Naccache 2001).

Increasingly, therefore, consciousness research relies on subjective reports as a defining criterion. Ideally, one should measure the extent of conscious perception on every single trial, possibly using a graded scale to capture even fine nuances of the percept (Del Cul et al. 2007; Sergent et al. 2005; Sergent and Dehaene 2004). For an identical objective stimulus, one may then contrast the brain activation observed when it is or is not subjectively seen.

The emphasis on subjective reporting goes against a long tradition in psychophysics and experimental psychology, which has emphasized the need for objective criteria based on signal-detection theory. According to this tradition, a masked stimulus is accepted as being subliminal only if performance on some direct task of stimulus perception falls to chance level (zero d-prime). There are several difficulties associated with this objective definition, however. First, it tends to overestimate conscious perception, as there are many conditions in which subjects perform better than chance, and yet deny perceiving any stimulus. Second, it requires accepting the null hypothesis of chance-level performance; usually d-prime never quite drops to zero, and whether it is significant or not depends merely on the number of trials dedicated to its measurement. Finally, performance can be at chance level for some tasks, but not others. Does above-chance performance on the former tasks count as evidence of conscious perception, or merely of subliminal processing? The issue seems unsolvable unless we have a good theory of which tasks can only be performed at a conscious level, and thus constitute appropriate objective measures of conscious access, and which tasks can operate under subliminal conditions.

By focusing first and foremost on subjective reports, we can avoid this somewhat Byzantine discussion of what constitutes a good subliminal stimulus. It is an empirical fact that, when subjects rate a stimulus subjectively as having been seen consciously, a major transition occurs such that the stimulus also becomes available for a variety of objective tasks. For instance, Figure 2.1 shows data from a masking paradigm (Del Cul et al. 2007) where subjects were asked, on every trial, to perform two tasks on a masked digit: (a) a subjective task of rating the stimulus visibility; (b) an objective, forced-choice task of deciding whether the stimulus was larger or smaller than five. As the interval between the target and mask increased, both subjective and objective performance increased in a nonlinear sigmoidal manner. Both sigmoids allowed for the definition of a threshold (placed at the inflection point). We found that these subjective and objective definitions of the consciousness threshold were virtually identical and highly correlated between subjects. Furthermore, both were degraded jointly in patients with schizophrenia or multiple sclerosis (Del Cul et al. 2006; Reuter et al. 2007). Interestingly, below this threshold, the objective and subjective tasks could be dissociated, as there was a proportion of

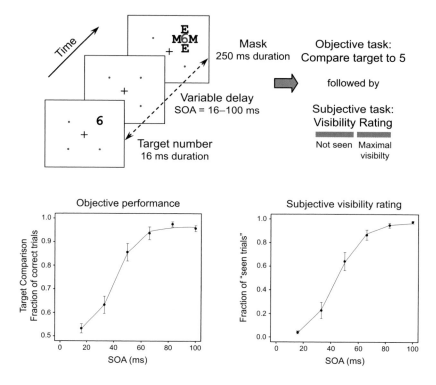

Figure 2.1   Example of a masking paradigm where objective and subjective measures concur to define a threshold for perceptual consciousness (after Del Cul et al. 2007). A digit is flashed at one of four parafoveal locations and is followed after a variable delay by a surrounding letter mask (top left panel). On each trial, participants are asked to perform an objective task (decide if the digit is larger or smaller than 5) and a subjective task (rate the stimulus visibility). Both measures concur: performance is low at short delays, but suddenly jumps to a high value above a threshold delay (around 50 ms). This method thus defines a range of "subliminal" (below-threshold) stimuli. SOA = stimulus onset asynchrony.

trials in which objective performance remained higher than chance, although subjects denied subjective perception.

In view of such results, the following operational definitions of conscious and nonconscious processing may be proposed. First, on a single-trial basis, priority should be given to subjective reports in defining what constitutes a "conscious" trial. Second, when averaging across trials, the threshold for conscious access may be identified with the major nonlinearity that occurs in both subjective and objective performance as the stimulus is progressively un-masked. Third, the presence of nonconscious processing can be inferred when-ever objective performance departs from subjective reports; for instance, by remaining above-chance in a region of stimulus space where subjective reports fall to zero.

The latter hypothesis lies at the heart of the *dissociation method*, which has been used by many others to separate conscious and nonconscious processing. For instance, masking conditions can be found that create a U-shaped curve for subjective perception as a function of target-mask interval. Other aspects of performance, such as response time and brain activity patterns, vary monotonically with the same stimulus parameter, thus clearly reflecting nonconscious stimulus processing (Haynes et al. 2005; Vorberg et al. 2003).

Subliminal Processing and Evidence Accumulation Models

A broad array of research has focused on the issue of the depth of subliminal processing of masked visual stimuli: to what extent is a masked stimulus that is reported subjectively as "not seen" processed in the brain? Here I present only a brief overview of this line of research (for a broader review, see Kouider and Dehaene 2007). The main goal is to examine these data in relation to models of decision making by evidence accumulation, which have proven highly successful in mathematical modeling of chronometric and neurophysiological data from simple psychophysical decisions (e.g., Laming 1968; Link 1992; Smith and Ratcliff 2004; Usher and McClelland 2001; Shadlen, this volume).

For the sake of concreteness, one such accumulation model is presented in Figure 2.2. This particular model was shown to capture much of what is known about simple numerical decisions and their neural bases (Dehaene 2007). While many variants can be proposed (see Smith and Ratcliff 2004), this model incorporates mechanisms that are generic to a variety of psychophysical tasks. To illustrate this, consider the task of deciding if a number, presented either as a set of dots or as an Arabic numeral, is smaller or larger than 10. The model assumes the following steps:

1. Visual perception of the stimulus.
2. Semantic coding along the appropriate dimension (here, numerosity).
3. Categorization of the incoming evidence in relation to the instructions. This is achieved by separating this continuum into pools of units, each favoring a distinct response (here, units preferring numbers larger than 10 and units preferring numbers smaller than 10).
4. Computation of a log likelihood ratio (logLR), a quantity which estimates the likelihood that response R1 or R2 is correct, given the sensory evidence.
5. Stochastic accumulation of the logLR over a period of time, until a threshold amount is obtained in one direction or the other.
6. Emission of a motor response when the threshold is exceeded.

Models of this form have been shown to capture the details of chronometric data, including the shape of response time (RT) distributions and speed-accuracy trade-offs. Within the context of conscious versus nonconscious

1. Visual perception

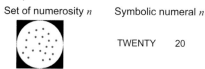

Set of numerosity *n*   Symbolic numeral *n*

                            TWENTY   20

2. Semantic coding by Log-Gaussian numerosity detectors

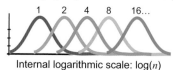

Internal logarithmic scale: log(*n*)

3. Categorization: formation of two pools of units

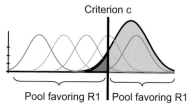

Pool favoring R1 ⎪ Pool favoring R1

4. Computation of log likelihood ratio (logLR)

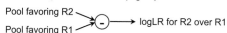

Pool favoring R2
Pool favoring R1 → logLR for R2 over R1

5. Stochastic accumulation of logLR, forming a random-walk process

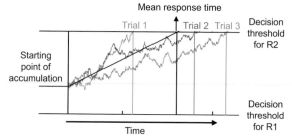

6. Application of a threshold and emission of a motor response

Figure 2.2   Proposed theoretical model of decision making in an objective numerical comparison task (for a full mathematical exposition, see Dehaene 2007). Subjects first encode each input number as a random variable on an internal continuum (top). The decision mechanism consists in accumulating evidence by adding up the log likelihood ratios (logLRs) for or against each of the two possible responses provided by successive samples of the random variable (middle). As a result, each trial consists in an internal random walk of the accumulated logLR (bottom). A response is emitted whenever the random walk reaches one of two response thresholds. Evidence reviewed in the present chapter suggests that all stages of the model can begin to operate in the absence of consciousness.

computation, a key question is: Which of the model's mechanisms can operate under subliminal conditions, and which cannot?

Subliminal Perception

Extensive research has demonstrated that a subliminal masked stimulus can be processed at the perceptual level. The main support comes from the *repetition priming* experiment, in which a subliminal prime is shown to facilitate the subsequent processing of an identical stimulus presented as a target. Priming is evidenced behaviorally as a reduction of response time on repeated trials compared to nonrepeated trials and neurally as a reduction in the amount of evoked brain activity (repetition suppression).

Repetition priming indicates that a subliminal stimulus can be registered perceptually. As illustrated in Figure 2.3, however, priming can occur at multiple levels. In extrastriatal cortex, priming is sensitive to the repetition of the exact same stimulus. In more anterior sectors of fusiform cortex, priming is more abstract and can resist a change in surface format, for example, when the same word is presented in upper case or lower case (Dehaene et al. 2001).

Subliminal Semantic Processing

At an even more abstract level, semantic subliminal priming has been observed, for example, in the left lateral temporal cortex for synonym words such as sofa/couch (Devlin et al. 2004) or for Japanese words presented in Kanji and Kana notations (Nakamura et al. 2005). Likewise, numerical repetition priming has been observed in bilateral intraparietal cortex when number words are presented in Arabic or word notations (Naccache and Dehaene 2001a). These observations have been confirmed by detailed behavioral studies (Naccache and Dehaene 2001b; Reynvoet et al. 2002). In terms of the model presented in Figure 2.2, they suggest that subliminal primes can partially bias the level of semantic coding.

The reality of subliminal semantic processing is confirmed by several empirical findings. Subliminal words can evoke an N400 component of the event-related potential, which depends on their semantic relation to a previously presented word (Kiefer 2002; Kiefer and Brendel 2006). Subliminal words that convey an emotion (e.g., rape, shark) can cause an activation of the amygdala (Naccache et al. 2005), and the threshold for their conscious perception is lowered, indicating that they receive distinct processing even prior to conscious access (Gaillard, Del Cul et al. 2006).

In many of these cases, brain activation evoked by a subliminal stimulus is much reduced compared to the activation evoked by the same stimulus under conscious perception conditions (Dehaene et al. 2001). However, there are

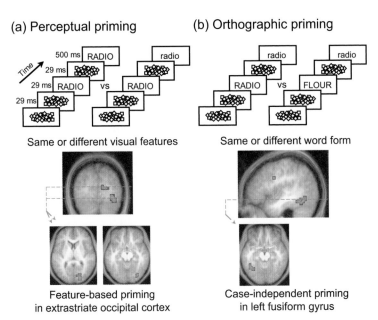

(a) Perceptual priming

(b) Orthographic priming

Same or different visual features

Same or different word form

Feature-based priming
in extrastriate occipital cortex

Case-independent priming
in left fusiform gyrus

Figure 2.3   Brain imaging evidence for nonconscious processing at multiple levels of word and digit processing. All experiments rely on the priming method (Naccache and Dehaene 2001a), which consists in examining whether a subliminal prime can modulate the processing of a subsequent conscious target. The nature of the prime-target relation changes the site of modulation of brain activation: (a) shared low-level visual features cause perceptual priming in extrastriate occipital cortex; (b) case-independent orthographic priming of words occurs in the left occipito-temporal "visual word form area" (Dehaene et al. 2001).

some cases in which a full-blown activation can be observed in the absence of conscious perception. In early visual areas, even heavily masked stimuli can produce essentially unchanged event-related responses in both fMRI (Haynes et al. 2005) and ERPs (Del Cul et al. 2007). In higher visual areas, large non-conscious responses have been observed under conditions of light masking, where invisibility is due to distraction by a secondary task (e.g., the attentional blink paradigm). Even a late (~400 ms) and abstract semantic event such as the N400 can be largely (Sergent et al. 2005) or even fully (Luck et al. 1996) preserved during the attentional blink.

Subliminal Accumulation of Evidence towards a Decision

Dehaene et al. (1998) and Leuthold (Leuthold and Kopp 1998) first showed that a subliminal stimulus can bias a decision all the way down to the response programming level. The paradigm used by Dehaene et al. (1998) is illustrated in Figure 2.3c, d. Subjects had to categorize numbers as being larger or smaller

(c) Semantic priming

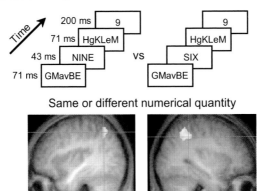

Same or different numerical quantity

Quantity priming in bilateral intraparietal sulci

(d) Motor congruity priming

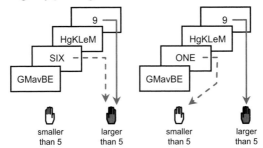

Same or different motor response

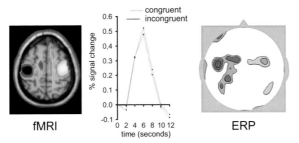

Response congruity effect in motor cortex

Figure 2.3 (continued)   (c) Repetition of a number, in Arabic or verbal notation, causes semantic priming in bilateral intraparietal sulci (Naccache and Dehaene 2001a); (d) congruence of the motor responses associated with the prime and target modulates motor cortex activity, as if motor representations accumulate partial evidence from the prime before accumulating the main evidence arising from the target (Dehaene et al. 1998).

than five by pressing a right- or left-hand button (the response mappings were assigned randomly and switched in the middle of the experiment). Unknown to the participants, a subliminal number was presented prior to each target. A congruity effect was observed: on congruent trials, where the prime fell on the same side as the target (e.g., 9 followed by 6, both being larger than 5), responses were faster than on incongruent trials where they fell on different sides of 5 (e.g., 1 followed by 6). This effect could be measured by fMRI and ERP recordings of the motor cortex as a partial accumulation of motor bias towards the response side elicited by the prime.

Thus, activation evoked by an unseen prime can propagate all the way down to the motor level. Within the context of the model presented in Figure 2.2, this implies that semantic coding of the stimulus, categorization by application of arbitrary instructions, and response selection by evidence accumulation can all proceed, at least in part, without conscious perception. Research by Vorberg et al. (2003) supports this conclusion well. Using primes shaped as arrows pointing left or right, Vorberg et al. showed that the behavioral priming effect increased monotonically with the time interval separating the prime from the mask (while conscious prime perception was either absent or followed a non-monotonic, U-shaped curve). Those results, presented in Figure 2.4, can be captured mathematically using an evidence accumulation model similar to the one presented in Figure 2.2. Vorberg et al's model supposes that the various response alternatives are coded by leaky accumulators which receive stochastic input: first from the prime, then from the target. The accumulators add up sensory evidence until a predefined threshold is reached, after which a response is emitted. Mathematical analysis and simulations show that this model can reproduce the empirical observation of a bias in response time. At long SOAs, the model predicts that primes can also induce a high error rate, especially if the response threshold is relatively low—a prediction which is empirically supported by the data.

Role of Instruction and Attention in Subliminal Processing

Subliminal processing was previously thought to be automatic and independent of attention. In recent years, however, several effects from top-down modulation on subliminal processing have been identified.

Modulation by Instructions

Task instructions readily alter the fate of subliminal stimuli. As just described, masked primes can elicit instruction-dependent activation in the motor cortex (Dehaene et al. 1998; Eimer and Schlaghecken 1998; Leuthold and Kopp 1998; Vorberg et al. 2003). Even details of the instructions provided to subjects, such as whether they are told that the targets consist of all numbers 1

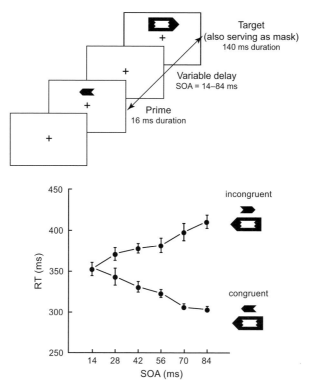

Figure 2.4 Evidence suggesting a partial accumulation of evidence from a nonconscious prime during a simple sensorimotor task (after Vorberg et al. 2003). Subjects classify target arrows as pointing right or left, while a masked prime also points left or right. A linear priming effect is seen: as the prime-target delay increases, congruent primes induce a monotonic speed-up of response times, while incongruent primes cause a monotonic slowing down. The slope of the effect is such that the difference in response time (RT) is essentially equal to the prime-target delay (SOA = stimulus onset asynchrony), suggesting that evidence is being continuously accumulated, first from the prime, then from the target.

through 9 or just the numbers 1, 4, 6 and 9, can affect subliminal priming (Kunde et al. 2003). Though still debated, those results suggest that the arbitrary stimulus-response mappings conveyed by conscious instructions can also apply to nonconscious stimuli. As noted above, within the framework of evidence accumulation models, this implies that an entire instruction set, reflected in how the stimulus is categorized and mapped onto responses, can be partially applied to a nonconscious stimulus.

Modulation by Executive Attention

Within-task changes in executive attention also seem to impact on subliminal processing. For instance, Kunde et al. (2003) studied the "Gratton effect," a strategic increase in executive control which follows Stroop interference trials. The effect is such that, if on trial $n-1$ subjects experience a cognitive conflict due to a Stroop-incongruent trial, then on trial n the Stroop effect is reduced, as if subjects somehow regain stronger control over the task (perhaps by focusing attention more tightly around the time of the target). Kunde et al. manipulated the consciousness of the conflict by presenting, on each trial, a subliminal or supraliminal prime followed by a conscious target. They observed that the Gratton effect could only be induced by a conscious trial (i.e., the conflict at trial $n-1$ had to be a conscious conflict). Once established, however, the increase in control applied to both subliminal and supraliminal trials: the effect of conflict at trial n was diminished, whether or not this conflict was consciously perceived. This suggests that executive attention, once modified by a conscious stimulus, can have an impact on subsequent subliminal processing.

Modulation of Subliminal Priming by Temporal Attention

An impact of temporal attention on subliminal processing was demonstrated by Naccache et al. (2002) in a numerical masked priming paradigm. They showed that subliminal priming was present when subjects could attend to the time of presentation of the prime-target pair, but vanished when stimuli could not be temporally attended. Kiefer and Brendel (2006) observed a similar effect in an experiment investigating the N400 potential elicited by masked words. Unseen masked words elicited a much larger N400 when they were temporally attended than when they were not.

In terms of evidence accumulation models, temporal attention effects may relate to the little-studied issue of how the accumulators are reset and opened. To operate optimally, the accumulators must be emptied before each trial, and evidence must only be accumulated once the stimulus is actually present. The above effects can be interpreted as showing that semantic and decision-related evidence arising from subliminal primes fails to be accumulated whenever it is presented outside of the temporal window when the target is expected. Alternatively, if accumulated, it is reset to zero and therefore cannot bias target processing.

Modulation by Spatial Attention

Kentridge et al. (1999, 2004) first reported that blindsight patient GY could use consciously perceived cues to enhance unconscious processing of visual targets. When a target was presented in his scotoma region, patient GY responded more quickly and accurately when it was validly cued by a consciously perceptible arrow pointing to it, than when he was invalidly cued. In both cases, he still claimed that he could not see the target. Modulation of subliminal priming by spatial attention was also observed in normal subjects (Lachter et al. 2004; Marzouki et al. 2007).

In summary, task preparation includes many different components, including attention to the relevant stimulus parameter (e.g., number) and to the likely location and presentation time of the stimulus, as well as preparation of a stimulus-response mapping and setting of executive-level parameters (e.g., response threshold). Evidence suggests that essentially all of these task-preparation components, once prepared for a conscious target, apply as well to a nonconscious target.

Recent Evidence for Extended Subliminal Processing

Recently, subliminal research has gone one step further and asked whether task-preparation processes themselves can be primed subliminally. The central issue is whether processes traditionally associated with a "central executive" system can also unfold in the absence of consciousness.

Pessiglione et al. (2007) demonstrated that one aspect of task setting—motivation—could be cued subliminally. Prior to each trial of a force-generation task, subjects were presented with conscious information about the amount of money they could earn on the subsequent trial: one penny or one pound. Unknown to them, each conscious monetary cue was preceded by a subliminal image which could be congruent or incongruent with the conscious image. This subliminal information modulated the subject's motivation, as evidenced by a modulation of both the applied force and the amount of activation of a bilateral ventral pallidal region known to convey reward anticipation information.

In a similar line of research, Mattler (2003) presented a series of experiments in which a square or diamond shape successively cued increasingly abstract aspects of the task: response finger, response hand, stimulus modality (auditory or visual), or the requested task (pitch or timbre judgment). For instance, in one experiment, subjects heard a variable sound which, if preceded by a square, had to be judged for its timbre and, if preceded by a diamond, had to be judged for its pitch. Unknown to the subject, each instruction cue was preceded by a masked prime which could be congruent or incongruent with the cue. Response times were systematically shorter on congruent trials and this effect increased with the prime-mask interval in a manner which was dissociated from the U-shaped curve for conscious perception. Thus, even task selection seemed to be biased by a subliminal cue.

Unfortunately, Mattler's (2003) results could also be interpreted as a conflict at a purely visual level of cue identification; that is, the measure response time included components of cue identification, task selection, and task execution, and the observed priming might have arisen from the perceptual component alone. To demonstrate firmly that a subliminal prime could affect task selection, Lau and Passingham (2007) resorted to functional imaging. They selected tasks of phonological versus semantic judgment on visual words that are associated with broadly different cortical networks. Using a design similar to Mattler's, they then showed that not only the response time but the entire task-related network was modulated up or down as a function of whether the subliminal prime was congruent or incongruent with the task information provided by the visible cue. This subliminal task-cueing effect was not sufficient to reverse the conscious task cue, but it did yield an increase in subjects' error rate.

One last paradigm of relevance to the present discussion was developed by van Gaal et al. (2007). They showed that a subliminal cue could fulfill the role of a "stop signal" requiring subjects to interrupt their ongoing response to a main task. Unconscious stop signals yielded a minuscule but still significant slowing down of response time and increase in errors. Thus, subliminal stimuli can trigger the first hints of a task interruption.

How can one interpret such high-level priming effects? One possibility is that, even at the "central executive" level, task selection and task control processes continue to operate according to rules of evidence accumulation, which can be biased by subliminal priming. According to the model illustrated in Figure 2.2, subjects select a motor response by forming two pools of units: those accumulating evidence for response R1 and those accumulating evidence for response R2. Perhaps the "central executive" consists of nothing but similar decision mechanisms organized in a control hierarchy (Koechlin et al. 2003). At a higher level, similar evidence accumulation processes would be involved in the selection of one of two tasks, T1 and T2. Those accumulators would accrue evidence provided by conscious cues, but also by subliminal cues. Sigman and Dehaene (2006) presented precisely such a model of task selection in a dual-task context. They showed how the time to select which task to perform added a variable duration to the overall response time which could be captured well by an accumulator model. It remains to be seen whether these ideas can be extended to an entire hierarchy of interacting decision systems, as proposed, for example, by Koechlin et al (2003).

Limits to Subliminal Processing

Given this wealth of evidence which indicates that subliminal processing can extend to a high cognitive level, one may reasonably ask if there are any limits to subliminal processing. Are there mental processes that can be executed only once conscious perception has occurred? This question naturally arises in relation to the evolutionary role of consciousness. Although the evidence remains fragmentary, several mental operations can be associated speculatively with conscious-level processing.

Durable and Explicit Information Maintenance

Priming experiments show that subliminal information tends to be short-lived: after about 500 ms, priming effects typically cease to be detectable (Greenwald et al. 1996; Mattler 2005). To bridge delays of a few seconds, information is thought to be stored in working memory by active populations of neurons, particularly in prefrontal cortex. When information reaches this working memory stage, Dehaene and Naccache (2001) have suggested that it is always consciously accessible. Kunde et al.'s (2003) work, reviewed above, fits nicely with this conclusion, since it shows that only the conscious variables of trial *n*–1 can be carried out to trial *n*. Similar evidence is provided by the trace-conditioning paradigm, in which conditioning across a temporal gap only occurs if subjects report being aware of the relations among the stimuli (Clark et al. 2002). Additional supporting data has been reviewed by Dehaene and Naccache (2001). Altogether, the evidence points to a crucial role of consciousness in bridging information across a delay.

Global Access and Novel Combinations of Operations

Consciousness has been suggested to play an essential role in the expression of novel behaviors that require putting together evidence from multiple sources (e.g., by confronting evidence spread across several trials). For instance, Merikle et al. (1995) studied subjects' ability to control inhibition in a Stroop-like task as a function of the conscious perceptibility of the conflicting information. Subjects had to classify a colored target string as green or red. Each target was preceded by a prime, which could be the word GREEN or RED. In this situation, the classical Stroop effect occurred: responses were faster when the word and color were congruent than when they were incongruent. However, when the prime-target relations were manipulated by presenting 75% of incongruent trials, subjects could take advantage of the predictability of the target from the prime to become faster on incongruent trials than on congruent trials, thus inverting the Stroop effect. Crucially, this strategic inversion occurred only when the prime was consciously perceptible. No strategic effect was observed when the word prime was masked (Merikle et al. 1995) or fell outside the focus of attention (Merikle and Joordens 1997). Here, only the classical, automatic Stroop effect prevailed. Thus, the ability to inhibit an automatic stream of processes and to deploy a novel strategy depended crucially on the conscious availability of information.

This conclusion may need to be qualified in the light of recent evidence, reviewed above, that is, task switching or task stopping can be modulated partially by subliminal cues (Lau and Passingham 2007; Mattler 2003; van Gaal et al. 2007). Note, however, that this evidence was always obtained under conditions of highly routinized performance. Subjects performed hundreds of trials with consciously perceived task cues before the same cues, presented subliminally, began to affect task choice. This is very different from the rapid deployment of novel strategies that, presumably, can only be deployed under conscious conditions.

Intentional Action

As noted by Dehaene and Naccache (2001), the spontaneous generation of intentional behavior may constitute a third property specifically associated with conscious perception. It is noteworthy that, in all of the above priming tasks, although subliminal primes modulate the response time to another conscious stimulus, they almost never induce a full-blown behavior in and of themselves. Only on a very small proportion of trials do subliminal primes actually cause overt responses. When they do, such trials are typically labeled as unintended errors by the subject (and by the experimenter).

As a related example, consider the case of blindsight patients (Weiskrantz 1997). Some of these patients, even though they claim to be blind, show an excellent performance in pointing to objects. As noted by Dennett (1992) and Weiskrantz (1997), a fundamental difference with normal subjects, however, is that blindsight patients never spontaneously initiate any visually guided behavior in their impaired field. Good performance can be elicited only by forcing them to respond to stimulation.

In summary, nonconscious stimuli do not seem to reach a stage of processing at which information representation enters into a deliberation process that supports voluntary action with a sense of ownership. If they do reach this stage, it is only with a trickle of activation that modulates decision time but does not determine the decision outcome.

Cerebral Bases of Conscious and Nonconscious Computations

The hypothesis that conscious information is associated with a second stage of processing that cannot be deployed fully for subliminal stimuli meshes well with recent experiments that have directly compared the brain activation evoked by conscious versus nonconscious stimuli. Many such experiments have been performed with fMRI, and they converge to suggest that, relative to a masked stimulus, an unmasked stimulus is amplified and gains access to high levels of activation in prefrontal and parietal areas (Dehaene et al. 2006; Dehaene et al. 2001; Haynes et al. 2005; for review and discussion, see Kouider et al. 2007). Most relevant to the present discussion are time-resolved experiments using ERPs or MEG that have followed the processing of a stimulus in time as it crosses or does not cross the threshold for conscious perception. My colleagues and I have performed such experiments under conditions in which invisibility was created either by masking (Del Cul et al. 2007; see also Koivisto et al. 2006; Melloni et al. 2007; van Aalderen-Smeets et al. 2006) or by inattention during the attentional blink (Gross et al. 2004; Kranczioch et al. 2003; Sergent et al. 2005). In both cases, we were able to analyze a subset of trials in which the very same stimulus was presented, but was or was not consciously perceived according to subjective reports.

The results were highly convergent in coarsely separating two periods of stimulus processing. During the first 270 ms, brain activation unfolded in an essentially unchanged manner whether or not the stimuli were consciously perceived. Strong visual activation was seen, quickly extending to the ventral temporal visual pathway. In the case of the attentional blink, the nonconscious activation extended even further in time, with very strong left lateral temporal activity around 400 ms plausibly associated with semantic-level processing (see also Luck et al. 1996). However, around 270 ms, an important divergence occurred, with a sudden surge of additional activation being observed on conscious trials only. Over a few tens of milliseconds, activation expanded into bilateral inferior and dorsolateral frontal regions, anterior cingulate cortex, and posterior parietal cortex. As shown in Figure 2.5, this activity was reduced drastically on nonconscious trials: only short-lived activation was seen, quickly decaying towards zero about 500 ms after stimulus presentation. By contrast, activation seemed to be amplified actively on conscious trials.

The parsing of brain activation into two stages— early activation by subliminal stimuli, followed by late global amplification and reverberation—seems to be a generic phenomenon that can be observed in various stimulus modalities, by a variety of methods, and in multiple species. Thus Victor Lamme and collaborators (2002), using electrophysiological recordings in macaque area V1, have distinguished early feed-forward versus late feedback responses. They found that only the latter were sensitive to attention and reportability. Using intracranial electrodes in human epileptic patients, my team has obtained evidence for a similar division in human subjects during subliminal versus conscious word reading (Gaillard, Naccache et al. 2006; Naccache et al. 2005). In many electrodes, subliminal words evoked only a first peak of activation whereas conscious words evoked a similar but magnified peak followed by a sustained period of activation.

To give yet a third example, Nieuwenhuis et al. (2001) used ERPs in humans to track error detection and compensation processes. When subjects made an undetected erroneous saccade, an early error-related negativity was observed over mesial frontal electrodes, presumably reflecting a nonconscious triggering of an anterior cingulate system for error detection. However, only when the error was detected consciously was this early waveform amplified and followed by a massive P3-like waveform associated presumably with the expansion of activation into a broader cortical and subcortical network.

A Global Workspace Model of Conscious Access

Jean-Pierre Changeux and I have suggested that these global self-amplifying properties of brain activation during conscious access can be accounted for by the concept of a "global workspace" (Dehaene and Changeux 2005; Dehaene and Naccache 2001; Dehaene et al. 2003). This model, which has been backed

S. Dehaene

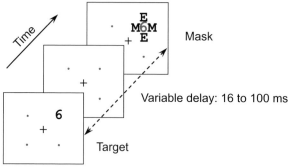

Mask

Variable delay: 16 to 100 ms

Target

1. Effects of target-mask delay

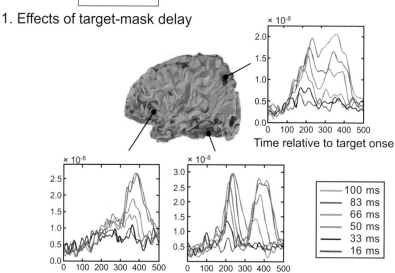

Time relative to target onse

	100 ms
	83 ms
	66 ms
	50 ms
	33 ms
	16 ms

2. Effects of target visibility at a fixed delay (50 ms)

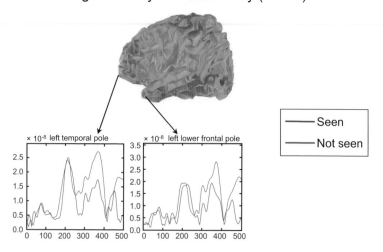

Seen

Not seen

up with explicit computer simulations of realistic thalamo-cortical networks, supposes that access to consciousness again corresponds to a form of accumulation of activation within a recurrently connected network. However, this accumulation is postulated to occur, not just locally, but within a highly distributed set of columns coding for the same object within distinct brain areas. These columns are interconnected in a reciprocal manner by distinct cortical "workspace neurons" with long-distance axons. As a result, an entire set of distributed brain areas can function temporarily as a single integrator, with a strong top-down component such that higher association areas send supportive signals to the sensory areas that first excited them.

Computer simulations show that such a network, when stimulated by a brief pulse of activation, presents complex dynamics with at least two distinct stages. In the first stage, activation climbs up the thalamo-cortical hierarchy in a feed-forward manner. As it does, the higher levels send increasingly stronger top-down amplification signals. If the incoming signal is strong enough, then at a certain point a dynamic threshold is crossed and activation becomes self-amplifying and increases in a nonlinear manner. During this second stage, the whole distributed assembly coding for the stimulus at multiple hierarchical levels then "ignites" into a single synchronously activated state. In peripheral neurons, this creates a late second peak of sustained firing. The corresponding brain state is illustrated schematically in Figure 2.6.

Why would this global brain state correspond to conscious access? Computer simulations show that once stimulus-evoked activation has reached highly interconnected associative areas, two important changes occur:

1. The activation can now reverberate for a long time period, thus holding information on-line for a duration essentially unrelated to the initial stimulus duration.
2. Stimulus information represented within the global workspace can be propagated rapidly to many brain systems.

Figure 2.5   Changes in brain activity associated with crossing the threshold for conscious perception during masking (after De Cul et al. 2007). The paradigm is described in Figure 2.1, and involves varying the delay between a digit and the subsequent mask. Event-related potentials are recorded with a 128-channel electrode net and reconstructed on the cortical surface with BrainStorm software. As the delay increases, rendering the stimulus increasingly visible, activation increases monotonically in posterior areas, then a threshold effect is seen. The late part of the activation (beyond 270 ms) suddenly increases nonlinearly in a sigmoidal manner once the delay exceeds a critical value which coincides with the threshold value for conscious perception. This nonlinear activation is highly global and occurs simultaneously in inferior and anterior prefrontal cortex as well as in posterior parietal and ventral occipito-temporal cortices. Even when the delay is fixed, the same results are seen when sorting the individual trials into seen versus not-seen (bottom panel): there is a clear separation between an initial period where activation is identical for seen and not-seen trials, and a later period (>270 ms) where activation suddenly re-increases globally on seen trials.

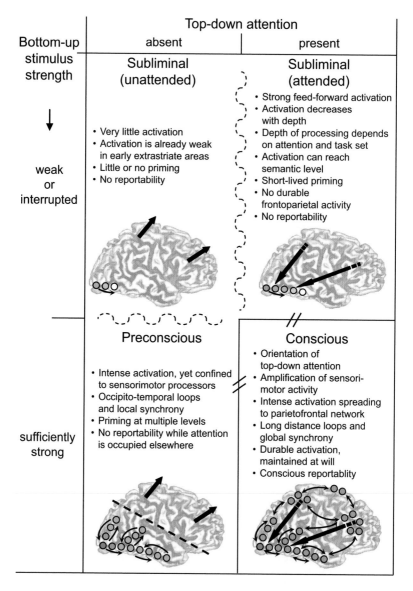

Figure 2.6 Theoretical proposal of a distinction between brain states of subliminal, preconscious, and conscious processing (after Dehaene et al. 2006). Conscious processing occurs when the accumulated stimulus-evoked activation exceeds a threshold and evokes a dynamic state of global reverberation ("ignition") across multiple high-level cortical areas forming a "global neuronal workspace," particularly involving prefrontal, cingulate and parietal cortices (bottom right). These areas can maintain the information on-line and broadcast it to a variety of other processors, thus serving as a central hub for global access to information—a key property of conscious states. Subliminal processing corresponds to a data-limited situation where only a trickle of

We argue that both properties are characteristic of conscious information processing. As noted above, the information can be maintained in time, buffered from fast fluctuations in sensory inputs, and can be shared across a broad variety of processes including evaluation, verbal report, planning, and long-term memory (Baars 1989).

Anatomically, the model postulates that workspace neurons are particularly dense in prefrontal, parietal, and anterior cingulate cortices, thus explaining why these regions are recurrently found to be associated with conscious access across various paradigms and modalities (Dehaene et al. 2006). However, according to the model, workspace neurons are also present to variable degrees in essentially all of the cortex, thus permitting essentially any active cortical contents to be brought together into a single brain-scale assembly. Indeed, it would seem likely that this long-distance network has been subject to a particular selective pressure in humans. A number of recent observations support this possibility, including (a) the disproportionate increase of prefrontal white matter volume in our species (Schoenemann et al. 2005), (b) the massive increase in dendritic branching and spine density in prefrontal cortex across the primate lineage (Elston 2003); and (c) the presence in anterior cingulate cortex of large projection neurons ("spindle cells") seemingly unique to humans and great apes (Nimchinsky et al. 1999).

Accounting for Subliminal Processing

The proposed workspace architecture separates, in a first minimal description, two computational spaces, each characterized by a distinct pattern of connectivity. Subcortical networks and most of the cortex can be viewed as a collection of specialized and automatized processors, each attuned to the processing of a particular type of information via a limited number of local or medium-range connections that bring to each processor the "encapsulated" inputs necessary to its function. On top of this automatic level, we postulate a distinct set of cortical workspace neurons characterized by their ability to send and receive projections to many distant areas through long-range excitatory axons, thus allowing many different processors to exchange information.

---

partial evidence is able to propagate through specialized cerebral networks, yet without reaching a threshold for global ignition and thus without global reportability (top line). The orientation and depth of subliminal processing may nevertheless depend on the top-down state of attention (top right). A distinct nonconscious state, preconscious processing, corresponds to a resource-limited situation where stimulus processing is blocked at the level of the global neuronal workspace while it is temporarily occupied by another task. A preconscious stimulus may be temporarily buffered within peripheral sensory areas and later accessed by the fronto-parietal system once it is released by its distracting task. In this case, information switches from nonconscious to conscious.

Can this model explain observations on subliminal processing? According to the proposed model, subliminal processing corresponds to a condition of specialized processing without global information accessibility (see Figure 2.6). A subliminal stimulus is a stimulus that possesses sufficient energy to evoke a feed-forward wave of activation in specialized processors, but it has insufficient energy or duration to trigger a large-scale reverberating state in a global network of neurons with long-range axons. As explained above, simulations of a minimal thalamo-cortical network (Dehaene and Changeux 2005) indicate that such a nonlinear self-amplifying system possesses a well-defined dynamic threshold. While it has been observed that activation exceeding a threshold level grows quickly into a full-scale ignition, a slightly weaker activation propagates forward, sometimes all the way into higher areas. It, however, loses its self-supporting activation and dies out quickly. Subliminal processing would correspond to the latter type of network state.

Let us examine briefly how this schematic model may account for the data reviewed in the preceding sections. We have seen that a masked visual stimulus that is not consciously reportable is nevertheless processed at multiple levels, including visual but also semantic, executive, and motor levels. These observations mesh well with the notion of an ascending wave of feed-forward activation that begins to accumulate within decision systems, but does not lead to a full-blown activation crossing the response threshold. Recent theorizing suggests that local neural assemblies recurrently interconnected by glutamatergic synapses with a mixture of AMPA and NMDA receptors can operate as accumulators of evidence (Wong and Wang 2006). The global workspace model suggests that such multiple integrators can operate in parallel during subliminal processing, each integrating evidence for or against their preferred stimulus. In priming experiments, where a subliminal stimulus is followed by a supraliminal target, this partial accumulation of evidence evoked by the prime would shift the baseline starting level of these accumulators, thus creating priming effects in response time, determined primarily by the congruity of the prime and target.

As long as the prime-based accumulation remains subthreshold, and therefore fails to trigger a global recurrent assembly, there is nothing in the global workspace model that prevents subliminal processing from occurring at any cognitive level, including higher-level control processes. However, the model predicts that only the most specialized processors, tightly attuned to the stimulus, should be capable of activating strongly to a subliminal stimulus. This prediction meshes well with the narrow localized activation measured by fMRI and intracranial recordings in response to subliminal words and digits (Dehaene et al. 2001; Naccache and Dehaene 2001a; Naccache et al. 2005). Note that, under the model's hypotheses, subliminal processing is not confined to a passive spreading of activation, independent of the subject's attention and strategies, as previously envisaged. On the contrary, whichever task and attentional set are prepared consciously, it can serve to orient and amplify the processing of a subliminal stimulus, even if its bottom-up strength remains insufficient for global ignition. This aspect of our model agrees with the many top-down influences on subliminal processing that have been observed experimentally.

Finally, the model predicts correctly that subliminal activation may be very strong within the first 100–300 ms after stimulus presentation, but progressively dies out in the next few hundreds of milliseconds as time elapses and as the stimulus reaches higher levels of representation. Such a decay of subliminal activation, both in time and in cortical space, has indeed been observed experimentally with high-density recordings of event-related potentials (Del Cul et al. 2007; see Figure 2.5). It can explain why only small behavioral influences of subliminal stimuli are measurable at higher cognitive levels (van Gaal et al. 2007; Mattler 2003), and why most if not all subliminal priming effects decay to a nonmeasurable level once the prime-target interval exceeds 500 ms (Mattler 2005). Only very rarely are subliminal effects seen beyond the range of a few seconds. My colleagues and I have suggested that when they do (Gaillard et al. 2007), it may be because the subliminal stimulus has caused structural changes (e.g., changes in synaptic efficacy) rather than it being due to lingering brain activity.

A Distinct State of Preconscious Processing

Simulations of the global workspace have revealed that global workspace ignition can also be prevented in a different manner, suggesting a distinct state of nonconscious processing that we have proposed to call *preconscious* (or potentially conscious, or P-conscious). Contrary to subliminal processing, where the incoming stimulus itself does not have enough energy or duration to trigger a supra-threshold reverberation of activation, preconscious processing corresponds to a neural process that potentially carries enough activation for conscious access, but is temporarily blocked from activating the global workspace due to its transient occupancy by another stimulus. Simulations have shown that such a competitive interaction for global access can occur when two stimuli are presented in short succession, in a paradigm akin to the "attentional blink." The first target (T1) creates a global workspace ignition, but while this global state is occurring, lateral inhibition prevents a second target (T2) from entering the workspace. Essentially, the global workspace acts as a central bottleneck (Chun and Potter 1995; Pashler 1994) whose occupancy by T1 deprives the T2-evoked neural assembly from its top-down support. The corresponding postulated brain state is illustrated schematically in Figure 2.6.

Computer simulations (Dehaene and Changeux 2005) suggest that during preconscious processing, T2 activation is blocked sharply at the central level; it can, however, be quite strong at peripheral levels of processing. It may excite resonant loops within medium-range connections that may maintain the representation of the stimulus temporarily active in a sensory buffer for a few hundreds of milliseconds. As a result, a preconscious stimulus is literally on the brink of consciousness and can compete actively for conscious access with other stimuli, including the currently conscious one. Furthermore, although temporarily blocked, a preconscious stimulus may later achieve conscious access once the central workspace is freed. This aspect of the model may correspond to the empirical observation of a "psychological refractory period" in behavioral dual-task performance (Pashler 1984; Sigman and Dehaene 2005), in which one task is put on hold while another task is being processed. The model assumes that the key difference between the psychological refractory period and attentional blink phenomena is the possibility of a lingering of T2-induced activation in peripheral circuits. T2 may never gain access to conscious processing if its preconscious representation is erased prior to the orienting of top-down attention (as achieved by masking in the attentional blink paradigm).

At present, only a few studies have examined brain activity during states where conscious access is prevented by top-down attentional competition, such as the attentional blink (for review, see Marois and Ivanoff 2005). Time-resolved experiments suggest that the initial activation by an unseen T2 can be very strong and essentially indistinguishable from that evoked by a conscious stimulus during a time window of about 270 ms (Sergent et al. 2005). The attentional blink then creates a sudden blocking of part of the activation starting around 270 ms, particularly in inferior prefrontal cortex (Sergent et al. 2005), and a global state of fronto-parietal synchrony indexed by the scalp P3 and by evoked oscillations in the beta range is prevented from occurring (Gross et al. 2004; Kranczioch et al. 2003). Other fMRI experiments also point to a distributed prefronto-parietal network as the main locus of the bottleneck effect in competition paradigms, consistent with the global workspace model (Dux et al. 2006; Kouider et al. 2007).

Conclusion: Conscious Access as a Solution to von Neumann's Problem?

The purpose of this chapter was to survey the rich cognitive neuroscience literature on nonconscious processing and to establish links with evidence accumulation models. The main generalizations that I have proposed to draw from these observations are the following:

1. *Subliminal processing* corresponds to a state of partial accumulation of evidence within multiple sensory, semantic, executive, and motor networks, yet without reaching a full-blown decision threshold.

2. Nonconscious processing can also occur in a distinct state of *preconscious processing,* where evidence accumulation can proceed normally within posterior sensory and semantic networks while being blocked from

accessing anterior networks due to competition with another attended mental representation.

3. *Conscious access* is associated with the crossing of a dynamic threshold beyond which the stimulus activation reverberates within a global fronto-parietal network. The sensory representation of the stimulus can thus be maintained online and be used for higher-level executive processes, such as reasoning and decision making.

I end with a final speculative note on one of the possible functions of consciousness in evolution. In his 1958 book, *The Computer and the Brain*, von Neumann asked how a biological organ such as the brain, where individual neurons are prone to errors, could perform multistep calculations. He pointed out that in any analogical machine, errors accumulate at each step so that the end result quickly becomes imprecise or even useless. He therefore suggested that the brain must have mechanisms that discretize the incoming analogical information, much like the TTL or CMOS code of current digital chips is based on a distinction of voltages into high (between 4.95 and 5 volts) versus low (between 0 and 0.05 volts).

Tentatively, I surmise that the architecture of the "conscious workspace" may have evolved to address von Neumann's problem. In the human brain, one function of conscious access would be to control the accumulation of information in such a way that information is pooled in a coherent manner across the multiple processors operating preconsciously and in parallel, and a discrete categorical decision is reached before being dispatched to yet other processors. By pooling information over time, this global accumulation of evidence would allow the inevitable errors that creep up during analog processing to be corrected or at least to be kept below a predefined probability level. Many decision models already postulate such an accumulation of evidence within local brain systems such as the oculo-motor system (see, e.g., Shadlen, this volume). The role of the conscious global workspace would be to achieve such accumulation of evidence in a unified manner across multiple distributed brain systems and, once a single coherent result has been obtained, to dispatch it back to essentially any brain processor as needed by the current task. This architecture would permit the execution of a multistep mental algorithm through successive, consciously controlled steps of evidence accumulation followed by result dispatching. The latter proposal is consistent with recent findings from the "psychological refractory period" paradigm, where response time in a dual-task situation was shown to result from a temporal succession of multiple non-overlapping stochastic accumulation periods (Sigman and Dehaene 2005, 2006).

While clearly speculative and in need of further specification, the proposed architecture seems to combine the benefits of two distinct computational principles: massive parallel accumulation of evidence at a nonconscious level, followed by conscious broadcasting of the outcome permitting the operation of the human brain as a slow serial "Turing machine."

References

Baars, B. J. 1989. A Cognitive Theory of Consciousness. Cambridge, MA: Cambridge Univ. Press.

Chun, M. M., and M. C. Potter. 1995. A two-stage model for multiple target detection in rapid serial visual presentation. *J. Exp. Psychol.: Hum. Perc. Perf.* **21(1)**:109–127.

Clark, R. E., J. R. Manns, and L. R. Squire. 2002. Classical conditioning, awareness, and brain systems. *Trends Cogn. Sci.* **6(12)**:524–531.

Dehaene, S. 2007. Symbols and quantities in parietal cortex: Elements of a mathematical theory of number representation and manipulation. In: Sensorimotor Foundations of Higher Cognition, ed. P. Haggard and Y. Rossetti. Oxford: Oxford Univ. Press, in press.

Dehaene, S., and J. P. Changeux. 2005. Ongoing spontaneous activity controls access to consciousness: A neuronal model for inattentional blindness. *PLoS Biol.* **3(5)**:e141.

Dehaene, S., J. P. Changeux, L. Naccache, J. Sackur, and C. Sergent. 2006. Conscious, preconscious, and subliminal processing: A testable taxonomy. *Trends Cogn. Sci.* **10(5)**:204–211.

Dehaene, S., and L. Naccache. 2001. Towards a cognitive neuroscience of consciousness: Basic evidence and a workspace framework. *Cognition* **79**:1–37.

Dehaene, S., L. Naccache, L. Cohen, D. L. Bihan, J. F. Mangin et al. 2001. Cerebral mechanisms of word masking and unconscious repetition priming. *Nat. Neurosci.* **4(7)**:752–758.

Dehaene, S., L. Naccache, G. Le Clec'H, E. Koechlin, M. Mueller et al. 1998. Imaging unconscious semantic priming. *Nature* **395**:597–600.

Dehaene, S., C. Sergent, and J. P. Changeux. 2003. A neuronal network model linking subjective reports and objective physiological data during conscious perception. *Proc. Natl. Acad. Sci.* **100**:8520–8525.

Del Cul, A., S. Baillet, and S. Dehaene. 2007. Brain dynamics underlying the non-linear threshold for access to consciousness. *PLoS Biol.*, **5(10)**:e260.

Del Cul, A., S. Dehaene, and M. Leboyer. 2006. Preserved subliminal processing and impaired conscious access in schizophrenia. *Arch. Gen. Psychiatry* **63(12)**:1313–1323.

Dennett, D. C. 1992. Consciousness Explained. London: Penguin.

Devlin, J. T., H. L. Jamison, P. M. Matthews, and L. M. Gonnerman. 2004. Morphology and the internal structure of words. *Proc. Natl. Acad. Sci.* **101(41)**:14,984–14,988.

Dux, P. E., J. Ivanoff, C. L. Asplund, and R. Marois. 2006. Isolation of a central bottleneck of information processing with time-resolved fMRI. *Neuron* **52(6)**:1109–1120.

Eimer, M., and F. Schlaghecken. 1998. Effects of masked stimuli on motor activation: Behavioral and electrophysiological evidence. *J. Exp. Psychol.: Hum. Perc. Perf.* **24(6)**:1737–1747.

Elston, G. N. 2003. Cortex, cognition and the cell: New insights into the pyramidal neuron and prefrontal function. *Cerebral Cortex* **13(11)**:1124–1138.

Gaillard, R., L. Cohen, C. Adam, S. Clémenceau, M. Baulac et al. 2007. Subliminal words durably affect neuronal activity. *Neuroreport* **18(15)**:1527–1531.

Gaillard, R., A. Del Cul, L. Naccache, F. Vinckier, L. Cohen et al. 2006. Nonconscious semantic processing of emotional words modulates conscious access. *Proc. Natl. Acad. Sci.* **103(19)**:7524–7529.

Gaillard, R., L. Naccache, P. Pinel, S. Clemenceau, E. Volle et al. 2006. Direct intracranial, fmri, and lesion evidence for the causal role of left inferotemporal cortex in reading. *Neuron* **50(2)**:191–204.

Greenwald, A. G., S. C. Draine, and R. L. Abrams. 1996. Three cognitive markers of unconscious semantic activation. *Science* **273(5282)**:1699–1702.

Gross, J., F. Schmitz, I. Schnitzler, K. Kessler, K. Shapiro et al. 2004. Modulation of long-range neural synchrony reflects temporal limitations of visual attention in humans. *Proc. Natl. Acad. Sci.* **101(35)**:13,050–13,055.

Haynes, J. D., J. Driver, and G. Rees. 2005. Visibility reflects dynamic changes of effective connectivity between V1 and fusiform cortex. *Neuron* **46(5)**:811–821.

Kentridge, R. W., C. A. Heywood, and L. Weiskrantz. 1999. Attention without awareness in blindsight. *Proc. Roy. Soc. Lond. B* **266(1430)**:1805–1811.

Kentridge, R. W., C. A. Heywood, and L. Weiskrantz. 2004. Spatial attention speeds discrimination without awareness in blindsight. *Neuropsychologia* **42(6)**:831–835.

Kiefer, M. 2002. The N400 is modulated by unconsciously perceived masked words: Further evidence for an automatic spreading activation account of N400 priming effects. *Brain Res. Cogn. Brain Res.* **13(1)**:27–39.

Kiefer, M., and D. Brendel. 2006. Attentional modulation of unconscious "automatic" processes: Evidence from event-related potentials in a masked priming paradigm. *J. Cogn. Neurosci.* **18(2)**:184–198.

Koechlin, E., C. Ody, and F. Kouneiher. 2003. The architecture of cognitive control in the human prefrontal cortex. *Science* **302(5648)**:1181–1185.

Koivisto, M., A. Revonsuo, and M. Lehtonen. 2006. Independence of visual awareness from the scope of attention: An electrophysiological study. *Cereb. Cortex* **16(3)**:415–424.

Kouider, S., and S. Dehaene. 2007. Levels of processing during non-conscious perception: A critical review of visual masking. *Phil. Trans. Roy. Soc. Lond. B,* **362(1481)**:857–875.

Kouider, S., S. Dehaene, A. Jobert, and D. Le Bihan. 2007. Cerebral bases of subliminal and supraliminal priming during reading. *Cereb. Cortex* 17(9):2019–2029.

Kranczioch, C., S. Debener, and A. K. Engel. 2003. Event-related potential correlates of the attentional blink phenomenon. *Brain Res. Cogn. Brain Res.* **17(1)**:177–187.

Kunde, W., A. Kiesel, and J. Hoffmann. 2003. Conscious control over the content of unconscious cognition. *Cognition* **88(2)**:223–242.

Lachter, J., K. I. Forster, and E. Ruthruff. 2004. Forty-five years after Broadbent (1958): Still no identification without attention. *Psychol. Rev.* **111(4)**:880–913.

Laming, D. R. J. 1968. Information Theory of Choice-Reaction Times. London: Academic Press.

Lamme, V. A., K. Zipser, H. and Spekreijse. 2002. Masking interrupts figure-ground signals in V1. *J. Cogn. Neurosci.* **14(7)**:1044–1053.

Lau, H. C., and R. E. Passingham. 2007. Unconscious activation of the cognitive control system in the human prefrontal cortex. *J. Neurosci.* **27(21)**:5805–5811.

Leuthold, H., and B. Kopp. 1998. Mechanisms of priming by masked stimuli: Inferences from event-related potentials. *Psychol. Sci.* **9**:263–269.

Link, S. W. 1992. The Wave Theory of Difference and Similarity. Hillsdale, NJ: Lawrence Erlbaum.

Luck, S. J., E. K. Vogel, and K. L. Shapiro. 1996. Word meanings can be accessed but not reported during the attentional blink. *Nature* **383(6601)**:616–618.

Marois, R., and J. Ivanoff. 2005. Capacity limits of information processing in the brain. *Trends Cogn. Sci.* **9(6)**:296–305.

Marzouki, Y., J. Grainger, and J. Theeuwes. 2007. Exogenous spatial cueing modulates subliminal masked priming. *Acta Psychol.* **126(1)**:34–45.

Mattler, U. 2003. Priming of mental operations by masked stimuli. *Perc. Psychophys.* **65(2)**:167–187.

Mattler, U. 2005. Inhibition and decay of motor and nonmotor priming. *Perc. Psychophys.* **67(2)**:285–300.

Melloni, L., C. Molina, M. Pena, D. Torres, W. Singer et al. 2007. Synchronization of neural activity across cortical areas correlates with conscious perception. *J. Neurosci.* **27(11)**:2858–2865.

Merikle, P. M., and S. Joordens. 1997. Parallels between perception without attention and perception without awareness. *Conscious Cogn.* **6(2–3)**:219–236.

Merikle, P. M., S. Joordens, and J. A. Stolz. 1995. Measuring the relative magnitude of unconscious influences. *Conscious. Cogn.* **4**:422–439.

Naccache, L., E. Blandin, and S. Dehaene. 2002. Unconscious masked priming depends on temporal attention. *Psychol. Sci.* **13**:416–424.

Naccache, L., and S. Dehaene. 2001a. The Priming Method: Imaging Unconscious Repetition Priming Reveals an Abstract Representation of Number in the Parietal Lobes. *Cereb. Cortex* **11(10)**:966–974.

Naccache, L., and S. Dehaene. 2001b. Unconscious semantic priming extends to novel unseen stimuli. *Cognition* **80(3)**:215–229.

Naccache, L., R. Gaillard, C. Adam, D. Hasboun, S. Clémenceau et al. 2005. A direct intracranial record of emotions evoked by subliminal words. *Proc. Natl. Acad. Sci.* **102**:7713–7717.

Nakamura, K., S. Dehaene, A. Jobert, D. Le Bihan, and S. Kouider. 2005. Subliminal convergence of Kanji and Kana words: Further evidence for functional parcellation of the posterior temporal cortex in visual word perception. *J. Cogn. Neurosci.* **17(6)**:954–968.

Nieuwenhuis, S., K. R. Ridderinkhof, J. Blom, G. P. Band, and A. Kok. 2001. Error-related brain potentials are differentially related to awareness of response errors: Evidence from an antisaccade task. *Psychophys.* **38(5)**:752–760.

Nimchinsky, E. A., E. Gilissen, J. M. Allman, D. P. Perl, J. M. Erwin et al. 1999. A neuronal morphologic type unique to humans and great apes. *Proc. Natl. Acad. Sci.* **96(9)**:5268–5273.

Pashler, H. 1984. Processing stages in overlapping tasks: Evidence for a central bottleneck. *J. Exp. Psychol.: Hum. Perc. Perf.* **10(3)**:358–377.

Pashler, H. 1994. Dual-task interference in simple tasks: Data and theory. *Psychol. Bull.* **116(2)**:220–244.

Pessiglione, M., L. Schmidt, B. Draganski, R. Kalisch, H. Lau et al. 2007. How the brain translates money into force: A neuroimaging study of subliminal motivation. *Science* **316**:904–906.

Reuter, F., A. Del Cul, B. Audoin, I. Malikova, L. Naccache et al. 2007. Intact subliminal processing and delayed conscious access in multiple sclerosis. *Neuropsychologia* **45(12)**:2683–2691.

Reynvoet, B., M. Brysbaert, and W. Fias. 2002. Semantic priming in number naming. *Qtly. J. Exp. Psychol.* **55(4)**:1127–1139.

Schoenemann, P. T., M. J. Sheehan, and L. D. Glotzer. 2005. Prefrontal white matter volume is disproportionately larger in humans than in other primates. *Nat. Neurosci.* **8(2)**:242–252.

Sergent, C., S. Baillet, and S. Dehaene. 2005. Timing of the brain events underlying access to consciousness during the attentional blink. *Nat. Neurosci.* **8(10)**:1391–1400.

Sergent, C., and S. Dehaene. 2004. Is consciousness a gradual phenomenon? Evidence for an all-or-none bifurcation during the attentional blink. *Psychol. Sci.* **15(11)**:720–728.

Sigman, M., and S. Dehaene. 2005. Parsing a cognitive task: A characterization of the mind's bottleneck. *PLoS Biol.* **3(2)**:e37.

Sigman, M., and S. Dehaene. 2006. Dynamics of the Central Bottleneck: Dual-task and task uncertainty. *PLoS Biol.* **4(7)**:e220.

Smith, P. L., and R. Ratcliff. 2004. Psychology and neurobiology of simple decisions. *Trends Neurosci.* **27(3)**:161–168.

Usher, M., and J. L. McClelland. 2001. The time course of perceptual choice: The leaky, competing accumulator model. *Psychol. Rev.* **108(3)**:550–592.

van Aalderen-Smeets, S. I., R. Oostenveld, and J. Schwarzbach. 2006. Investigating neurophysiological correlates of metacontrast masking with magnetoencephalography. *Adv. Cogn. Psychol,* **2(1)**:21–35.

van Gaal, S., K. R. Ridderinkhof, W. P. M. van den Wildenberg, and V. A. Lamme. 2007. Exploring the boundaries of unconscious processing: Response inhibition can be triggered by masked stop-signals. *J. Vision* **7(9)**:425.

von Neumann, J. 1958. The Computer and the Brain. London: Yale Univ. Press.

Vorberg, D., U. Mattler, A. Heinecke, T. Schmidt, and J. Schwarzbach. 2003. Different time courses for visual perception and action priming. *Proc. Natl. Acad. Sci.* **100(10)**:6275–6280.

Weiskrantz, L. 1997. Consciousness Lost and Found: A Neuropsychological Exploration. New York: Oxford Univ. Press.

Wong, K. F., and X. J. Wang. 2006. A recurrent network mechanism of time integration in perceptual decisions. *J. Neurosci.* **26(4)**:1314–1328.

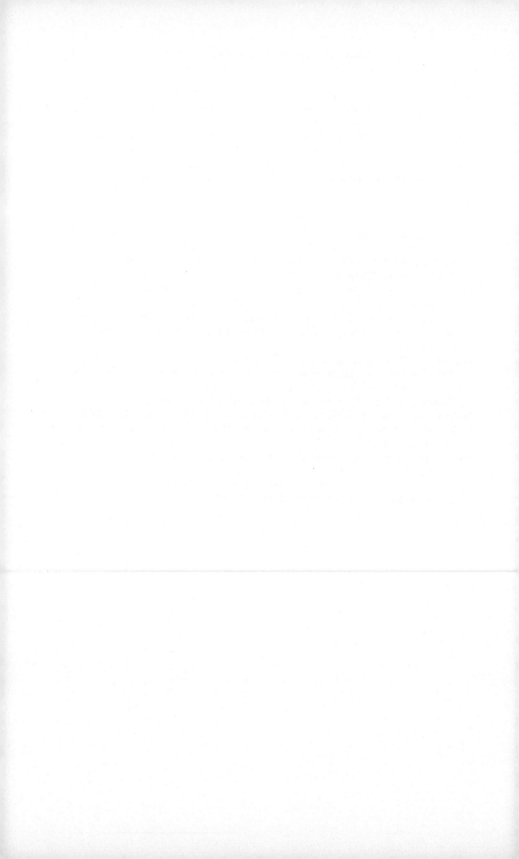

3

The Role of Value Systems in Decision Making

Peter Dayan

Gatsby Computational Neuroscience Unit, UCL, London WC1N 3AR, U.K.

Abstract

Values, rewards, and costs play a central role in economic, statistical, and psychological notions of decision making. They also have surprisingly direct neural realizations. This chapter discusses the ways in which different value systems interact with different decision-making systems to fashion and shape affectively appropriate behavior in complex environments. Forms of deliberative and automatic decision making are interpreted as sharing a common purpose rather than serving different or non-normative goals.

Introduction

There is perhaps no more critical factor for the survival of an organism than the manner in which it chooses between different courses of action or inaction. A seemingly obvious way to formalize choice is to evaluate the predicted costs and benefits of each option and pick the best. However, seething beneath the surface of this bland dictate lies a host of questions about such things as a common currency with which to capture the costs and benefits, the different mechanisms by which these predictions may be made, the different information that predictors might use to assess the costs and benefits, the possibility of choosing when or how quickly to act as well as what to do, and different prior expectations that may be brought to bear in that vast majority of cases when aspects of the problem remain uncertain.

In keeping with the complexity and centrality of value-based choice, quite a number of psychologically and neurally different systems are involved. These systems interact both cooperatively and competitively. In this chapter, I outline the apparent dependence of four decision-making mechanisms on four different value systems. Although this complexity might seem daunting, we will see that exact parallels can be found in ideas about how artificial systems such as robots might make choices, that the different systems capture rather natural trade-offs that are created by the statistical and computational complexities of optimal control, and that at least some of the apparent problems of choice actually arise from cases in which reasonable a priori expectations about the world are violated by particular experimental protocols.

I begin by describing a formal framework that derives from the field of reinforcement learning (Sutton and Barto 1998). Reinforcement learning mostly considers how artificial systems can learn appropriate actions in the face of rewards and punishments. For our purposes, however, it is convenient since it (a) originated in mathematical abstractions of psychological data, (b) has a proof-theoretic link to statistical and normative accounts of optimal control, and (c) lies at the heart of widespread interpretations of neurophysiological and neuroimaging data. I show the roles played by value-based predictions in reinforcement learning and indicate how different psychological and neurobiological ideas about decision making map onto roughly equivalent reinforcement learning notions.

Thereafter, I describe four different value systems and four different decision-making systems that arise naturally within this framework. Two of the decision makers—one associated with goal-directed or forward model-based control, the other associated with habitual control (Dickinson and Balleine 2001)—are well characterized neurally; the substrates of the other two are somewhat less clear. Equally, the anatomical (e.g., neuromodulatory) bases of two of the value systems are somewhat clearer than those of the other two. Different decision makers use value information directly and through learning in different ways; they also enjoy cooperative and competitive relations with each other. The extent to which these interactions might underlie some of the complexity in the data on choice is then considered. I conclude with a discussion of the key open issues and questions.

A few remarks at the outset: First, we would like to aim toward a theory of behavior, not just of "decisions," somehow more narrowly defined. That the systems involved in normative choice appear also to be implicated in the tics of a patient with Tourette's syndrome or the compulsions of one with obsessions suggest that we should not start by imposing arbitrary boundaries. Second, our analysis owes an important debt to Dickinson (e.g., 1994), who, adopting a view that originated with Konorski (1948, 1967), and together with his colleagues (e.g., Dickinson and Balleine 2001), has long worked on teasing apart the various contributions from different systems. Third, we will typically lump together information derived from rodent, monkey, and human studies. We are far from having a sufficiently refined understanding to be able sensibly to embrace the obviously large differences between these species. Finally, the limit on the number of citations has forced the omission of many highly relevant studies.

Reinforcement Learning and Dynamic Programming

The problem for decision making can be illustrated in the simple maze-like task in Figure 3.1. It is helpful to define a formalism which allows us to describe the external state of the subject ($x \in \{x_1, x_2, x_3\}$, its position in the maze), its internal state (m, mostly motivational factors such as hunger or thirst), its possible choices ($c \in \{L, R\}$), and a set of possible outcomes ($o \in \Omega = \{\text{cheese},$ nothing, water, carrots$\}$, but in general also including aversive outcomes such as shocks).

Immediate Outcomes

Let us first consider the case that the subject has just one choice to make at a single state, for instance x_3 in the maze. We write the probability of receiving outcome o given choice c as $O_{co}(x)$. This would be stochastic if, for instance, the experimenter probabilistically swaps the outcomes. To select which action to execute, the subject must have preferences between the outcomes. One important way to describe these preferences is through a utility function $u_o(m)$, which we call a native (or experienced) utility function (Kahneman et al. 1997). This should depend on the motivational state of the subject since, for instance, all else being equal, thirsty subjects will prefer the water, and hungry subjects, the cheese. Example utilities for all the outcomes are shown in Figure 3.1b.

   The native utility function quantifies the actual worth to the subject of the outcome. It is the first of the four value functions that we will consider overall. Given the utility, the subject could choose normatively the action that maximizes the expected utility of the choice, or, more formally, defining these as the Q values of choice c at environmental and motivational states x and m, respectively,

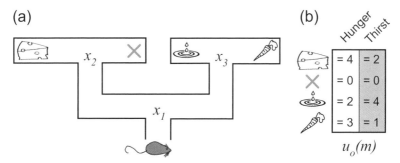

Figure 3.1   Maze task: (a) A simple maze task for a rat, comprising three choice points (x_1, x_2, x_3) and four outcomes ($o \in \{\text{cheese, nothing, water, and carrots}\}$). The rat has to run forward through the maze and must go left (L) or right (R) at each choice point. (b) Utilities $u_o(m)$ for the four outcomes are shown for the two motivational states, m = hunger and m = thirst. Figure adapted from Niv, Joel, and Dayan (2006).

$$Q_c(x, m) = \sum_o O_{co}(x)u_o(m), \tag{1}$$

it could choose:

$$c^*(x, m) = \mathrm{argmax}_c \left\{ Q_c(x, m) \right\}. \tag{2}$$

The systematic assignment of choices to states is usually called a *policy*, a term which comes from engineering. Policies can be deterministic (as here) or, as is often found experimentally, probabilistic, with the subject choosing all actions, but some (hopefully, the better ones) more frequently than others. One conventional abstraction of this stochastic choice is that the probability of executing action c is determined by competition between Q values, as in a form of Luce choice rule (Luce 1959) or softmax:

$$P(c; x, m) = \frac{\exp\left(\beta Q_c(x, m)\right)}{\sum_d \exp\left(\beta Q_d(x, m)\right)}. \tag{3}$$

Here, parameter $\beta > 0$ (sometimes called an inverse temperature) regulates the strength of the competition. If β is small, then choices that are worth very different amounts will be executed almost equally as often.

Straightforward as this may seem, there are conceptually quite different ways of realizing and learning such policies. These different methods are associated with different combinations of value and decision-making systems. Key combinations are described briefly here; the separate systems and their interactions will be discussed later.

1. Perhaps the simplest approach would be to implement Equations 1 and 2 directly by learning a so-called *forward model* $\hat{O}$ [note: hats are used to indicate estimated, approximate, or learned quantities]; that is, the consequences of each action, together with a way of estimating the utility of each outcome, $\hat{u}$. If the contributions can be accumulated, as in Equation 1, then each action could compete according to its estimated $\hat{Q}$ value (a form of predicted utility; Kahneman et al. 1997). Figure 3.2a shows how this works for the case of state x_3 in the maze. The neural substrate of this means of evaluating the worth of options is a second value system influencing choice. This will be related below to the psychological notion of a goal-directed controller implemented in the prefrontal cortex and dorsomedial striatum.

2. One alternative to the computational and representational costs of this scheme would be to try and learn the Q values directly and then only have those compete. This would obviate the need for learning and using O. Figure 3.2b shows these values, again for the case of x_3.

   A mainstay of psychology, the Rescorla-Wagner learning rule, which is equivalent to engineering's delta rule, suggests one way of doing this.

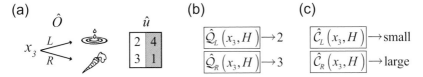

Figure 3.2   Decision making at x_3: (a) The forward model consists of $\hat{O}$ and $\hat{u}$. By exploring the explicit options, the subject can work out which action is best under which circumstance. (b) The $\hat{Q}$ values suffice to indicate the expected utilities for each action under a motivational state (in this case, hunger), but the provenance of these values in the actual outcomes themselves is not accessible. (c) An even more direct controller just specifies ordinal quantities $\hat{C}$ on which choice can be based; these numbers, however, lack anything like an invertible relationship with expected utilities. Figure adapted from Niv, Joel, and Dayan (2006).

According to this rule, the estimate $\hat{Q}_c(x, m)$ is represented, perhaps using a set of synaptic weights, and when action c is tried, leading to outcome o, the estimate is changed according to the prediction error:

$$\hat{Q}'_c(x, m) = \hat{Q}_c(x, m) + \alpha \left[u_o(m) - \hat{Q}_c(x, m) \right], \tag{4}$$

where α is called a learning rate (or associability). This rule has a normative basis and will often lead to $\hat{Q} = Q$, at least on average. There is good evidence that a prediction error closely related to this is represented in the activity of dopamine neurons (Montague et al. 1996; Schultz 1998).

The structure that expresses estimates like $\hat{Q}_c(x, m)$ is actually the third of the value systems that plays a role in decision making. Such values are sometimes called *cached* (Daw et al. 2005) because they cache information actually observed about future outcomes in the form of expected utilities.

The nature of the dependence on the motivational state m is a critical facet of cached values (see Dayan and Balleine 2002). In general, there is ample evidence for state dependence in learning and recall (i.e., m might indeed be involved in the representation of the $\hat{Q}$ values). However, consider the case that a subject learns $\hat{Q}$ values in one motivational state (e.g., hunger, as in Figure 3.2b). Since these values are simply numbers, utilities that are divorced from their bases in actual outcomes, they can be expected to generalize promiscuously, certainly more so than values from the forward model. In particular, if they generalize to other motivational states such as thirst, then the subjects may continue to favor actions leading to food, even though this is inappropriate. To put it another way, there may be no way to move from the Q values appropriate to hunger to the ones suitable for thirst without explicit relearning. This type of inflexibility is indeed a hallmark of behavioral habits, as we explore in more detail below.

3.   An even simpler scheme would be to use a choice mechanism such as that in Equation 2, but to observe that the policy only requires that the

value used in the argmax associated with action $c^*(m, x)$ has to be numerically larger than the values associated with all the other actions, and not that it actually satisfies Equation 1. Figure 3.2c demonstrates this, using $\hat{C}_c(x, m)$ for the action values. Learning rules for such values are closely related to the psychological notion of stimulus-response learning, with a choice being stamped in or reinforced by large delivered utilities. We treat these action values as also being cached, since they share critical characteristics with the Q values (e.g., they are only indirectly sensitive to motivational manipulations).

In short, there are different mechanisms, all of which can be used to achieve the same ostensive goal of optimizing the net expected value. The differences will become apparent when aspects of the motivational state that pertained during training are different from those during the test. Understanding how the different systems generalize is therefore critical. Bayesian ideas are rapidly gaining traction as providing general theories of this, encouraging careful consideration of prior expectations, here in the nature of any or all of O, u, Q, and c as well as the internal representations of x and m underlying these functions. I will argue that such priors play a central role in everything from Pavlovian conditioning (arising from a prior over actions appropriate to predictions of reward or punishment) to learned helplessness (a prior over the nature of the controllability of an environment).

Delayed Outcomes

One important characteristic of many choice problems is that the outcome may not be provided until a whole sequence of actions has been executed. In the maze shown in Figure 3.1, this is true for state x_1, as either action only gets the subject to x_2 or x_3, and not directly to any of the outcomes. In fact, many outcomes may be provided along a trajectory and not just a single one at the end. In simple (Markovian) environments like the maze, it is possible to formalize trajectories by considering transitions from one state x to others y whose probabilities $T_{xy}(c)$ may depend on the action chosen c.

A key definitional problem that arises is assessing the worth of a delayed outcome. Various schemes for doing so have been suggested in economics and psychology. One idea is *discounting*, with an outcome o that will be received in the future after time t, having a reduced net present value of $u_o(m) \times f(t)$, where $f(t) = \exp(-\gamma t)$ might be exponential or $f(t) = 1/(1 + \gamma t)$ hyperbolic ($\gamma > 0$). Under discounting, it becomes advantageous to advance outcomes with positive utilities and delay those with negative utilities.

Exponential discounting is akin to using a form of interest rate. It turns out that there are natural extensions to the definition of Q values that are suitable for trajectories (Watkins 1989), and necessitating only a small change to the learning rule in Equation 4. Indeed, much of the data about the neural basis of value systems depends on these extensions.

Although hyperbolic discounting generally fits behavioral data more proficiently, it is not clear how this might be implemented without imposing implausible requirements on memory for learning. Hyperbolic discounting infamously leads to temporal inconsistencies (see Ainslie 2001). For instance, if $\gamma = 1 \text{ s}^{-1}$, then although a reward of 4 units that arrives in 10 s would be preferred to one of 3 units in 9 s, after 8 seconds has passed, the reward of 3 units, which would now arrive in 1 s, would be preferred to the reward of 4 units, which would arrive in a further 2 s. The latter pattern, in which a larger, but later reward is rejected in favor of a smaller, but earlier one, is called *impulsive*.

An alternative method for handling delayed outcomes is to optimize the *rates* at which rewards are received and costs avoided. Most of the consequences of this are too complex to describe here; however, in this scheme a key role is played by the fourth value system, which evaluates and predicts the long-run average rate (ρ) of the delivery of utility. The rate is the sum of all the utility received over a long period of time (from all sources), divided by that time period. The rate turns out to matter most when we consider optimizing the choice of not just *which* action, but also its alacrity, speed or vigor, given that the cost of acting quickly is taken into account (Niv, Daw et al. 2006; Niv, Joel, and Dayan 2006).

Four Value Systems

Having introduced the four value systems above, I will now summarize some of their properties. Note, in particular, the distinction between the true utilities $u_o(m)$ and true Q values $Q_c(x, m)$ that depend on them, and the various estimates (distinguished using hats) which depend in different ways on the various underlying learned quantities. As will be apparent, many uncertainties remain.

Native Values

The actual utility (or experienced utility, in terms of Kahneman et al. 1997) $u_o(m)$ of an outcome in a motivational state m (or at least the most immediate neural report of this) should ground all methods of choice. Berridge and Robinson (1998) discuss extensive evidence about the existence of a so-called *liking* system, which reports on the motivational state-dependent worth of an outcome. Although its exact anatomical substrates are not completely clear, for food reward, liking has been suggested as being mediated by structures such as the primary taste system in the brainstem; further, neurons in the hypothalamus, for instance, have the ability to sense certain aspects of the internal state of an animal (e.g., hydration), and thus could play an important role. Nuclei in the pain system, such as the periacqueductal gray, may play a similar role in the mediation of primary aversion (i.e., disliking). Opioids and benzodiazepines can act to boost liking and reduce disliking, perhaps by manipulating this value.

Forward-model Values

The second value system involves learning and using a forward model of the probabilities $\hat{O}$ of the outcomes (and, in the case of trajectories, the transitions $\hat{T}$) consequent on a choice, together with the motivational state-dependent utility $\hat{u}$ of those outcomes (Figure 3.2a). This involves the use of a model in the service of computing a predicted utility (Kahneman et al. 1997). There is evidence in various species that prefrontal areas (notably dorsolateral prefrontal cortex, the dorsomedial striatum, and the insular cortex) are involved in this sort of model-dependent predictions of future outcomes (and future states). The nature and substrate of the assessment of the state-dependent utility $\hat{u}$ is less clear, and various suggestions have been made about the psychological and neural mechanisms involved. For instance, one idea involves *incentive learning* (Dickinson and Balleine 2001); namely, that subjects learn the utilities from direct experience and the observed native utility. Another notion is that of a *somatic marker*; crudely that the body itself (or a cortical simulacrum thereof) is used to evaluate the native utility of a predicted outcome via a mechanism of top-down influence (Damasio et al. 1991).

One interesting question for these schemes concerns the motivational state m used to make the assessments. If this is the subject's current motivational state, but the prediction is about an outcome that will be obtained in a different motivational state, then the prediction might be wrong. In discussing "hot" and "cold" cognition, Loewenstein (1996) makes just such a point.

Cached Values

The Q values (Watkins 1989) discussed above and shown in Figure 3.2b can be seen as alternative estimates of predicted utilities (Kahneman et al. 1997). Unlike the native or forward model-based values, these Q values pay no direct allegiance to their provenance in terms of particular outcomes. This turns out to have distinct computational benefits for choice, particularly in the case of optimizing actions over whole trajectories. However, as has already been discussed, it has problems coping efficiently with changes to the environment or motivational state.

In the trajectory case, there is an important role for the cached value $V(x, m)$ of the state x in motivational state m, which is defined by averaging the choices over the policy, as either

$$V(x,m) = Q_{c'}(x,m) \qquad \text{given Equation 2, or} \qquad (5)$$

$$= \sum_c P(c; x, m) Q_c(x, m) \text{ given Equation 3.} \qquad (6)$$

Estimates $\hat{V}$ can be learned using a learning rule similar to that in Equation 4.

There is strong evidence for the involvement of the phasic release of the neuromodulator dopamine in the appetitive aspects of learning these cached values (e.g., Montague et al. 1996; Schultz 1998), and for the basolateral nucleus of the amygdala, the orbitofrontal cortex, and regions of the striatum in representing the $\hat{V}$ and $\hat{Q}$ values. This has all been reviewed extensively elsewhere (e.g., O'Doherty 2004; Balleine and Killcross 2006), including in its ascription by Berridge and Robinson (1998) to the second of their two systems influencing choice ("wanting," which complements liking). The reader is referred to these excellent sources.

There is rather less agreement about how the aversive components of cached utilities are represented and manipulated, although there are ample data on the involvement of the amygdala and insula. An important psychological idea is that of opponency, between appetitive and aversive cached value systems. Indeed, some of the best psychological evidence for the existence of outcome-independent value systems, such as Q values, comes from facets of opponency. For instance, the *non*delivery of an expected *shock* can play some of the critical roles through learning of the delivery of an *un*expected *reward* (see Dickinson and Balleine 2001). It has been suggested that another neuromodulator, serotonin, has a starring role in the cached aversive system (Daw et al. 2002), but most of the evidence is rather circumstantial.

There may be a critical anatomical and functional separation between the systems associated with representing the cached values of states $\hat{V}$ and those representing the cached $\hat{Q}$ values (O'Doherty 2004). This would be particularly important if cached action values like those considered in Figure 3.2c are employed, as these are further divorced from the utilities.

Long-run Average Value

The final notion of value is the long-run average utility ρ. This is important when it is the average utility per unit time that must be optimized, which is indeed the case for large classes of psychological experiments in such things as free operant schedules, for which rates of responding (i.e., choices about the times at which to act) are more central than choices between punctate actions. In the context of the maze, this might translate to the speed of running rather than the choice of which direction to run.

The importance of the long-run average value in controlling response rates has only fairly recently been highlighted, notably in the work of Niv, Daw et al. (2006) and Niv, Joel and Dyan (2006). They point out the link between ρ and the opportunity cost for behaving slothfully. When ρ is big and positive, animals should act faster, since every idle moment is associated directly with a greater amount of lost (expected) utility. This helps explain why animals that are highly motivated by the expectation of receiving large rewards per unit time perform all actions quickly (and often not just those actions that lead directly to the reward).

In principle, ρ could be realized in either a forward model-based or a cache-based manner. However, Niv, Daw et al. (2006) suggest that the existing evidence, again for rewards rather than punishments, may favor an assignment of ρ to the tonic activation of dopaminergic neurons.

Again, less work has been done on the nature and realization of long-run average negative values. It is notable that various forms of depression have been postulated as depending in some way on stress and excessive affective negativity. We might expect these to be associated with a form of anergia (i.e., actions slowed are expected punishments postponed). However, more sophisticated effects of prior expectations appear to be at work in other paradigms used to capture aspects of depression, such as learned helplessness.

Four Decision Makers

As outlined above, these four value systems contribute in various ways to the different structures involved in decision making. Indeed, most of the evidence about the value systems derives from observations of choices that are inferred to depend on values of one sort or another. In this section, I briefly describe first the decision-making systems, and then some critical aspects of their interaction.

Goal-directed Control

The forward model is the most straightforward control mechanism. It was discussed in the description of Figure 3.2a. Choices are based on approximate evaluations ($\hat{u}$) of predicted ($\hat{O}$) outcomes. If the evaluation system $\hat{u}$ is sensitive to motivational state, then so will be the choice of action.

Figure 3.3a shows the extension of Figure 3.2a to the case of the full maze. The main difference is that the search process starts at x_1 and includes the use of $\hat{T}$ to work out which states follow which actions until outcomes are reached. By searching to the end of the tree, the subject can favor going left at x_1 when hungry, but right at x_1 when thirsty. This motivational dependence of control, which itself is a function of the motivational dependence of $\hat{u}$, is why this controller is typically deemed to be *goal-directed*. Since choices are based on search through the tree, which may be considered to be working-memory intensive and deliberative (see Sanfey et al. 2006), this controller distributes information in exactly the correct way. For instance, if the subject is hungry, but when it visits x_2 it discovers that the path to the cheese is blocked, then the next time x_1 is visited, the appropriate choice of action (going right) can be made,

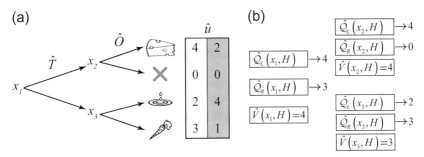

Figure 3.3 Complete maze task: (a) Goal-directed control uses a forward model of the transitions $\hat{T}$, the outcomes $\hat{O}$ and the utilities $\hat{u}$ to predict the values. (b) Cached control uses $\hat{Q}$ (and $\hat{V}$) values to quantify the worth of each action (and state) without modeling the underlying cause of these values. Figure adapted from Niv, Joel, and Dayan (2006).

since the new, impoverished consequence of going left can be calculated. This is a hallmark of the sort of sophisticated, cognitive control whose investigation was pioneered by Tolman (1948).

As mentioned, there is evidence for the involvement of dorsolateral prefrontal cortex and dorsomedial striatum in goal-directed control (Balleine 2005), perhaps because of the demands on working memory posed by forward search in the tree. The representation of $\hat{u}$, however, is less clear.

Habitual Control

Figure 3.3b is the extension of Figure 3.2b to the case of the full maze and shows the complete set of cached $\hat{V}$ and $\hat{Q}$ values for the case of hunger. These are actually the optimal values in the sense that they relate to the optimal choice of action at each state in the maze. As mentioned above, these values can be learned directly from experience. However, the cached values lack the flexibility of the forward model-based values, in particular not being based on knowledge, or estimates, of the actual outcomes. Therefore, behavior at x_3 may not change immediately with a change in motivational state from hunger to thirst, and the behavior at x_1 may not change immediately when the subject learns about the impossibility of turning left at x_2. These inflexibilities are the psychological hallmarks of automatic, habitual control (Sanfey et al. 2006).

One key feature for learning cached values in the case of trajectories is that the value of a state, or a prediction of this value, becomes a surrogate for the utilities that will arise for outcomes delivered downstream of that state. In the maze, for instance, assuming that the subject already knows to turn left there, state x_2 is worth $V(x_2, H) = 4$ in the case of hunger. This makes state x_2 a conditioned reinforcer (see Mackintosh 1983). Discovering this on turning left at x_1 can help reinforce or stamp in that choice at x_1. In the case of rewards, it is a learning rule that arises from this that has been validated in the activity of dopamine neurons, the concentration of dopamine at its striatal targets, and even the fMRI BOLD signal in humans undergoing simple conditioning tasks for primary or secondary reward (Montague et al. 1996; Schultz 1998; O'Doherty 2004). The combination of learning predictions and using those predictions to learn an appropriate policy is sometimes called the actor–critic learning rule (Sutton and Barto 1998).

These and other studies suggest that habitual control depends strongly on dorsolateral regions of the striatum (Balleine 2005). This region is subject to dopaminergic (and serotonergic) neuromodulation, and there is evidence from pharmacological studies that these neuromodulators influence the learning of appropriate actions.

Episodic Control

Both goal-directed and habitual controllers can be seen as learning appropriate actions through the statistical process of measuring the correlations between actions and either outcomes or the utilities of those outcomes. An apparently more primitive scheme, called an episodic controller, would be simply to repeat wholesale any action or sequence of actions that has been successful in the past (Lengyel and Dayan 2007). This requires a structure that can store the successful actions, putatively a job for an episodic memory, plus a way of coupling ultimate success to storage or consolidation within this memory. Although different interpretations are possible, there is indeed evidence in rats and humans that the hippocampus, a critical structure for episodic memory, whose storage appears to be under rich neuromodulatory control, may indeed have a key role to play (Poldrack and Packard 2003).

Pavlovian Control

The three controllers described thus far encompass ways of making, or at least learning to make, essentially arbitrary choices in light of the outcomes to which they lead. They are sometimes called instrumental controllers, since they favor actions that are instrumental in achieving rewards or getting to safety. This sort of choice may, however, just be a thin layer of icing on the overall cake of control (Breland and Breland 1961). Inbuilt, instinctive mechanisms, which have been programmed by evolution, specify vast swathes of appropriate actions in the direct face of particular appetitive or aversive outcomes (Mackintosh 1983). This is particularly apparent in the response to clear and present dangers; such defensive and aggressive responses even appear to enjoy a topographic organization along an axis of the dorsal periacqueductal gray (Keay and Bandler 2001). It is also apparent in the appetitive (licking) and aversive (gapes) responses to the direct provision of primary rewards that Berridge and Robinson (1998) used to measure the extent of liking, as well as perhaps in consummatory responses, such as the drinking behavior of a pigeon faced with a water dispenser or its eating behavior faced with grain in a hopper.

More critically, however, there is also a range of inbuilt responses to *predictions* of future rewards or punishments, which may be considered to come from a Pavlovian controller. These responses are emitted even though they may be immaterial (or indeed, as will be seen below, antagonistic) to the delivery of the outcomes. Very crudely, one component of these responses is outcome-independent, including approach and engagement to predictors associated with positive utilities and withdrawal and disengagement from predictors associated with negative utilities. For instance, pigeons will approach or peck a key whose illumination is temporally predictive of the delivery of food or water at another part of the experimental chamber; rats will move away from a stimulus that predicts the delivery of a shock. A second component is outcome-dependent; that is, the detailed topography of the keypeck is dependent on whether the pigeon expects food or water.

In view of these findings, it is likely that there are multiple Pavlovian controllers, with outcome-dependent responses arising from the predictions of something akin to the forward model, and outcome-independent reactions arising from something more like cached values. Indeed, exactly the same anatomical and pharmacological mechanisms seem to play similar roles, and it may be that Pavlovian values arise from the systems discussed above. However, the different classes of Pavlovian responses seem not to be separated as readily using motivational manipulations, and the distinctions between the different controllers is less well understood.

Pavlovian control is important since most tasks that are designed to test instrumental controllers also create Pavlovian contingencies (Mackintosh 1983). In the maze of Equation 1, for instance, how do we know if hungry animals run from x_1 to x_2 because they have had the choice of going left stamped in by the utility available (an instrumental explanation) or because they have learned to predict the appetitive characteristic of $\hat{V}(x_2) > 0$, and to emit an inbuilt approach response to stimuli or states associated with positive utility (a Pavlovian one)? In fact, a *reductio ad absurdum* exists: since Pavlovian responses have likely been designed over evolution to be appropriate to the general environmental niche occupied by the subjects, experimenters can arrange it such that the Pavlovian response is instrumentally inappropriate. A famous case of this is negative automaintenance: Consider the autoshaping experiment mentioned above, in which pigeons come to peck keys simply because they are illuminated a short while before food or water is presented. If an additional, instrumental, contingency is imposed, such that no food or water will be provided on any trial on which the pigeon pecks the illuminated key, the pigeons continue to peck the key to some degree, despite the adverse effect of this pecking on their earnings. Many foibles of control and choice can be interpreted in terms of untoward cooperation and competition between Pavlovian and instrumental control (Dayan et al. 2006).

Interactions among the Systems

It is natural to ask what benefits could accrue from the existence of multiple, different decision-making systems and, indeed, to question how the new problem for choice they pose collectively might be solved; that is, choice between the choosers rather than between different possible actions.

Instrumental Competition

The first three decision makers at least share the common notional goal of making choices that will maximize predicted utilities. They base their choices on distinct value systems, which are differentially accurate in given circumstances. Daw et al. (2005) suggested that goal-directed and habitual controllers lie at two ends of a rough spectrum, trading off two sources of uncertainty: ignorance and computational noise. This trade-off is not unique to animals, but rather affects all decision makers. Daw et al. (2005) suggested that uncertainty should also be the principle governing the choice between the decision makers.

The goal-directed controller makes best use of information from the world, propagating findings at one state (e.g., a newfound inability to turn left at x_2) immediately to affect choice at other states (enabling the subject to choose to turn right at x_1). By contrast, information propagates between the in a more cumbersome manner over learning, and thus incorrect or inefficient behaviors (at states like x_1) may persist for a number of trials. In fact, one possible use for the reactivation of activity during sleep or quiet wakefulness is the consolidatory process of propagating information to eliminate any inaccuracy. In general, the goal-directed controller can be expected to be more accurate early in learning and after environmental change. Its use of $\hat{u}$ also makes it more reliable in the face of change to the motivational state.

Nevertheless, the goal-directed controller only gains this flexibility at the expense of computationally intractable and, at least in animals, noisy, computations. The task of explicitly searching the tree of choices is tough, since the number of branches and leaves of a tree typically grows very quickly with its depth. Keeping accurate track of the intermediate states and values is impossible for deep trees, and the resulting inaccuracies are a source of noise and uncertainty that removes therefore some of the benefits of goal-directed control. Note that if computational noise can be reduced through the application of (cognitive) effort or processing time, then forms of effort- or time-accuracy trade-offs may ensue (e.g., Payne et al. 1988).

Computational intractability has inspired the integration of goal-directed and habitual control in artificial systems. For instance, game-playing programs, such as the chess player Deep Blue, typically perform explicit search, but without reaching the leaves of the tree (where one or another player will be known to have won). Instead, they use an evaluation function to measure the worth of the positions on the board discovered through searching the tree.

This evaluation function is exactly analogous to the $V(x, m)$ function discussed above. As before, the ideal evaluator would report something akin to the probability of winning, starting from position x. Indeed, some of the earliest ideas in reinforcement learning stem from the realization that the tree search defines a set of consistency conditions for the evaluations, and that inconsistencies can be used to learn or improve evaluators (Sutton and Barto 1988).

Daw et al. (2005) suggest that the goal-directed and habitual systems should keep track of their own respective uncertainties. Then, as is standard in Bayesian decision theoretic contexts, the controllers' estimates should be integrated in a way that depends on their uncertainties. Calculating the uncertainties actually poses severe computational challenges of its own, and it is likely that approximations will be necessary. Daw et al. (2005) demonstrate that a very simple version of uncertainty-based competition sufficed to account for the data on the transition from goal-directed to habitual control that is routinely observed over the course of behavioral learning. This transfer is signaled by the different motivational sensitivities of the two controllers, which, in turn, comes from their dependence on different value systems. It occurs because after substantial experience, the uncertainty in the habitual controller, which stems from its inefficient use of information, is reduced below the level of the computational noise in the goal-directed system. Daw et al. (2005) interpret various psychological results by noting that the extent to which uncertainty favors one or another system depends on the depth of the tree (shallow trees may permanently favor goal-directed control) as well as the (approximate) models of uncertainty that each controller possesses.

The episodic controller can also fit into this general scheme for uncertainty-based utility and competition. Repeating a previously successful action is likely to be optimal in the face of substantial uncertainty and costly exploration. This suggests that the episodic controller should be most beneficial at the very outset of learning, even before the goal-directed controller. Experimental data on this are presently rather sparse (Poldrack and Packard 2003).

Pavlovian Competition

The Pavlovian controller is somewhat harder to locate within this apparently normative interaction between the instrumental controllers. It is difficult, for example, to see the logic behind the finding in negative automaintenance that pigeons will *learn* to emit actions (pecking the illuminated key because of its temporal association with the delivery of food) that are explicitly at odds with their instrumental ambitions (i.e., denying them food). More strikingly, learning may be based on exactly the same forward-modeling and cached value systems that underlie the instrumental decision makers.

One way to think about this is as an illusion of choice. Some perceptual illusions can be seen as arising when a particular observation is constructed in a way that violates statistical expectations or priors based either on evolutionarily specified characteristics of the natural sensory environment, or on characteristics that have been acquired over a lifetime of experience. The systems engaged in perceptual inference must weigh the evidence associated with a particular scene against the overwhelming evidence embodied by these priors. Illusions can result when the latter wins. Similarly, it is indeed generally appropriate to approach and engage with predictors of positive utility, and it is mainly in artificial experimental circumstances that this has negative consequences. Breland and Breland (1961) present an extensive and entertaining description of various other cases that can be seen in similar terms.

The task for us becomes one of understanding the net effects of the interaction between Pavlovian and instrumental control. Approach and engagement responses triggered by positive values could lead to the same sort of boost for a nearly immediately available rewarding outcome that underlies the impulsivity inherent in hyperbolic discounting (for a recent example, see McClure et al. 2004). Concomitantly, it could underlie indirectly the whole range of commitment behaviors that have been considered by proponents of this sort of discounting (e.g., Ainslie 2001).

Withdrawal responses caused by predictions of aversive outcomes can be equally important and, at least in experimentally contrived conditions, equally detrimental. However, perhaps not unreasonably, the range of Pavlovian responses to threat appears to be much more sophisticated than that to reward, with a need to engage flight (definitive withdrawal) or fight (definitive approach) under conditions that are only fairly subtly different. Nevertheless, it has been suggested (De Martino et al. 2006) that the framing effect, in which presenting equivalent choices as losses rather than gains makes them apparently less attractive, could well arise from Pavlovian withdrawal. Similarly, one can argue that Pavlovian responses might bias the sort of deliberative evaluation performed using a forward model, by inhibiting the exploration of paths that might have negative consequences and boosting paths that might have positive consequences. Various biases like these are known to exist, and indeed are systematically disrupted in affective diseases such as depression.

The last interaction is called Pavlovian-to-instrumental transfer, or PIT. This is the phenomenon whereby a subject engaging in an instrumental action to get an outcome will act more quickly or vigorously upon presentation of a Pavlovian predictor of that outcome, or indeed any other appetitive outcome that is relevant to the subject's current motivational state. The boost from predictors of the same outcome (called specific PIT) is greater than that of a different, though motivationally relevant, outcome (general PIT). The obverse phenomenon, in which a predictor of an aversive outcome will suppress ongoing instrumental behavior for rewards, is actually the standard way that the strengths of Pavlovian predictors of aversive outcomes are measured. One view of general PIT is that the Pavlovian cues might affect the prediction of the long-run average value ρ and, as discussed above, thereby change the optimal behavioral vigor (Niv, Joel, and Dayan 2006). A mechanism akin to this was interpreted as playing a key role in controlling the vigor with which habits are executed. This was argued as being necessary since the general motivational insensitivity of habits limits other ways of controlling habitual vigor.

Open Issues

There are many open issues about the nature of the individual systems and their interactions. In particular, the nature of the predicted utility $\hat{u}_o(m)$ in the forward-model value, and especially its dependence on motivational state m and relationship to the native "liking" value $u_o(m)$, are distressingly unclear. Equally, the coupling between forward-model mechanisms and neuromodulators is somewhat mysterious—a fact that is particularly challenging for the models designed to optimize the average rate of utility provision. Subjects have also been assumed to know what actions are possible, although this in itself might require learning that could be particularly taxing.

I would like to end by pointing to various issues that relate to the broader themes of this Ernst Strüngmann Forum.

Generalization and Value

I have stressed issues that relate to generalization: the way that information learned in one motivational state generalizes to another one, and generalization of facts learned in one part of an environment (e.g., the futility of going left at x_2) to other parts (the choice of going right at x_1). The issue of generalization in learning functions such as $\hat{Q}_c(x, m)$ is a large topic itself, raising many questions about things such as the representations of the states x and m that determine these values.

Foremost to generalization is prior expectations. Subjects can have prior expectations about many facets of the world, which then translate into prior expectations about all the unknown aspects of the problem (particularly T and O). Take, for instance, the phenomenon of learned helplessness, which is an animal and human model of depression (e.g., Maier 1984). In learned helplessness, two subjects are yoked to receive exactly the same shocks. One subject (the "master") can terminate the shock by its actions, whereas the other (the "yoke") cannot; it just experiences whatever length of shock the master experiences. In generalization tests to other tasks (or other environments), the master subjects perform like controls; however, the yoked subjects show signs that resemble depression, notably an unwillingness to attempt to choose actions to improve their lot. One interpretation (Huys and Dayan, pers. comm.) is that the yoked subjects generalize to the test, the statistical structure, which indicates that actions cannot be expected to have reliable or beneficial effects. Given this expectation, it is not adaptive to search for or to attempt appropriate actions, which is exactly the behavioral observation. Thus predictions about likely values and value structures can exert a strong influence on the whole interaction between a subject and its environment.

Conscious and Unconscious Control

A major theme at this Forum was the relationship between conscious and unconscious decision making. Without wishing to pass judgment on consciousness, we might think that the former has more to do with deliberative processing; the latter with automatic control. If we consider forward-model schemes to be deliberative and habitual ones automatic, then within the instrumental systems described herein, there appears to be a seamless integration with a single intended target. The Pavlovian controller can disturb this normativity, but it may also be based on deliberative and automatic evaluation mechanisms, each of which might disturb its matched instrumental controller. Our view is thus perhaps not completely consistent with some two-systems accounts, for instance, those that attribute a shorter timescale of discounting to the automatic rather than the deliberative system (McClure et al. 2004).

Deliberation, however, could clearly be much more complicated than the sort of rigid search that we have considered through a known tree. There are many choices inherent in the search process itself, and these are presumably the products of exactly the same sorts of mechanisms and rules that have been developed for externally directed actions. Understanding how they all work together as well as the way that biases in different systems affect the overall choice, are key areas for future exploration. To belabor one example, I have argued that amorphous and poorly understood tasks likely favor the episodic controller. However, since it is explicitly not designed on the principles of statistical averaging, which underlie the forward model and the habit system, this controller will most likely have a difficult time integrating statistical information correctly. This could lead to large biases in choice, given only moderate numbers of examples.

Conclusions

I have sketched an account of the influences of different systems involved in the assessment of value on different systems involved in making choices. Value systems, and therefore the behavioral systems they support, vary according to the nature and origin of their sensitivity to the motivational state of a subject, its knowledge about its environment, as well as their intrinsic timescales. Decision-making systems vary in related ways, bringing different information to bear on largely similar concerns. Instrumental controllers work together in a harmonious manner, whereas it is significantly more challenging to account for and understand Pavlovian control.

Acknowledgments

I am very grateful to my many collaborators in the work described here, notably Bernard Balleine, Nathaniel Daw, Yael Niv, John O'Doherty, Máté Lengyel, Ben Seymour, Quentin Huys, Ray Dolan, and Read Montague. I specially thank Nathaniel Daw, Yael Niv, and Ben Seymour for detailed comments on an earlier draft. I also thank Christoph Engel, Wolf Singer, and Julia Lupp for organizing the workshop, and to them, the members of Groups 1 and 2, Jon Cohen, and Eric Johnson for helpful comments. Funding was from the Gatsby Charitable Foundation.

References

Ainslie, G. 2001. Breakdown of Will. Cambridge: Cambridge Univ. Press.

Balleine, B. W. 2005. Neural bases of food-seeking: Affect, arousal and reward in corticostriatolimbic circuits. *Physiol. Behav.* **86**:717–730.

Balleine, B. W., and S. Killcross. 2006. Parallel incentive processing: An integrated view of amygdala function. *Trends Neurosci.* **29**:272–279.

Berridge, K. C., and T. E. Robinson. 1998. What is the role of dopamine in reward: Hedonic impact, reward learning, or incentive salience? *Brain Res. Rev.* **28**:309–369.

Breland, K., and M. Breland. 1961. The misbehavior of organisms. *Am. Psychol.* **16**:681–684.

Damasio, A. R., D. Tranel, and H. Damasio. 1991. Somatic markers and the guidance of behavior: Theory and preliminary testing. In: Frontal Lobe Function and Dysfunction, ed. H. S. Levin, H. M. Eisenberg, and A. L. Benton, pp. 217–229. New York: Oxford Univ. Press.

Daw, N. D., S. Kakade, and P. Dayan. 2002. Opponent interactions between serotonin and dopamine. *Neural Networks* **15**:603–616.

Daw, N. D., Y. Niv, and P. Dayan. 2005. Uncertainty-based competition between prefrontal and dorsolateral striatal systems for behavioral control. *Nature Neurosci.* **8**:1704–1711.

Dayan, P., and B. W. Balleine. 2002. Reward, motivation and reinforcement learning. *Neuron* **36**:285–298.

Dayan, P., Y. Niv, B. J. Seymour, and N. D. Daw. 2006. The misbehavior of value and the discipline of the will. *Neural Networks* **19**:1153–1160.

De Martino, B., D. Kumaran, B. Seymour, and R. J. Dolan. 2006. Frames, biases, and rational decision-making in the human brain. *Science* **313**:684–687.

Dickinson, A. 1994. Instrumental conditioning. In: Animal Learning and Cognition, ed. N. Mackintosh, pp. 45–79. San Diego: Academic Press.

Dickinson, A., and B. Balleine. 2001. The role of learning in motivation. In: Stevens' Handbook of Experimental Psychology, vol. 3: Learning, Motivation and Emotion, 3rd ed., ed. C.R. Gallistel, pp. 497–533. New York: Wiley.

Kahneman, D., P. Wakker, and R. Sarin. 1997. Back to Bentham? Explorations of experienced utility. *Qtly. J. Econ.* **112**:375–406.

Keay, K. A., and R. Bandler. 2001. Parallel circuits mediating distinct emotional coping reactions to different types of stress. *Neurosci. Biobehav. Rev.* **25**:669–678.

Konorski, J. 1948. Conditioned Reflexes and Neuron Organization. Cambridge: Cambridge Univ. Press.

Konorski, J. 1967. Integrative Activity of the Brain: An Interdisciplinary Approach. Chicago: Univ. of Chicago Press.

Lengyel, M., and P. Dayan. 2007. Hippocampal contributions to control: The third way. Neural Information Processing Systems conference.

Loewenstein, G. 1996. Out of control: Visceral influences on behavior. *Org. Behav. Hum. Dec. Proc.* **65**:272–292.

Luce, R. D. 1959. Individual Choice Behavior: A Theoretical Analysis. New York: Wiley.

Mackintosh, N. J. 1983. Conditioning and Associative Learning. Oxford: Oxford Univ. Press.

Maier, S. F. 1984. Learned helplessness and animal models of depression. *Prog. Neuropsychopharm. Biol. Psych.* **8**:435–446.

McClure, S. M., D. I. Laibson, G. Loewenstein, and J. D. Cohen. 2004. Separate neural systems value immediate and delayed monetary rewards. *Science* **304**:503–507.

Montague, P. R., P. Dayan, and T. J. Sejnowski. 1996. A framework for mesencephalic dopamine systems based on predictive Hebbian learning. *J. Neurosci.* **16**:1936–1947.

Niv, Y., N. D. Daw, D. Joel, and P. Dayan. 2006. Tonic dopamine: Opportunity costs and the control of response vigor. *Psychopharm.* doi:10.1007/s00213-006-0502-4.

Niv, Y., D. Joel, and P. Dayan. 2006. A normative perspective on motivation. *Trends Cogn. Sci.* **8**:375–381.

O'Doherty, J. P. 2004. Reward representations and reward-related learning in the human brain: Insights from neuroimaging. *Curr. Opin. Neurobiol.* **14**:769–776.

Payne, J. W., J. R. Bettman, and E. J. Johnson. 1988. Adaptive strategy selection in decision making. *J. Exp. Psychol.: Learn. Mem. Cogn.* **14**:534–552.

Poldrack, R. A., and M. G. Packard. 2003. Competition among multiple memory systems: Converging evidence from animal and human brain studies. *Neuropsychologia* **41**:245–251.

Sanfey, A. G., G. Loewenstein, S. M. McClure, and J. D. Cohen. 2006. Neuroeconomics: Cross-currents in research on decision-making. *Trends Cogn. Sci.* **10**:108–116.

Schultz, W. 1998. Predictive reward signal of dopamine neurons. *J. Neurophys.* **80**:1–27.

Sutton, R. S., and A. G. Barto. 1998. Reinforcement Learning. Cambridge, MA: MIT Press.

Tolman, E. C. 1948. Cognitive maps in rats and men. *Psychol. Rev.* **55**:189–208.

Watkins, C. J. C. H. 1989. Learning from delayed rewards. Ph.D. thesis, Univ. of Cambridge.

4

Neurobiology of Decision Making

An Intentional Framework

Michael N. Shadlen, Roozbeh Kiani,
Timothy D. Hanks, and Anne K. Churchland

Howard Hughes Medical Institute, Department of Physiology and Biophysics,
University of Washington Medical School, Seattle, WA 98195–7290, U.S.A.

Abstract

The aim of statistical decision theories is to understand how evidence, prior knowledge, and values lead an organism to commit to one of a number of alternatives. Two main statistical decision theories, signal-detection theory and sequential analysis, assert that decision makers obtain evidence—often from the senses—that is corrupted by noise and weigh this evidence alongside bias and value to select the best choice. Signal-detection theory has been the dominant conceptual framework for perceptual decisions near threshold. Sequential analysis extends this framework by incorporating time and introducing a rule for terminating the decision process. This extension allows the trade-off between decision speed and accuracy to be studied, and invites us to consider decision rules as policies on a stream of evidence acquired in time. In light of these theories, simple perceptual decisions, which can be studied in the neurophysiology laboratory, allow principles that apply to more complex decisions to be exposed.

The goal of this chapter is to "go beyond the data" to postulate a number of unifying principles of complex decisions based on our findings with simple decisions. We make speculative points and argue positions that should be viewed as controversial and provocative. In many places, a viewpoint will merely be sketched without going into much detail and without ample consideration of alternatives, except by way of contrast when necessary to make a point. The aim is not to convince but to pique interest.

The chapter is divided into two main sections. The first suggests that an intention-based framework for decision making extends beyond simple perceptual decisions to a broad variety of more complex situations. The second, which is a logical extension of the first, poses a challenge to Bayesian inference as the dominant mathematical foundation of decision making.

A Common Framework

Progress in understanding the neurobiology of decision making stems from simple experimental paradigms. Several pivotal studies (reviewed in Gold and Shadlen 2007) have emphasized tasks in which decision making reduces to a choice among actions. These studies have exploited the fact that when a decision bears on a particular act, the steps toward formation of the decision (i.e., the decision process) affect the neurons in the higher-level association areas of the brain that are identified with motor planning. Here, we suggest that the success of this enterprise is a consequence of a principle of brain organization, and we explore some of the extensions of these principles.

Intentional Organization

Information flow in the brain is effectively channeled into structures that are organized in terms of behavior. To a visual neuroscientist, it might seem that the point of visual processing is to elaborate more complex features and scene properties, as well as to generalize over invariants for purposes of object classification and recognition. Although the initial stages of visual processing can be considered automatic and oriented toward extraction of features, we think it is mistaken to assume that the goal of visual processing is the automatic extraction of such features. Viewed from the perspective of decision making, information in the sensory cortex merely supplies evidence bearing on propositions. The way this evidence is organized—the transformation of information and the functional architecture in support of maps—facilitates and constrains the accessibility of this evidence. We would be mistaken, however, to identify the representation of the sensory data as giving rise directly to perception (He et al. 1996; Naccache et al. 2002; Jiang et al. 2006). Perception, like decision making, arises by asking and answering questions that bear on specific propositions. Importantly, evidence-gathering mechanisms are organized in the brain in association with structures that control the body. This constrains the possible meanings of information and connects the analysis of vision to embodied perception, affordances, and intentionality (Gibson 1950; Merleau-Ponty 1962; Churchland et al. 1994; Rizzolatti et al. 1997; Clark 1997; O'Regan and Noë 2001; Cisek 2007).

Lessons from the Intraparietal Sulcus

Let us consider the organization of the posterior parietal lobe of the rhesus monkey.

Sensory modality specific.   The posterior/lateral bank of the intraparietal sulcus seems to receive predominantly visual input. The regions anterior and medial to it receive somatosensory and proprioceptive input. The more anterior parts of the sulcus (toward the temporal lobe) appear to receive auditory input (Poremba et al. 2003). Based on connectivity with frontal structures and input from sensory structures, the emerging picture is a regional organization (cm scale) respecting sensory modality and an area organization (mm scale) respecting modes of motor function (Petrides and Pandya 1984; Cavada and Goldman-Rakic 1989; Lewis and Van Essen 2000a, b; Colby and Goldberg 1999).

Gnosis versus praxis. Neurologists recognize that loss of parietal function leads to a loss of appreciation for the significance of contralateral space. The frame of reference for the designation "contralateral" can be the visual field, body, or an external landmark such as an object. Importantly, it is the knowledge of space (gnosis), not the ability to move around in the space (praxis), that is affected, at least at a gross level (Critchley 1953).

At a finer level of resolution (e.g., millimeters), it is becoming clear that the areas comprising this part of the brain have more specific associations with motor regions. The lateral intraparietal area (LIP), for example, is connected to structures involved in moving the gaze and therefore probably also in shifting spatial attention. Neurons in this area seem to be concerned with places in space, especially when the place contains a potential target of an eye movement. The parietal reach region (PRR), which is only millimeters away from LIP, is connected to frontal lobe structures involved in reaching movements. Its neurons respond to places in extrapersonal space, especially when the place contains a potential target of a reach. The anterior intraparietal region (AIP) connects to frontal lobe structures that control the shape of the hand. Neurons in AIP respond to the shapes of objects. Although there is heterogeneity of neuron response preferences in each of these areas, there is an emerging support for the concept that these areas associate visual information with particular modes of utilizing that information (Anderson and Buneo 2002; Scherberger and Andersen 2007; Scherberger et al. 2003; cf. Levy et al. 2007).

The three parietal areas—LIP, PRR and AIP—are not motor in the traditional sense: their activity does not cause an immediate movement of a body part, nor do they encode movement parameters such as force, velocity, or tension. Instead, we think they allow us to know that something is present as well as an intended purpose. Their activity might be viewed as an interrogation or query of the evidence in the visual cortex. They effectively construe this information as evidence for (or against) embodied hypotheses and propositions—statements about what the body might do to its world. We refer to this as an "intentional architecture" for information flow. It does not provide answers to complex problems in perception (e.g., constancies, segmentation, binding of parts of objects into wholes) but it does tell us where in the brain we might look for neural correlates of these capacities, and it adds constraints to problems in perception that could pave the way to progress (e.g., Shadlen and Movshon 1999).

We know far less about regions of the parietal lobe that receive predominantly auditory information (Poremba et al. 2003). It seems reasonable to predict that further research will expose the organization of the parietal lobe as being in the service of gathering specific forms of information (i.e., particular sensory submodalities) to guide potential action.

Challenges and Extensions to Intentional Architecture

When a decision about a state of the world necessitates a particular action, it may not be surprising to some that a slightly elaborated sensorimotor integration area, like LIP, might represent the evolving decision variable. However, we should be surprised by this! After all, we do not feel as if we make decisions with our eye movements but instead make decisions about the stimulus and then communicate the outcome of the decision in whatever way we are instructed. We decide that motion is rightward, for example, and then communicate this by making an eye movement, pushing a button, or making a verbal response.

If decisions are made by neurons that are connected to specific action modalities, then there are at least three challenges: First, if a decision can be made by eye, hand, or verbal response, what prevents these systems from reaching different decisions? Second, the design seems wasteful: why not make the decision in some central spot and allow a "central executive" to deliver the answer to whatever motor modality is used to communicate the outcome? Third, how do we make a decision if the mode of response is not specified ahead of time?

Agreement is natural. In many instances, decisions are determined by the evidence from the environment or the noisy evidence in sensory maps. If different effector systems examine the same evidence, they will naturally reach the same conclusion. This statement rests on an assumption about the source of variability in the decision process, an assumption that is likely to hold when accuracy is valued. Recall that for difficult perceptual decisions, the variations in choice rendered from trial to trial are explained by considering the signal and noise affecting the decision. As long as the noise is in the stimulus or in the sensory representation, it will explain the choice. Therefore, even if several decision makers work in parallel, as long as they access the same evidence, they will reach the same decision. This is because both the signal and the noise that determine the outcome of a single decision can be traced to the sensory evidence. If eye, hand, and language access the same evidence, they reach the same conclusion, correct or incorrect.

This is actually a quantitative argument. It boils down to an analysis of the noise contributions in brain regions that represent momentary evidence and areas that represent the decision variable. When accuracy is a desired goal, evidence is allowed to accumulate before the decision is terminated with a choice. Consequently, the noise introduced by neurons that represent the decision variable (e.g., neurons in LIP) does not contribute substantially to the error rate. In contrast, under speed stress, the decision terminates after very little averaging. In these circumstances, noise at the level of the decision makers can actually affect which choice is made. In that case it ought to be possible for different motor response modalities to reach different decisions, which, in the absence of further coordination among the response modalities, would result in incongruent responses. However, coordination of responses is feasible, and there is plenty of information in the decision outcome to provide a basis for it. For example, different modalities may reach their decisions at different times, and we might know that the first process to terminate could be an outlier and choose to delay until a few more systems weigh in.

One might argue that this parallel intentional architecture is inefficient. That may be true from the perspective of energy conservation, but it seems highly efficient to us from an evolutionary perspective. It allowed our brains to develop complex higher functions (contingency, deliberation) using a minor variation on a theme already developed for sensorimotor integration. No new wiring scheme was required!

In any case, our experiments tell us that when the action mode is known in advance, the high-level intentional structures represent partial information. If there were a central executive, it seems to pass on its deliberations to neurons concerned with motor planning while the decision evolves (Gold and Shadlen 2000, 2003; Spivey et al. 2005). Thus, it does not act as a central executive in that setting.

Abstract decisions. It is not difficult to understand how the intentional architecture can be extended to explain abstract decisions. In fact it helps to consider a simple case: a perceptual decision among two alternatives performed in a setting in which the action used to communicate the decision is not specified until after the decision is made.

Consider a monkey trained to decide between leftward and rightward motion of a random dot kinematogram. This is the same task as the one used to study neurons in LIP except for one important difference: there are no choice targets shown during the period of motion viewing. The monkey will ultimately communicate a choice by making an eye movement to a target, but it does not know where they will appear. When they do appear, one is red and the other is green. The monkey is trained to make an eye movement to the red target if the motion is rightward and to the green if it is leftward.

Monkeys can perform this task about as well as the version of the task described in our earlier work. When they do, it is clear that they have decided about right- or leftward direction and not which way they will make an eye movement. Indeed, on each trial, the monkey seems to embrace the proposition, "right" or "left." In this case, structures in the oculomotor pathways do not represent a decision variable. Instead, the brain seems to make the kind of abstract decision that does not involve intention. Or does it?

To picture this decision process, consider the accumulation of evidence toward a commitment to a plan, only here it is not a plan to make a particular eye movement but instead to select a red or a green target when they appear. We can think of the motion as instructing the implementation of a rule: when two targets appear, make an eye movement toward the red (or green) one. We have no trouble imagining neurons that accumulate evidence toward implementing this plan or rule, and we can imagine that this rule is enacted by selecting the appropriate circuits in the brain that allow a simple sensorimotor decision to ensue. Choose a target for an eye movement based on its color. This is just a decision to make a certain kind of decision.

Functional and anatomical considerations. Where would we expect to find such neurons? They should be in areas of the brain that project to the association areas. A reasonable candidate for the neurons in the red/green motion task are the parts of the dorsolateral prefrontal cortex (area 46) that project to area LIP (Cavada and Goldman-Rakic 1989). Neurons with the requisite properties have been found in this area, but experimental evidence is not all that compelling in our view. The problem with the experiments is that there is currently no way to sample neurons in A46 efficiently, based on their projection pattern to LIP (or other areas).

Although our hypothesis is not able to be tested at the present, there is some support for the idea that some A46 neurons carry on the kind of computations we have in mind. Wallis et al. (2001) described neurons in A46 that represent rules, and we have shown in one monkey that some neurons in A46 accumulate evidence for direction in this task (Gold and Shadlen 2001b). However, we view these studies with healthy skepticism because there is no obvious clustering of response patterns in A46 indicative of a functional architecture. Thus the reports (including ours) are based on a small fraction of randomly encountered neurons that happen to bear on the hypothesis. This concern about electrophysiology in A46 is not limited to the study of decision making.

Nonetheless, there are many parts of the association cortex in the nonhuman primate that map other association areas. They could achieve the computation we are proposing. The important conceptual point is that the computations underlying abstract decisions, which are not tied to specific actions, are probably similar formally to the computations we have studied in a simpler context: accumulation of information for a purpose and the representation of a plan to enact. In this case, the plan is to implement a rule.

If-then logic. Let us take this one step further. Consider that the plan of action is to enable a variety of circuits, not just one eye movement to red/green, but also several possible rules. This is then a means to establish a nested logical flow. It is a way for the brain to implement an if-then logic. Indeed, it does not seem improbable to consider that more areas that map the areas that select the sensorimotor circuits allow further nesting of this if-then logic. We are only hinting at the variety of functions that this functional architecture could achieve. Our main point is that the intentional architecture studied in simple decision-making tasks is likely to share common features and principles with the brain architecture that gives rise to complex functions. Figure 4.1 illustrates this scheme. The 25 million years of evolution between macaque and humans has probably served to expand the cortical mantle in the service of this nested intentional architecture. This seems far more likely to have occurred than the evolution of brand new principles of neural computation.

Value-based Decisions

Our research on perceptual decisions has focused on the way the brain combines evidence across time as well as from multiple sources. We have also studied the effect of prior probability in these tasks and see a clear connection (in our human studies) with asymmetric reward schedules, which should also promote a bias. These studies emphasize decisions that are based primarily on the evidence. Value-based decisions, on the other hand, emphasize the component of decision making that is predicated on weighting alternatives based on expected utility. These are often the types of decisions that mimic foraging for food.

It is not controversial to assert that, at the level of formalisms, evidence- and value-based decisions are fundamentally similar. Just about any theory of decision making posits that the decision variable or the criterion to which it is subjected is affected by values placed on the choices and their probable outcomes. How similar is the neurobiology in these cases? We argue that it is likely to be very similar. This is controversial for two reasons. First, the kinds of quantities that are involved in value-based decisions are poorly understood and seem to be quite different from the kind of information that is represented in the visual cortex. Second, the patterns of behavior observed in value-based decisions are thought by many to require a stage of strategic (i.e., deliberate) randomness in the decision-making process. We believe that this is incorrect and perhaps misguided.

Quantities in Value-based Decisions

All decisions are ultimately decisions about value. In evidence-based decisions, the value is in being correct. As such, value is implicitly represented in the decision variable (DV) and the criterion that is applied to it. In this way, the quantities that underlie the decision itself are similar in the two situations. What differ are the sources of signals that inform those quantities.

The representation of value and its association with places, features, foods, etc. seems to be conveyed by dedicated structures. Evidence from several groups point to the orbitofrontal cortex (OFC). A recent study from Padoa-Schioppa and Assad (2006) asserts that the value or utility of a potentially

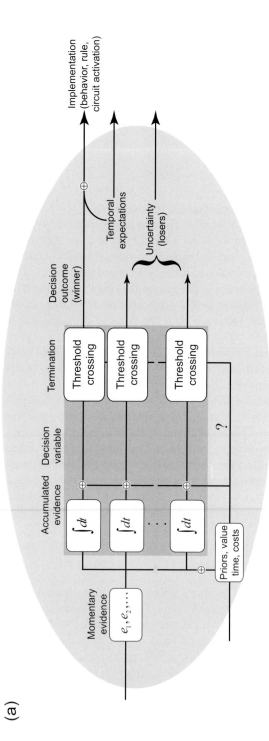

Figure 4.1 An intentional architecture for decision making. (a) Components of a basic decision module. The main input is the evidence bearing on the choices. Other inputs include information about prior probability, the rewards and penalties associated with the choices, and costs associated with elapsed time and sampling. The evidence is integrated in time to form a decision variable. A choice is rendered by a threshold crossing of one of the processes as it races against the decision variable representing the competing choices. Other inputs, such as prior information and costs, either contribute to the decision variable or adjust the threshold. The main output is a signal that identifies the winner for purposes of guiding a response or subsequent behavior. Other outputs include a representation of the degree of confidence and possibly a representation of revised temporal expectations (e.g., by when should an action pay off).

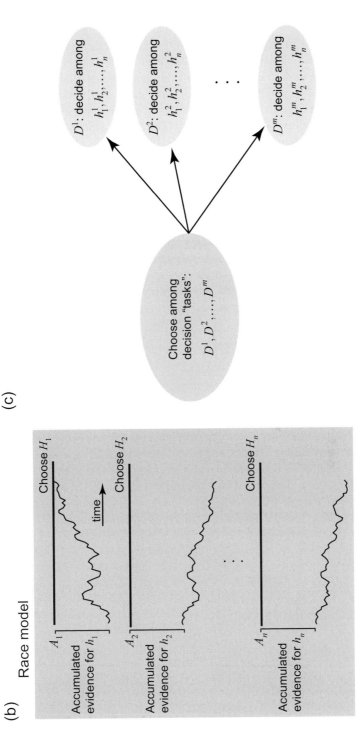

Figure 4.1 (continued) (b) The machinery underlying the decision module. (c) Generalization of the basic module to higher-order decisions. Multiple modules operate in a cascading fashion to make "decisions about decisions." This can be viewed as deciding which task to pursue.

rewarding experience is represented in units that would combine naturally with evidence: the firing rate encodes a quantity that contributes linearly to choice preference in units of log odds (see also Deaner et al. 2005; Gold and Shadlen 2001a). Thus the basic framework for making decisions is likely to be preserved. On the other hand, elucidation of mechanism will force us to study processes in brain regions like the OFC, anterior cingulate cortex, amygdala, and striatum, which presumably represent valence and establish termination rules (McCoy and Platt 2005; McCoy et al. 2003; Paton et al. 2006; Lo and Wang 2006; Kawagoe et al. 2004; Watanabe et al. 2003; Tremblay and Schultz 1999; Hikosaka and Watanabe 2000; Montague and Berns 2002).

We note one final point, which is also relevant to the following section: The kinds of quantities that contribute to the DV (and criteria for terminating) are not limited to evidence, priors, and value of reward or punishment. They also include premiums and penalties for taking time, for exploration, or for persisting. How a premium for exploration is calibrated against evidence is an open question, but it is likely to be no more mysterious than the standard mix of ingredients in decisions. In the end, all quantities in the DV add in units of a common currency, namely spike rate.

Randomness (of Choice) Arises from Noise Not Strategy

The conversion from DV to the expression of choice is commonly treated differently for evidence- and value-based decisions. Here, however, is a peculiar distinction, which we think is incorrect: less than perfect performance is attributed to noise in evidence-based decisions but to probabilistic behavioral response in value-based decisions. Consider a binary decision between options A and B. In both evidence- and value-based decisions, a DV summarizes the merits of A relative to B. For one type of decision, the DV is based mainly on evidence; for the other it is based primarily on utilities. We have already pointed out that a single framework (and a common neurobiology) can accommodate both DVs. The DV has some relationship with probability.

Both evidence- and value-based decisions appear to be stochastic from the point of view of the experimentalist. The sigmoid curve in Figure 4.2 could describe the probability that a monkey chooses rightward as a function of the strength of motion evidence to the right, or it could describe the probability of choosing the red location based on the experienced value of this choice as inferred from recent history of food collection. Neither behavior appears stochastic for extreme values of the *x*-variable. Near the middle of the graph, however, the responses are distributed probabilistically. Indeed a sequence of answers—especially from a practiced and highly motivated subject—appears nearly indistinguishable from the sequence of heads and tails produced by a weighted coin. Current theories of evidence- and value-based decisions diverge in their accounts of the neurobiological mechanism underlying this phenomenon.

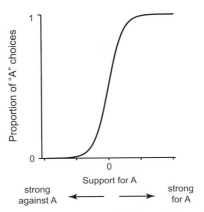

Figure 4.2   Choice function. The support might be evidence for choice "A" or an expected value that is associated with "A."

For value-based decisions, the brain represents a quantity related to relative utility of one of the choices. It is assumed that this value is explicitly converted to a probability, which then governs a process that is formally identical to flipping a coin (Figure 4.3). The specific mathematical operations are not important to the argument here, save for one: there is a conversion of a number (or vector) to a probability. For two choices this is like inverting a logistic to a parameter p (and $1-p$), which is realized as a random event (a so-called Bernoulli trial). For more than two choices, the idea naturally extends to inversion of a vector to a multinomial parameter $p_1, p_2, ..., p_n$, also realized as a random event. Thus, even when the relative utility of one choice is registered by the brain as the better choice, it is not always selected. Contrast this to the following.

For evidence-based decisions, the DV represents a quantity related to the likelihood that one proposition is true. Rather than converting this to a probability, the brain simply makes the best choice it can. Again, the details of the computation are not important. If the quantity is proportional to the log likelihood ratio, then zero marks the criterion at which evidence favors one or the other choice. However, any quantity that is monotonically related to relative likelihood will do, as long as it is accompanied by the appropriate criterion. The randomness to the behavior results because the DV is noisy. This is consistent with all accounts of neurophysiology, especially in the regime in which decisions are difficult; that is, a weak rightward stimulus gives rise to a representation of evidence that is noisy. Although a perfect transducer would always favor a right- over leftward direction, the fact is that on some fraction of trials, the brain represents a value with the wrong sign relative to the criterion.

Contrast the two ideas: in value-based decisions, the brain knows what the better option is but behaves randomly, depending on how much better the option is. In evidence-based decisions, the brain makes the best choice it can, based on the available evidence, which may be faulty. Is this distinction artificial or real?

(a)

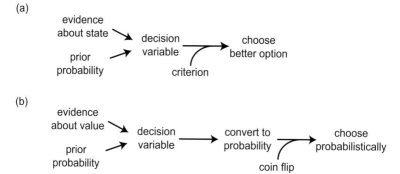

(b)

Figure 4.3   Components of simple decisions. (a) Flow used to explain perceptual- and evidence-based decisions. A decision variable is established from the evidence. A criterion is applied to achieve the best choice. The notion of "best" incorporates valuation, which is commonly incorporated in the criterion. (b) Flow used to explain value-based decisions. The choice is a realization of a random event (coin flip) to match a probability. We are critical of this concept.

We propose that such a distinction does not exist in the brain. The representation of a DV is noisy, whether it is constructed from sensory evidence or from knowledge of reward values. This is a fact of neurobiology (Softky and Koch 1993; Shadlen and Newsome 1994, 1998). This noise underlies the apparent randomness of choices in both evidence- and value-based decisions. Thus the neurobiology of these two types of decision is similar, and the seemingly stochastic behavioral response in neither of them is due to an explicit random number generator in the brain. In addition to the noise in the DV, there are other sources that contribute to the variability of behavioral responses. For instance, the subject often tries to reach a balance between exploitation of the existing knowledge and exploration of new possibilities. Exploration is more prominent in value-based decisions when the reward values can change (e.g., Sugrue et al. 2004). A tendency to explore the environment should not be mistaken with a deliberate randomization of behavior; it should just remind us of the complexity of the decision process. The DV can incorporate the anticipated costs and dividends associated with exploration and persistence. The random number generator in Figure 4.2 should be regarded as a mathematical convenience, rather than a neurally motivated computational principle, to lump multiple sources of variability together. Indeed, it spells out the wrong principle.

What led to the idea of a random stage in value-based decisions? The main reason was an absence of noise in psychological theories. Signal/noise relations have a long tradition in sensory physiology (Hecht and Mintz 1939; Barlow et al. 1971; Parker and Newsome 1998) and in psychophysics (Green and Swets 1966; Cohn et al. 1975; Tanner 1961; Thurstone 1959; Link 1992), but they are generally absent from psychological theories of choice (Luce 1959; Herrnstein 1961; Herrnstein and Vaughan 1980; Kahneman 2002, but see Manski 1977).

Absent noise, some sort of random number generator seems to be required. Enthusiasm for inclusion of a random number generator in the mechanism of value-based decisions is also partly rooted in game theory (Dorris and Glimcher 2004; Glimcher 2003, 2005; Lee et al. 2004; Lee et al. 2005; Barraclough et al. 2004). The optimal strategy in competitive games often necessitates random behavior to stop an intelligent opponent from exploiting predictable patterns in one's own behavior. However, such omniscient opponents are rarely present in real-life situations. In fact, the behavior of subjects in value-based decisions can often be successfully characterized by the history of subjects' decisions and payoffs even for competitive games (Lee et al. 2005; Barraclough et al. 2004; Corrado et al. 2005; Lau and Glimcher 2005). We argue that in these successful behavioral models the random number generator can be replaced by noisiness in the representation of evidence and value via a DV.

Summary of Generalized Intentional Framework

The intentional framework that we have characterized extends to a broad variety of decision-making situations using a cascade of the basic machinery that has been uncovered through studies of simpler decisions. In simple perceptual decisions, sensory neurons provide evidence about the current status of the external environment. This evidence is accumulated into a DV in structures that are associated with particular plans of action which would instantiate the outcome of the decision, should it come out one way or another (gray-shaded region of Figure 4.1). Such instantiation might be an immediate behavior, enactment of a behavioral rule (e.g., if-then logic), or more generally, activation of a specific neural circuit. The DV also incorporates information about prior probability, value, temporal costs, and any other factors that bear on the decision. The underlying machinery of this is simply a race model where the process that reaches the bound first results in the implementation of the corresponding decision outcome. There can be as many processes as necessary to underlie the possible decision outcomes. Furthermore, there can be cascades of decisions, where the outcome of one determines the nature of a subsequent deliberation through the appropriate circuit activation.

The basic building blocks of a decision establish a functional architecture, which in turn hints at the critical neurobiology. As shown in Figure 4.1, there must be accumulators: neurons whose rate of discharge depends on the history of the moment-by-moment fluctuations in the evidence furnished by sensory neurons. Many of the cells that demonstrate persistent activity, which is thought to play a role in working memory, motor planning, representation of context, etc., may also be capable of acting as accumulators. Such cells are ubiquitous in the association cortex.

To establish a termination rule or bound, there must be neurons that can sense a level crossing in the accumulators. These neurons can use temporal and reward-related information to set and implement the appropriate level. This is presumably achieved by the basal ganglia, perhaps in concert with its targets, the substantia nigra pars reticulata, the thalamus, and their targets (ultimately the neocortex). Other structures that represent value are also likely to partici-pate (e.g., ventral tegmentum, nucleus accumbens, amygdala, OFC).

The decision ends in a signal that stimulates another structure into action. In the case of simple real-time RT tasks, this might be neurons that generate movements of body parts; in other cases it might be a structure that activates another decision (Figure 4.1c). Further, we think that at least two other signals must accompany the declaration of the decision outcome. There must be some degree of confidence associated with the content and some prediction of the expected time that the decision should lead to an action, anticipated outcome, reward, or punishment. Little is known about the neurobiological correlates of these putative signals. We will not discuss the anticipated time signal except to say that it seems essential for a variety of functions, including learning. The "confidence" signal might also play a role in learning, but as discussed in the next section, it seems essential to negotiate between competing decisions or to interpolate rationally when the outcome from separate decision processes must be combined.

Decision Making Is Not Bayesian Inference

The relationship between Bayesian inference and decision making has held center stage in theorizing about the neural mechanisms for choice behavior. We question the wisdom of this paradigm. In particular, we focus on an impor-tant distinction between the Bayesian approach and what we term "decision as intention." The idea stems from the intentional architecture concept discussed above. That architecture suggests that decisions are not made in the abstract about states of the world but instead guide a choice among a discrete set of possible behaviors.

It may be sensible to preface the argument with a short list of caveats. Our argument is not anti-Bayesian. Indeed it endorses many of the key components of Bayesian decision making, as will be clear. It is not concerned with the na-ture of probability; it is not an embrace of the frequentist school of probability theory. It is instead a critique of the notion that posterior probability distribu-tions are calculated explicitly, represented and used to guide decisions.

The Bayesian Paradigm: "Decision As Inference"

Any sensible formulation of the problem of decision making must consider at least three main factors: (a) evidence pertaining to choices, (b) prior knowl-edge about states of the world, and (c) costs and rewards associated with the decision. The Bayesian paradigm assumes that the brain represents a posterior probability distribution over the possible states of the world. Decisions, actions, estimates, and confidence ratings all stem from this posterior.

Within this framework, decisions among discrete hypotheses are regarded as a special case of inference. In the context of decision making, the posterior is used to forecast expected cost and benefit associated with the consequences of each choice. The latter calculation can take a variety of forms, which incorporate different assumptions about utility, but all involve evaluation in light of the probable states of the world as represented by the posterior. For simple decisions among N alternatives, "decision as inference" postulates that decisions arise by placing criteria on the quantities calculated from posteriors.

The key to the Bayesian paradigm is that the posterior is used to achieve the projected prediction of utility. It is an independent entity, which can be used for a variety of purposes. We do not question the merit of this perspective in general, but we do question its direct application to the neurobiology of decision making; that is, whether the brain actually represents posterior probability distributions.

A Critique of the Data in Support of the Representation of Posterior Probabilities

The main experimental evidence in support of the explicit representation of posterior probability distributions involves integration of evidence from diverse sources. These are behavioral studies in perception and motor control (Ernst and Banks 2002; Rosas et al. 2005; Mamassian and Landy 2001; Landy et al. 1995; Trommershauser et al. 2005; Yuille and Bulthoff 1996; Knill and Saunders 2003; Kording and Wolpert 2004a; Brainard and Freeman 1997; van Ee et al. 2003; Kersten 1999; Kersten and Yuille 2003; Kersten et al. 2004). For example, when a subject is asked to judge the angle α of an object in space based on disparity and texture cues (i.e., binocular depth and perspective), the judgments reflect information from both sources, weighted in accordance with the relative reliability of the two sources. To achieve this, the brain must keep track of at least two numbers per cue: an estimate bearing in the decision and the degree of uncertainty/reliability.

The brain can achieve this in a number of ways. Clearly, if the brain represents two posterior probability distributions over possible angles,

$$P\left(\alpha \middle| e_{disparity}\right) \text{ and } P\left(\alpha \middle| e_{texture}\right), \tag{1}$$

it can combine these distributions to obtain

$$P\left(\alpha \middle| e_{disparity}, e_{texture}\right). \tag{2}$$

This is not necessarily as simple as multiplying the distributions, as will be discussed below (see section, "Conditional Dependencies Render Bayesian

Inference Impractical"). That is the Bayesian approach. A simpler idea is to use each source as a decision maker. Rather than combining probabilities over all possible values of angle, the brain makes two choices based on disparity and texture, respectively, and takes a weighted average based on the level of uncertainty, reliability, or confidence. Different weighting schemes translate into different valuations on error (see Kording and Wolpert 2004b). Thus, it is broadly consistent with Bayesian decision making. However, the approach is less versatile than the full representation of posterior probability distributions. We do not know how the brain actually solves a cue combination task such as the one described. Our point is simply that it need not represent posterior probability distributions explicitly to do so.

We are unaware of an experimental result that would necessitate a representation of posterior probability distributions over a simpler shortcut like combining estimates in accordance with their uncertainties. Also we do not know how the brain estimates uncertainty, reliability, and confidence. Some insights are forthcoming, however, from experiments that test the mechanism underlying the combination of evidence with prior probability in simple two-choice decisions (Shadlen et al. 2006b).

Decision Making from Decision Variables, Not Posteriors

Decisions are made by placing a criterion on a DV, which is a quantity that is calculated from diverse ingredients: evidence, priors, costs. At face value, this statement is compatible with decision making as Bayesian inference. Indeed, everything we are about to say about DVs can be translated to quantities that we could calculate in the Bayesian framework. Nonetheless, biology need not calculate the DV by an algorithm that adheres to a particular set of operations even if, in some cases, there is functional equivalence with the results produced by these operations. In particular, our experiments lead us to suspect that the brain does not represent posteriors explicitly.

We focus on three observations that arise in the study of decisions based on the sequential sampling of evidence: (a) the nature and necessity of a termination rule; (b) constraints imposed on the decision process by a finite set of choices; and (c) the simplification of conditional dependencies. All three may be viewed as heuristics that arise naturally in the framework of sequential sampling of evidence.

In a Decision Variable, Probability Is Not Dissociated from Other Terms

In most circumstances, decisions are not based on all the available evidence but instead incorporate a termination rule, thereby deciding based on some *quantum satis* of belief. This is beneficial when there is value associated with saving time or when there is cost associated with gathering evidence. Indeed these are the situations we face in almost all circumstances, for instance, to move from one decision to the next. By controlling the time spent on each decision, we can maximize reward per unit time. In these settings, a decision rule must specify the mapping of DV to choice, and a stopping rule must determine when to terminate the process. In some cases, the stopping rule and the decision rule operate on the same DV. The DV, or a race among several DVs, mediates both the outcome of the process (i.e., the choice) and the time that the process terminates.

The class of bounded accumulator models (Figure 4.1b) has been applied to a variety of decisions in perception, cognition, cryptography, quality control, and economics (Link 1992; Wald 1947; Smith and Ratcliff 2004; Ratcliff and Rouder 1998, 2000; Good 1979; Karlin and Taylor 1975). It has roots in optimality theory and is deeply connected to Bayesian inference (Wald and Wolfowitz 1947; Jaynes 2003; Bogacz et al. 2003; McMillen and Holmes 2006; Ma et al. 2006). In our studies of perceptual decisions using random dot motion, bounded accumulation explains the speed and accuracy of choice in human and nonhuman primate subjects. There is considerable experimental support for the computations: accumulation of noisy evidence and a termination bound in the responses of neurons in parietal cortex and elsewhere (for reviews, see Gold and Shadlen 2007; Shadlen et al. 2006a).

The simplest version of bounded accumulation is Wald's sequential probability ratio test (SPRT) (Wald 1947; Wald and Wolfowitz 1947). We will explain its connection to Bayesian decision making and use it to highlight the ways that the neural mechanisms depart from the Bayesian ideal. In SPRT, there are just two choices among states, s_1 and s_2. As each piece of evidence e_i arrives, it is converted to a log likelihood ratio (logLR),

$$\log\left[p\left(e_i|s_1\right)/p\left(e_i|s_2\right)\right], \tag{3}$$

and added to the accumulation. The process stops when the accumulated logLR reaches a predefined positive or negative bound. The process is Bayesian in the sense that we are using this term: the posterior probability is explicitly represented in the DV. The bounds are the log of the posterior odds,

$$\log\left[p\left(s_1|e_1,...,e_n\right)/p\left(s_2|e_1,...,e_n\right)\right], \tag{4}$$

and the same holds for the partial sums (e.g., the first m samples of evidence). In this simple case, the DV, the stopped DV and the termination rule would all satisfy the desire for an explicit representation of posterior probabilities. For example, if there were two sources of evidence bearing on the decision, we could combine estimates from the two terminated processes by adding log posterior odds, determined by their respective stopping rules. The SPRT can incorporate priors and loss functions without compromising this feature.

More commonly, however, a termination rule tends to render the posterior probability far less accessible, even for a simple binary choice. The main reason for this is that there is often missing information, which precludes the conversion of evidence to units of logLR. The motion discrimination task is an example. Consider a decision between $s_1 = up$ and $s_2 = down$. Assume the evidence to the decision maker is a sample of a difference in firing rates from two populations of neurons: one responds more when motion is upward whereas the other responds more when motion is downward. A single piece of momentary evidence, e_i, is the difference in the two spike rates (upward minus downward) measured in some brief epoch Δt. Positive values of this difference favor upward. These assumptions are supported by experimental findings (Ditterich et al. 2003; Huk and Shadlen 2005).

To carry out SPRT, we would convert the e_i to logLR based on our knowledge of the two sampling distributions, the probability of observing the possible values of e_i under s_1 and s_2, and therein lies the problem. Even in this simple experiment, we cannot do this because of one additional detail: there are a variety of stimulus strengths. For each decision, not only is the direction of motion randomized, so too is the intensity of the motion (i.e., the percentage of random dots that move coherently from one video frame to the next). Therefore, the sampling distributions depend on this motion strength.

For example, when motion is weak, a small positive difference, say $e = 1$ sp/s, often occurs for either direction of motion. It is only slightly more likely when motion is upward. Therefore, the logLR for up is only slightly larger than 0: weak evidence for upward motion. In contrast, when the motion is strong, the same $e = 1$ sp/s constitutes strong evidence. Consider, when motion is strongly downward, it would be a rare occurrence for the upward preferring neurons to respond more strongly than the downward preferring neurons. Therefore, the logLR for upward is a value much larger than 0. To make the conversion from evidence to logLR, the brain would need to know the motion strength. However, it does not know this at the beginning of the trial. This example illustrates why SPRT cannot be properly implemented. In a task with stimuli of varying difficulty, there is no unique relationship between evidence and logLR. Thus, there is no proper way to implement SPRT.

For the purpose of making a decision about direction, the motion strength is a nuisance parameter. From the perspective of Bayesian inference, one would like to marginalize out this variable. This proves to be difficult in general and imprudent in this case (and many like it). Impracticality results from the requirement of solving integrals, a problem that is well known to Bayesians but not the crux of our argument. We wish to emphasize a different point that arises in the context of sequential sampling. For this experiment, the nuisance parameter remains fixed for all samples until a decision is made. The brain cannot know the value of the motion strength at the beginning of viewing, but it can exploit the fact that it is the same for all samples of evidence.

There are two points. First and most germane to the argument here, it would be unwise to marginalize motion strength to its expectation over all possible stimuli. That would only make sense if each sample of evidence were drawn from the larger pool of all possible motion strengths at each time step Δt. This, however, is not the case: until a decision is completed, the evidence is drawn from a particular source associated with just one motion strength. Second, the assumption of a stationary nuisance parameter over the time course of the decision—in this case justified, but a heuristic more generally—can be exploited. For example, as time passes, if the decision has not terminated, it is probably because the motion strength is low. The brain appears to exploit this knowledge (Shadlen et al. 2006b). In theory, it is possible to develop a Bayesian inference framework that exploits the information about the passage of time, but it would be extremely cumbersome (e.g., involving elapsed time in the conversion of firing rates to probability).

Whenever different stimulus strengths are possible, the termination bound no longer represents the log of the posterior odds. It does so only in a convoluted sense. It is the log of the posterior odds of a correct choice at each of the motion strengths. As shown in Figure 4.2, the subject typically answers correctly when motion is stronger. Thus the bound does not have a unique mapping to log posterior odds. Instead, the stopping rule is to terminate when the DV—the accumulated firing rate difference—reaches a critical level. This is what the physiology indicates, and it explains with a single rule both the reaction times and the error rates in the motion experiments. This success comes at a cost, however. In contrast with Bayesian inference, there is no explicit representation of posterior probability.

Value and Utility Are Time Dependent

How do we interpret the stopping rule? If the DV does not represent posterior probability, then the bound is not a level of posterior probability. Nonetheless, there is an insight from SPRT that might be exploited. Assuming that the nuisance parameter(s) are fixed for a trial (by which we mean a decision on a stream of evidence), then at least in principle, one could apply SPRT. That means that any bound is a log posterior odds. What is missing is the magnitude of the setting. Again, we do not know the value of the bound in units of log posterior odds, because we do not know the nuisance parameters. However, we can adjust it to achieve a desired policy (e.g., maximum utility per unit time).

In some instances, like the random dot motion task, elapsed time conveys information about the nuisance parameters. In general, as time elapses, it is increasingly likely that the stimulus is low coherence. Indeed there are probably many instances in which less reliable evidence leads to slower accumulation toward a decision bound (a counterexample is when unreliability is caused by a change in variance rather than signal strength). If this is known (or assumed), then whatever the value of bound was in units log posterior odds at early times, it is worth less as time passes. It follows that the representation of expected value (or utility) is time dependent.

We have tested this idea directly in experiments in which the prior probability of up or down is manipulated in a block of trials. Briefly, a fixed prior is incorporated in the DV dynamically as elapsed time effectively discounts the posterior that would be represented by the terminated DV (Shadlen et al. 2006b). This heuristic is likely to be both useful and appropriate when there is reason to believe that the nuisance parameters are stationary over the time spanned by a single decision.

The important point is that a terminated DV lacks a unique, straightforward mapping to a posterior. We have illustrated this using binary decisions with nuisance parameters—aspects of the sources of evidence that affect the conversion to logLR. The problem is likely to be worse with more than two choices because a multidimensional SPRT is not uniquely specified (see McMillen and Holmes 2006; Bogacz et al. 2006). Thus the main feature of Bayesian inference, the posterior probability, is absent. It can be approximated with knowledge of nuisance parameters and/or elapsed time, but it is not represented explicitly nor is it accessible.

The Constraint on the Choice Space Is Not Trivial

The argument in this section is a natural extension of the "intentional architecture" introduced earlier in this chapter. When we process information in general, but especially in the context of making a decision, we construe it as evidence that bears on a set of competing hypotheses. At first glance, this statement seems perfectly compatible with decision making as Bayesian inference. However, the neurobiology suggests that the framework tends to dissipate any meaningful notion of a posterior probability distribution. In the end, this is because the neural architecture is concerned with a limited choice space; that is, the repertoire of possible actions, intentions, and "decisions about decisions."

Placing criteria on posteriors (or their transformed functions of expected value and utility) only approximates a decision process in which termination rules apply. To illustrate the concept with a simple case, consider the decision of whether direction of motion, θ, is to the left or right. The Bayesian inference approach is to represent the posterior $P(\theta \mid observations)$ and to simply choose left or right based on which is more likely (or to satisfy some other loss function besides accuracy). The question we raise here is how knowledge of the space of possible choices affects the decision process.

Placing priors on the possible states is an appealing approach, but it too has limitations. Here we start with the prior that $P(\theta)=0$, $\forall\ \theta\neq left\ or\ right$. Using Bayes's rule, the posterior can only achieve nonzero probability at left and right. This approach remains Bayesian inference because it asserts an explicit representation of the posterior, $P(\theta)$, although there are only two possible values for which this posterior can be nonzero. We think this approach leads to difficulties for termination of the decision process, as described below.

The rules for termination are affected by the choice space. This poses a deeper problem. For example, knowledge that there are 2 or 4 or 8 possible choices affects the policy governing when to terminate decisions. This can probably be formulated as Bayesian inference, but it is not parsimonious and it is ultimately wanting. Above, we explained why a bound is not a posterior when there are different degrees of reliability associated with the members of a class of items upon which a decision is to be made. The same argument applies here, but there is an interesting extension. If the termination rule were to be based on a relative degree of belief, we would have to imagine adjusting this value differently for different N and for different stimulus strengths. A termination rule based on $P(\theta \mid observations)$ is cumbersome when the reliability of the evidence (observations) is not known. Such a termination rule is also inconsistent with experimental results: achieving a criterion on uncertainty or posterior probability cannot explain a performance function—the error rates as a function of evidence quality (e.g., strength of motion).

The intended goal of the decision process can be achieved without representing the posteriors. The brain can exploit regularities that arise under sequential sampling. For example, as described above, the reliability of the evidence may not be known, but it is presumed to be stationary during evidence gathering. The brain can also exploit time-dependent factors. For example, the longer the decision process takes, the lower the quality of evidence. The effect of time and stationary evidence on the outcome of the decision process is affected by the number of choices. These factors can be easily incorporated in a decision variable toward an intended goal (i.e., the intentional framework) without any need for explicit representation of the posterior probability. More importantly, the experimental data suggests that the brain uses a decision variable that governs both choice and decision time, effectively abandoning the exact posterior in favor of something simpler and more efficient that satisfies the intentions.

Conditional Dependencies Render Bayesian Inference Impractical

Even without nuisance parameters, it is far from straightforward to compute a posterior for a large class of even simple decisions. To compute a posterior, it is often necessary to combine probabilities from sources of evidence that arrive in a stream, $e_1, e_2, e_3, \ldots$. If the likelihoods, $P(e_i \mid S_j)$, are known, and in particular if they are independent, then the posterior $P(S \mid e_1, e_2, e_3, \ldots)$ can be calculated using Bayes's rule. However, for a wide class of decisions, even when $e_1, e_2, e_3, \ldots$ are sampled independently, they are not independent, conditional on S. Hence the likelihoods are not independent! Here we wish to make three points: (a) this is a common situation, (b) the sequential sampling poses obstacles to representing the true likelihood, (c) the brain does not appear to respect this reality but instead presumes conditional independence.

This last heuristic might have interesting implications for so-called irrational decision making.

Conditional dependence.   Often we gather evidence bearing on some state of the world, S, that holds as true or false. For example, S might be left- or rightward, and the evidence we gather is a sample of motion energy taken from a video display or the spikes from direction selective neurons in the visual cortex. In this case, if the samples are independent, then they are also conditionally independent. In contrast, there are many types of decisions in which the evidence we gather has a bearing on S: Will I arrive at Frankfurt on time? There are separate factors to sample (e.g., weather in Seattle, weather in Frankfurt, traffic patterns, airline labor issues, airplane equipment failures, a terrorist event, etc.) that are presumably independent. They are not sampled conditionally on S = "on time" or S = "late" but instead bear on that outcome.

The situation is so common that it might come as a surprise to discover that it is largely ignored in standard applications, at least the ones we know. For example, in the theory of signal detection, it is assumed that if the $e_1, e_2, e_3,\ldots$ are sampled independently, such that $P(e_1, e_2) = P(e_1)P(e_2)$, then the likelihoods are conditionally independent: $P(e_1, e_2 \mid S) = P(e_1 \mid S)P(e_2 \mid S)$. This is a natural assumption because we think of sampling evidence under conditions where one state holds. That is the case for the sequential sampling of evidence about direction of motion in the preceding examples. On any one trial, motion is, for example, either up or down. If the evidence samples are independent, then they are also conditionally independent, because they are always sampled under one condition (up or down). However, that is exactly what is not true in situations in which samples of evidence affect S.

We are not arguing that it is impossible to learn statistical dependencies. For example, every medical student develops an intuition about whether the joint occurrence of headache and fever bear on the possibility of meningitis in a manner that is not predicted by the product of their likelihoods. What we are saying is that conditional independence does not hold in a variety of circumstances when at face value there is no obvious reason to suspect this. The variant of the so-called "weather prediction" task studied by Yang and Shadlen (2007) provides one example. These issues are discussed in more detail in the supplementary material to that paper.

It is hard (but not impossible) to accommodate conditional dependencies in a decision variable.   In principle, a DV and termination rule ought to be able to incorporate conditional dependencies, but it is costly. To put it simply, there is no easy update rule and no way to exploit marginal probabilities. This problem is especially severe under sequential sampling of evidence. The same piece of evidence will affect the current estimate of probability differently depending on what other evidence has arrived.

A relevant experiment.   We trained monkeys to make predictions about the location of a reward based on observing a sequence of four shapes. Each shape affects the probability of the outcome (reward at the red or green target). Our findings suggest that in these experiments, the brain gathers evidence under an assumption of conditional independence. In other words, it takes the observations associated with outcomes and makes the correct inference that they have independent effects on outcome. It, however, makes the incorrect inference that the probabilities of the observations are independent from one another, conditional on the outcome. Thus each shape increases or decreases the decision variable by a fixed amount, regardless (approximately) of when it appears in the sequence and regardless (again approximately) of what other shapes were displayed before it (Yang and Shadlen 2007).

Implications and Speculations

The arguments above raise new questions about decision making and the underlying neurobiology. Here are some examples.

The Traffic Cop Problem

The intentional architecture discussed earlier resolves several long-standing problems in perception, mainly by casting them as chimeras. For example, there is no need for a central interpreter of information—the so-called homunculus or little man that sits in the brain and makes sense of the data. Similarly, the "combinatorial explosion" that supposedly arises when trying to assemble the atoms of vision (small receptive fields) into coherent percepts vanishes. Both of these problems are seen to arise from a mistaken assumption that the data stream gives rise to one out of a vast set of possible interpretations. Instead, according to the intentional architecture, the data only bear evidence on a finite (large perhaps, but manageable) set of hypotheses that are currently under consideration. Admittedly, this creates a new set of problems.

What is it that establishes the question that the brain is asking about the data? What establishes the set of hypotheses? What establishes the intention or list of possible intentions at any moment? We do not know the answer to these questions, but we suspect they will turn out to be more tractable than the problems they replace. For example, the organism learns which tasks to consider—decisions about decisions—based on conceptual cues. Perhaps we forage in a landscape of possible tasks using mechanisms similar to the ones that underlie value-based decisions in a landscape of potential sources of nutrition and predators.

Agency without a Central Executive

Begin with the premise that value-based and perceptual decisions are mediated by a common framework. Consider decisions about choice of task as a problem akin to foraging. Instead of looking for a tree with better fruit, we are searching a task space for a better project. Recall that abstract decisions are simply decisions about which questions sensorimotor-like structures should be asking of the evidence. Thus, searching for the right question is like looking for the right task. It is a value-based decision where the search is for a task that is likely to pay off in some way. There are probably costs and dividends associated with exploration, exploitation, and perseverance. Thus looking for the right questions is just another kind of decision.

This is the way the animal exercises its own rapport with the world. It is what the philosophers refer to as agency. However, what we have described (albeit vaguely) can operate without any explicit awareness of the steps. It can have the kind of automaticity that is referred to as subconscious. From the outside, it has all the qualities of purposeful, autonomous choice. When we are aware of these choices, we express ownership of our behavior and experience our "free will." What we do in the subconscious version of this, however, is not capricious and thus just as much a candidate for free will. After all, as long as the choices are not capricious, they are expressions of the relative weights the brain assigns to evidence, value, and policy (e.g., balancing time pressure against deliberation).

It should be obvious that the neural computations discussed earlier should be capable of achieving these foraging decisions. Although we do not know as much about the neurobiology of value-based decisions as we do about evidence-based decisions, the key ingredients are not mysterious. For example, termination rules lead to a switch of task rather than an action. On the other hand, we do not have a good idea about what neural events occur that distinguish the awareness of a foraging decision from the ones we make "unconsciously."

One possibility is that awareness is just a decision to activate the circuits that mediate "actions" (e.g., engaging items in the world, reporting, forming narrative internally, and interrogating). Thus when a subconscious process of decision making leads to a choice to engage, we experience the world (or an item in it) as consciously attended. We are aware. Indeed, the establishment of consciousness after sleep, anesthesia, or coma might be regarded as an unconscious decision to engage the world at all (Shadlen and Kiani 2007).

Extensions of the Foraging Idea

Bistability and Rivalry

There are examples of perceptual phenomena that seem like they might be mediated by the kinds of mechanisms at play in this "foraging" mode of query.

If we approach problems in visual recognition as a set of queries (e.g., How should I hold my hand to grasp this object? If I move this edge, which bit will move with it? Should I scrutinize this further? Does this appeal to me?) then we can think about the brain perseverating away at the analysis of a scene that contains features worthy of further query. We can also consider the possibility of the brain abandoning this immediate set of queries to search for alternatives.

It seems that we experience something like this search for alternatives when we view bistable figures and when we experience binocular rivalry. Perhaps the study of rivalry might expose some of the computational principles that are common to value-based decisions that resemble "foraging." It might be fruitful to compare and contrast standard foraging behavior with the intervals between perceptual alternations, including regularities in the sampling schedules brought on by differences in the salience of competing images.

Mental Disorders

This is a rather large leap, but it seems possible that some mental disorders may be better understood from the perspective of decision making. Consider the two primary ways that we might expect foraging to fail. It could favor exploration at the expense of deliberation and deeper interrogation of evidence pertaining to the task at hand (i.e., the current workspace). This would lead to peripatetic behavior, flightiness, and deficits in concentration. The other failure mode is too little exploration. This would appear as a lack of interest in things external to the current workspace. Severely autistic children meet this description (Kanner 1973). Perhaps some of the odd expertise exhibited by some autistic patients (typically mild autism) reflects a lack of exploration. Perhaps a brain that tends to be stuck in the deliberative exploitation of the current workspace tends to acquire expertise.

Concluding Remarks

This essay should be regarded as a speculative exercise. We have tried to elaborate a set of principles that have been elucidated in the experiments on the neurobiology of decision making in nonhuman primates. Naturally, these experiments (reviewed in Gold and Shadlen 2007) use simple paradigms suitable for laboratory investigations in animal subjects. We have extracted key insights from these investigations and extrapolated beyond the data to demonstrate how a simple architecture might underlie the wonderfully complex landscape of human decision making. We have tried to paint a picture of functional architecture that is aimed primarily at choosing among possible actions. We extended this principle to choices among possible tasks or decisions. Among other things, we think this perspective hints at the way in which the bigger cerebral cortex in humans provides the basis for higher cognitive functions.

The functional architecture is also a computational architecture. Viewed from this perspective, we question the popular wisdom that the brain operates as an information-processing device that performs probabilistic inference. These points are likely to be regarded as controversial (or just plain wrong) by many readers. We are less wed to the conclusions than to the motivation: decisions among possible courses of action invite us to formulate inference differently than the formulations derived from probability theory and statistics (Jaynes 2003). If our tone was overly polemical, it was not intended to be so. We do not see ourselves as anti-Bayesian. Indeed, in many instances the brain's decision variables can be seen as a way to implement aspects of Bayesian decision making.

Ours is not an argument against Bayesian inference but an embrace of the intentional architecture. The goal of information processing is not to identify content or estimate parameters but to answer questions concerning choices among possible actions, including posing the next question.

Acknowledgments

We are grateful to Mehrdad Jazayeri, Peter Meilstrup and Tianming Yang for input and discussions. We thank the organizers of the Ernst Strüngmann Forum and the members of the working group on the neural basis of decision making for comments and many insights. Our research is supported by the Howard Hughes Medical Institute, the National Eye Institute (EY11378), the National Institute of Drug Abuse (DA022780), the National Center for Research Resources (RR00166), and the James S. McDonnell Foundation.

References

Andersen, R. A., and C. A. Buneo. 2002. Intentional maps in posterior parietal cortex. *Ann. Rev. Neurosci.* **25**:189–220.

Barlow, H. B., W. R. Levick, and M. Yoon. 1971. Responses to single quanta of light in retinal ganglion cells of the cat. *Vision Res. Suppl.* **3**:87–101.

Barraclough, D. J., M. L. Conroy, and D. Lee. 2004. Prefrontal cortex and decision making in a mixed-strategy game. *Nature Neurosci.* **7(4)**:404–410.

Bogacz, R., E. Brown, J. Moehlis, P. Holmes, and J. D. Cohen. 2006. The physics of optimal decision making: A formal analysis of models of performance in two-alternative forced choice tasks. *Psychol. Rev.* **113**:700–765.

Bogacz, R., J. M. Moehlis, E. T. Brown, P. Holmes, and J. D. Cohen. 2003. Neural mechanisms for decision optimization. In: 2003 Abstract Viewer/Itinerary Planner, Program No. 197.6. Washington DC: Society for Neuroscience.

Brainard, D. H., and W. T. Freeman. 1997. Bayesian color constancy. *J. Opt. Soc. Am. A* **14(7)**:1393–1411.

Cavada, C., and P. Goldman-Rakic. 1989. Posterior parietal cortex in rhesus monkey: II. Evidence for segregated corticocortical networks linking sensory and limbic areas with the frontal lobe. *J. Comp. Neurol.* **287**:422–445.

Churchland, P. S., V. S. Ramachandran, and T. J. Sejnowski. 1994. A critique of pure vision. In: Large-Scale Neuronal Theories of the Brain, ed. C. Koch and J. L. Davis, pp. 23–60. Cambridge, MA: MIT Press.

Cisek, P. 2007. Cortical mechanisms of action selection: The affordance competition hypothesis. *Phil. Trans. Roy. Soc. Lond. B* **362**:1585–1599.

Clark, A. 1997. Being There: Putting Brain, Body, and World Together Again. Cambridge, MA: MIT Press.

Cohn, T. E., D. G. Green, and W. P. Tanner. 1975. Receiver operating characteristic analysis. Application to the study of quantum fluctuation in optic nerve of Rana pipiens. *J. Gen. Physiol.* **66**:583–616.

Colby, C. L., and M. E. Goldberg. 1999. Space and attention in parietal cortex. *Ann. Rev. Neurosci.* **22**:319–349.

Corrado, G.S., L. P. Sugrue, H. S. Seung, and W. T. Newsome. 2005. Linear-nonlinear-Poisson models of primate choice dynamics. *J. Exp. Anal. Behav.* **84(3)**:581–617.

Critchley, M. 1953. The Parietal Lobes. New York: Hafner Publ. Co.

Deaner, R. O., A. V. Khera, and M. L. Platt. 2005. Monkeys pay per view: Adaptive valuation of social images by rhesus macaques. *Curr. Biol.* **15(6)**:543–548.

Ditterich, J., M. Mazurek, and M. N. Shadlen. 2003. Microstimulation of visual cortex affects the speed of perceptual decisions. *Nature Neurosci.* **6**:891–898.

Dorris, M. C., and P. W. Glimcher. 2004. Activity in posterior parietal cortex is correlated with the relative subjective desirability of action. *Neuron* **44(2)**:365–378.

Ernst, M. O., and M. S. Banks. 2002. Humans integrate visual and haptic information in a statistically optimal fashion. *Nature* **415(6870)**:429–433.

Gibson, J. J. 1950. Perception of the Visual World. Boston: Houghton Mifflin.

Glimcher, P. W. 2003. Decisions, Uncertainty, and the Brain: The Science of Neuroeconomics. Cambridge, MA: MIT Press.

Glimcher, P. W. 2005. Indeterminacy in brain and behavior. *Ann. Rev. Psychol.* **56**:25–56.

Gold, J. I., and M. N. Shadlen. 2000. Representation of a perceptual decision in developing oculomotor commands. *Nature* **404(6776)**:390–394.

Gold, J. I., and M. N. Shadlen. 2001a. Neural computations that underlie decisions about sensory stimuli. *Trends Cogn. Sci.* **5**:10–16.

Gold, J. I., and M. N. Shadlen. 2001b. Neural correlates of an abstract perceptual decision in monkey area 46. *Soc. Neurosci. Abstr.* **27**:237.6.

Gold, J. I., and M. N. Shadlen. 2003. The influence of behavioral context on the representation of a perceptual decision in developing oculomotor commands. *J. Neurosci.* **23(2)**:632–651.

Gold, J. I., and M. N. Shadlen. 2007. The neural basis of decision making. *Ann. Rev. Neurosci.* **30**:535–574.

Good, I. J. 1979. Studies in the history of probability and statistics. XXXVII A.M. Turing's statistical work in World War II. *Biometrika* **66(2)**:393–396.

Green, D. M., and J. A. Swets. 1966. Signal Detection Theory and Psychophysics. New York: Wiley.

He, S., P. Cavanagh, and J. Intriligator. 1996. Attentional resolution and the locus of visual awareness. *Nature* **383(6598)**:334–337.

Hecht, S., and E. U. Mintz. 1939. The visibility of single lines of various illuminations and the retinal basis of visual resolution. *J. Gen. Physiol.* **22**:593–612.

Herrnstein, R. J. 1961. Relative and absolute strength of response as a function of frequency of reinforcement. *J. Exp. Anal. Behav.* **4**:267–272.

Herrnstein, R. J., and W. Vaughan. 1980. Melioration and behavioral allocation. In: Limits to Action: The Allocation of Individual Behavior, ed. J. Staddon, pp. 143–176. New York: Academic Press.

Hikosaka, K., and M. Watanabe. 2000. Delay activity of orbital and lateral prefrontal neurons of the monkey varying with different rewards. *Cerebral Cortex* **10(3)**:263–271.

Huk, A. C., and M. N. Shadlen. 2005. Neural activity in macaque parietal cortex reflects temporal integration of visual motion signals during perceptual decision making. *J. Neurosci.* **25(45)**:10,420–10,436.

Jaynes, E. T. 2003. Probability Theory: The Logic of Science. Cambridge: Cambridge Univ. Press.

Jiang, Y., P. Costello, F. Fang, M. Huang, and S. He. 2006. A gender- and sexual orientation-dependent spatial attentional effect of invisible images. *Proc. Natl. Acad. Sci.* **103(45)**:17,048–17,052.

Kahneman, D. 2002. Nobel prize lecture: Maps of bounded rationality: A perspective on intuitive judgment and choice. In: Nobel Prizes 2002. Nobel Prizes, Presentations, Biographies, and Lectures, ed. T. Frangsmyr, pp. 419–499. Stockholm: Almquist and Wiksell Intl.

Kanner, L. 1973. The birth of early infantile autism. *J. Autism Child Schizophr.* **3(2)**:93–95.

Karlin, S., and H. M. Taylor. 1975. A First Course in Stochastic Processes, 2nd ed. Boston, MA: Academic Press.

Kawagoe, R., Y. Takikawa, and O. Hikosaka. 2004. Reward-predicting activity of dopamine and caudate neurons: A possible mechanism of motivational control of saccadic eye movement. *J. Neurophys.* **91(2)**:1013–1024.

Kersten, D. 1999. High-level vision as statistical inference. In: The Cognitive Neurosciences, ed. M. S. Gazzaniga, pp. 353–363. Cambridge, MA: MIT Press.

Kersten, D., P. Mamassian, and A. Yuille. 2004. Object perception as Bayesian inference. *Ann. Rev. Psychol.* **55**:271–304.

Kersten, D., and A. Yuille. 2003. Bayesian models of object perception. *Curr. Op. Neurobiol.* **13(2)**:150–158.

Knill, D. C., and J. A. Saunders. 2003. Do humans optimally integrate stereo and texture information for judgments of surface slant? *Vision Res.* **43(24)**:2539–2558.

Kording, K. P., and D. M. Wolpert. 2004a. Bayesian integration in sensorimotor learning. *Nature* **427(6971)**:244–247.

Kording, K. P., and D. M. Wolpert. 2004b. The loss function of sensorimotor learning. *Proc. Natl. Acad. Sci.* **101(26)**:9839–9842.

Landy, M. S., L. T. Maloney, E. B. Johnston, and M. J. Young. 1995. Measurement and modeling of depth cue combination: In defense of weak fusion. *Vision Res.* **35(3)**:389–412.

Lau, B., and P. W. Glimcher. 2005. Dynamic response-by-response models of matching behavior in rhesus monkeys. *J. Exp. Anal. Behav.* **84(3)**:555–579.

Lee, D., M. L. Conroy, B. P. McGreevy, and D. J. Barraclough. 2004. Reinforcement learning and decision making in monkeys during a competitive game. *Cogn. Brain Res.* **22**:45–58.

Lee, D., B. P. McGreevy, and D. J. Barraclough. 2005. Learning and decision making in monkeys during a rock-paper-scissors game. *Cogn. Brain Res.* **25**:416–430.

Levy, I., D. Schluppeck, D. J. Heeger, and P. W. Glimcher. 2007. Specificity of human cortical areas for reaches and saccades. *J. Neurosci.* **27(17)**:4687–4696.

Lewis, J. W., and D. C. Van Essen. 2000a. Corticocortical connections of visual, senso-rimotor, and multimodal processing areas in the parietal lobe of the macaque mon-key. *J. Comp. Neurol.* **428(1)**:112–137.

Lewis, J. W., and D. C. Van Essen. 2000b. Mapping of architectonic subdivisions in the macaque monkey, with emphasis on parieto-occipital cortex. *J. Comp. Neurol.***428**(1):79–111.

Link, S. W. 1992. The Wave Theory of Difference and Similarity. Hillsdale, NJ: Lawrence Erlbaum.

Lo, C. C., and X. J. Wang. 2006. Cortico-basal ganglia circuit mechanism for a decision threshold in reaction time tasks. *Nature Neurosci.* **9(7)**:956–963.

Luce, R. D. 1959. Individual Choice Behavior: A Theoretical Analysis. New York: Wiley.

Ma, W. J., J. M. Beck, P. E. Latham, and A. Pouget. 2006. Bayesian inference with probabilistic populaton codes. *Nature Neurosci.* **9(11)**:1432–1438.

Mamassian, P., and M. S. Landy. 2001. Interaction of visual prior constraints. *Vision Res.* **41(20)**:2653–2668.

Manski, C. 1977. The structure of random utility models. *Theory and Decision* **8**:229–254.

McCoy, A., J. Crowley, G. Haghighian, H. Dean, and M. Platt. 2003. Saccade reward signals in posterior cingulate cortex. *Neuron* **40(5)**:1031–1040.

McCoy, A. N., and M. L. Platt. 2005. Risk-sensitive neurons in macaque posterior cin-gulate cortex. *Nature Neurosci.* **8(9)**:1220–1227.

McMillen, T., and P. Holmes. 2006. The dynamics of choice among multiple alterna-tives. *J. Math. Psychol.* **50**:30–57.

Merleau-Ponty, M. 1962. Phenomenology of Perception. London: Routledge and Kegan Paul Ltd.

Montague, P. R., and G. S. Berns. 2002. Neural economics and the biological substrates of valuation. *Neuron* **36(2)**:265–284.

Naccache, L., E. Blandin, and S. Dehaene. 2002. Unconscious masked priming depends on temporal attention. *Psychol. Sci.* **13(5)**:416–424.

O'Regan, J. K., and A. Noë. 2001. A sensorimotor account of vision and visual con-sciousness. *Behav. Brain Sci.* **24(5)**:939–973.

Padoa-Schioppa, C., and J. A. Assad. 2006. Neurons in the orbitofrontal cortex encode economic value. *Nature* **441(7090)**:223–226.

Parker, A. J., and W. T. Newsome. 1998. Sense and the single neuron: Probing the physiology of perception. *Ann. Rev. Neurosci.* **21**:227–277.

Paton, J. J., M. A. Belova, S. E. Morrison, and C. D. Salzman. 2006. The primate amyg-dala represents the positive and negative value of visual stimuli during learning. *Nature* **439(7078)**:865–870.

Petrides, M., and D. N. Pandya. 1984. Projections to the frontal cortex from the poste-rior parietal region in the rhesus monkey. *J. Comp. Neurol.* **228**:105–116.

Poremba, A., R. C. Saunders, A. M. Crane, M. Cook, L. Sokoloff et al. 2003. Functional mapping of the primate auditory system. *Science* **299(5606)**:568–572.

Ratcliff, R., and J. N. Rouder. 1998. Modeling response times for two-choice decisions. *Psychol. Sci.* **9**:347–356.

Ratcliff, R., and J. N. Rouder. 2000. A diffusion model account of masking in two-choice letter identification. *J. Exp. Psychol. Hum. Perc. Perf.* **26(1)**:127–140.

Rizzolatti, G., L. Fogassi, and V. Gallese. 1997. Parietal cortex: From sight to action. *Curr. Op. Neurobiol.* **7**:562–567.

Rosas, P., J. Wagemans, M. O. Ernst, and F. A. Wichmann. 2005. Texture and haptic cues in slant discrimination: Reliability-based cue weighting without statistically optimal cue combination. *J. Opt. Soc. Am. A. Opt. Image Sci. Vis.* **22(5)**:801–809.

Scherberger, H., and R. A. Andersen. 2007. Target selection signals for arm reaching in the posterior parietal cortex. *J. Neurosci.* **27(8)**:2001–2012.

Scherberger, H., M. A. Goodale, and R. A. Andersen. 2003. Target selection for reaching and saccades share a similar behavioral reference frame in the macaque. *J. Neurophys.* **89(3)**:1456–1466.

Shadlen, M. N., T. D. Hanks, A. K. Churchland, R. Kiani, and T. Yang. 2006a. The speed and accuracy of a simple perceptual decision: A mathematical primer. In: Bayesian Brain: Probabilistic Approaches to Neural Coding, ed. K. Doya et al., pp. 209–237. Cambridge, MA: MIT Press.

Shadlen, M. N., T. D. Hanks, M. E. Mazurek, R. Kiani, T. Yang et al. 2006b. The brain uses elapsed time to convert spike rate to probability. Program No. 605.6. Neuroscience Meeting Planner Atlanta: Soc. for Neuroscience.

Shadlen, M. N., and R. Kiani. 2007. Neurology: An awakening. *Nature* **448(7153)**: 539–540.

Shadlen, M. N., and J. A. Movshon. 1999. Synchrony unbound: A critical evaluation of the temporal binding hypothesis. *Neuron* **24(1)**:67–77.

Shadlen, M. N., and W. T. Newsome. 1994. Noise, neural codes and cortical organization. *Curr. Op. Neurobiol.* **4**:569–579.

Shadlen, M. N., and W. T. Newsome. 1998. The variable discharge of cortical neurons: Implications for connectivity, computation and information coding. *J. Neurosci.* **18**:3870–3896.

Smith, P. L., and R. Ratcliff. 2004. Psychology and neurobiology of simple decisions. *Trends Neurosci.* **27(3)**:161–168.

Softky, W. R., and C. Koch. 1993. The highly irregular firing of cortical cells is inconsistent with temporal integration of random EPSPs. *J. Neurosci.* **13(1)**:334–350.

Spivey, M. J., M. Grosjean, and G. Knoblich. 2005. Continuous attraction toward phonological competitors. *Proc. Natl. Acad. Sci.* **102(29)**:10,393–10,398.

Sugrue, L. P., G. S. Corrado, and W. T. Newsome. 2004. Matching behavior and the representation of value in the parietal cortex. *Science* **304(5678)**:1782–1787.

Tanner, W. P. Jr. 1961. Physiological implications of psychophysical data. *Ann. NY Acad Sci.* **89**:752–765.

Thurstone, L. L. 1959. The Measurement of Values. Chicago: Univ. Chicago Press.

Tremblay, L., and W. Schultz. 1999. Relative reward preference in primate orbitofrontal cortex. *Nature* **398**:704–708.

Trommershauser, J., S. Gepshtein, L. T. Maloney, M. S. Landy, and M. S. Banks. 2005. Optimal compensation for changes in task-relevant movement variability. *J. Neurosci.* **25(31)**:7169–7178.

van Ee, R., W. J. Adams, and P. Mamassian. 2003. Bayesian modeling of cue interaction: Bistability in stereoscopic slant perception. *J. Opt. Soc. Am. A* **20(7)**:1398–1406.

Wald, A. 1947. Sequential Analysis. New York: Wiley.

Wald, A., and J. Wolfowitz. 1947. Optimum character of the sequential probability ratio test. *Ann. Math. Statist.* **19**:326–339.

Wallis, J. D., K. C. Anderson, and E. K. Miller. 2001. Single neurons in prefrontal cortex encode abstract rules. *Nature* **411**:953–956.

Watanabe, K., J. Lauwereyns, and O. Hikosaka. 2003. Neural correlates of rewarded and unrewarded eye movements in the primate caudate nucleus. *J. Neurosci.* **23(31)**:10,052–10,057.

Yang, T., and M. N. Shadlen. 2007. Probabilistic reasoning by neurons. *Nature* **447(7148)**:1075–1080.

Yuille, A., and H. H. Bulthoff. 1996. Bayesian decision theory and psychophysics. In: Perception as Bayesian Inference, ed. D. C. Knill and W. Richards, pp. 123–162. Cambridge: Cambridge Univ. Press.

5

Brain Signatures of Social Decision Making

Kevin McCabe[1] and Tania Singer[2]

[1]Center for the Study of Neuroeconomics, George Mason
University, Fairfax, VA 22030, U.S.A.
[2]Institute for Empirical Research in Economics,
University of Zurich, 8006 Zurich, Switzerland

Abstract

Over the last decade much progress has been made in the study of social decision making. From economics and game theory, tasks have been defined to study the strategic interaction involving trust (the investment/trust game) and negotiation (the ultimatum game). From cognitive neuroscience and neuroeconomics, areas of the brain have been identified that allow individuals to share affective (empathy) or abstract mental (ToM) states. Activities in these areas of the brain are also found to be correlated with the strategies that people use in the economic games. Current research hopes to explain general principles of cortical computation that can explain the role of shared mental content in shaping the strategic decisions of interacting players.

Introduction

Humans stand out in the quantity, quality, and the variety of social decisions made; indeed, human success depends critically on how social decisions unfold. In this chapter, we explore the evidence for unique brain signatures involved in social decision making. For purposes of this article, a brain signature for a given functional capacity is a consistent set of BOLD response activations that occurs when this function is being utilized in a number of different tasks. What the BOLD response measures and how it should be interpreted has been the focus of numerous other papers and is not pursued here. For our purposes, we think of these brain signatures as being relatively large, at least in terms of BOLD response, binding sites for the integrative computation of the requisite function. Two brain signatures stand out because of their functional role in sharing the world with others: empathy (i.e., the ability to share another person's emotion) and mentalizing (i.e., the ability to share another person's mental states such as beliefs and goals).

Evolutionary pressures have endowed human beings with the capability of sharing emotional and intentional perspectives with others, in part because it enhances our inclusive fitness and in part because we all build the same neuronal machinery to process and respond to experience. However, while empathy and mentalizing allow us to understand others better, we do so imperfectly as we cannot directly share their brains' activations but can instead only indirectly experience this as simulations or activations in our own brains. Since our abilities are subject to error, their use introduces new and different risks into our lives.

One reason why our social interaction is risky is because at any point in time we are motivated by a mixture of incentives that sometimes leads us to compete and at other times induces us to cooperate. In studying the brain signatures of social decision making, game theory has turned out to be useful in providing both simple decision scenarios for social interactions and a quantitative approach to studying how incentives, information, and social knowledge influence the strategies that should be chosen to optimize one's social interaction. From a game theoretic perspective, the strategies that should be chosen are those that determine the Nash equilibrium of the game.

A simple example of a two-person game in extensive form is shown in Figure 5.1a. The game is depicted as a tree, which begins at the top node (known as a decision node) and progresses through other decision nodes until a terminal node is reached. Notice that each terminal node has two numbers: the top number is the payoff to player 1; the bottom node is the payoff to player 2. The number just to the left of each node indicates which player (1 or 2) is making a choice at that node. In our example, player 1 makes the first decision. The nodes are connected by branches that are identified by labels on the immediate right. When we speak about a player's move, we refer to the branch they choose. For example, a play of the game might be (L, left) resulting in each player getting 50, while another play of the game might be (L, right, rR) resulting in both players getting 20. Let us now discuss the strategies of players and the Nash equilibrium of the game.

A pure strategy is a choice of branch at each decision node of the game. Player 1 has the following four pure strategies: $X = \{(L, rL), (L, rR), (R, rL), (R, rR)\}$. Player 2 has only two pure strategies: $Y = \{\text{left}, \text{right}\}$. We will call x player 1's choice of strategy and y player 2's choice of strategy. Furthermore, we will call $P(x, y)$ player 1's payoff and $Q(x, y)$ player 2's payoff. If, for example, $x = (L, rL)$ and $y = \text{right}$, then $P(x, y) = 30$ and $Q(x, y) = 60$. We can now define a Nash equilibrium (NE) in pure strategies, for this game as a choice of strategies x' and y', such that, $P(x', y') \geq P(x, y')$ for all $x \in X$, and $Q(x', y') \geq Q(x', y)$ for all $y \in Y$. Here is one NE of the game: $x' = (R, rR)$ and $y' = \text{right}$, resulting in a payoff of 40 for both. Notice that neither player can do better by unilaterally changing his or her strategy. Here is another NE of the

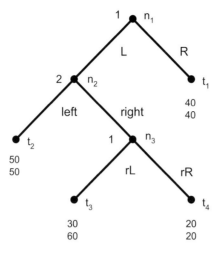

Figure 5.1 An extensive form game is played by two decision makers (DM), has three decision nodes (n_1–n_3) and four terminal nodes (t_1–t_4). Payoffs for each DM are shown as a column vector at each terminal node, with the top payoff going to DM1 and the bottom payoff going to DM2. Decision makers are assumed to prefer larger payoffs. DM1 moves first by moving left (L) or right (R). If DM1 moves right, the game ends, and each person receives 40. If DM1 moves left, then DM2 has the opportunity to move left or right. If DM2 moves left, the game ends, and each person receives 50. If DM2 moves right, then DM1 must choose between rL and rR. Either choice ends the game with the payoffs shown. Game theory assumes that DM will take into account each other's analysis of the game. In particular, at n_3 DM1 should prefer 30 to 20 and thus choose rL. Reaching this conclusion, DM2 should choose right at n_2 preferring 60 to 50. Therefore, DM1, should conclude that it is best to move R at node n_1 getting 40 instead of 30. Such an analysis fails to take into account the insult DM1 may feel upon reaching n_3 and the subsequent desire to punish DM2 by moving to t_4.

game: $x' = $ (L, rR) and $y'=$ left, resulting in a payoff of 50 for both. It is easy to see that $x = $ (L, rL) and $y = $ right is not a NE, since player 1 does better switching to $x = $ (R, rL) and getting 40 instead of 30.

Since there are two Nash equilibria for this game, which is more likely to be played? Using backwards induction to solve the game, we can construct a set of strategies (x^*, y^*) for our players by asking what would be the optimal action at each stage of the game given what we found was optimal at later stages. Starting with the last move by player 1 we see that rL is better than rR. So we can construct part of player 1's strategy as $x^* = $ (?, rL). Given this knowledge it is clear that player 2 should choose right over left; thus, player 2's strategy is now $y^* = $ right. Now we see that player 1 should move R in the first stage, resulting in the strategy $x^* = $ (R, rL). It is easy to see that x^*, y^* constructed this way is a NE of the game, but it is the only NE of the game that requires our players to have rational expectations with respect to each other's backwards induction of the game.

Games similar to the one above have been run as laboratory experiments (McCabe et al. 1996, 2003). Notice the (50, 50) NE is thought by game theorists to be less rational, since it requires player 1 to be willing to punish by playing rR when he or she would be better off playing rL. When subjects play the game similar to the one above, only with an anonymous counterpart, 90% of the data converged to either the (40, 40) or (50, 50) NE. Furthermore, when the game is repeated, we see an increase in the likelihood of the (50, 50) outcome; however, we also see an increase in defections (i.e., move right by player 2), which are frequently met by punishments (i.e., rR by player 1). These experiments tell us that although NE is useful in predicting behavior in strategic games, our usual game theoretic models of rationality must be modified to account for how people *actually* play the game.

One important brain system that is not directly social, but which plays an important role in social decision making, is the goal-related system of the brain. This extensive neural system allows the individual to choose among goals, form strategies (also called policies), and take actions to reach a given goal and learn from experience how to update one's strategy to reach the goal better the next time.

To see the relationship between the goal-directed decision making and social decision making, we can replace player 2 in the game in Figure 5.1 by a random move due to Nature. In particular, let q be the probability that Nature picks left, and let $(1 - q)$ be the probability that Nature picks right. If player 1 knows q, then player 1 can simply pick the strategy x^{**} that maximized the expected payoff $E(x^{**}, q) = qP(x^{**}, \text{left}) + (1 - q)P(x^{**}, \text{right})$. In this case, $x^{**} = x^*$ whenever $q \leq \frac{1}{2}$. For $q > \frac{1}{2}$, player 1 should adopt the strategy (L, rL).

When q and payoffs are unknown and must be learned from experience, some of the key neural components of this system have been identified. Both single-cell firing studies (Schultz et al. 1997) and bold signatures of functional activity (O'Doherty et al. 2003) have identified the activity of dopamine neurons in the ventral and dorsal striatum as playing a key role in temporal difference learning, while neurons in the dorsal striatum in holding elements of the strategy need to be updated. Furthermore, the dopamine-gating hypothesis (O'Reilly et al. 1999) explains how dopamine can be used to gate prefrontal activity to evaluate and/or change goals.

Two Systems for Social Decision Making

Neural systems for social decision making interact with our neural systems for goal-directed behavior in two ways: by making another person the goal of our behavior and by taking into account others, either as cooperators or as competitors, in reaching the goals that we desire.

Mentalizing

Over the last several decades, research in developmental psychology, social psychology, and cognitive neuroscience has focused on the human ability to have a "theory of mind" or to "mentalize" (e.g., Frith and Frith 2003); that is, to make attributions about the mental states (desires, beliefs, intentions) of others. This ability is absent in monkeys and only exists in a rudimentary form in apes (Povinelli and Bering 2002). It develops in humans by about age 4–5 and is impaired in autistic individuals. The lack of a theory-of-mind in most autistic children could explain their observed failures in communication and social interaction.

Theory-of-mind (ToM) has been defined as both a linguistic construct (i.e., differentiating bilateral from trilateral mental representations) and a cognitive construct (i.e., mental simulation of cognitive representation); however, it is often defined operationally as whether or not an observer can infer the false beliefs of another person, or whether or not an interacting participant in a game can infer another player's goal or intentions. In one version of the false beliefs task, a child is observed to watch the experimenter put a favorite toy in a cupboard positioned on the right side of the room. The child then leaves the room, and the experimenter moves the toy to the left cupboard. A subject, who has observed everything, is then asked: When the child returns to the room, where will he go to get the toy? An autistic subject is likely to say the left cupboard, since this is where the toy was last placed. A normal subject over roughly the age of four, however, will respond by saying the right cupboard, because he knows this is where the child thinks that the toy is.

Autistic individuals who lack ToM are also deficient in shared attention (i.e., the ability to attend to their mutual attention, with someone else, on a shared object, third party, or experience). Such shared attention is important for mutual knowledge, as it is thought to solve the recursive problem of knowing what the other knows (or what game theorists call "common knowledge"): "I know that you know that I know…X." The example of ToM reasoning in the false beliefs task above is said to be offline because it is used by a third-person observer. One interpretation is that the observer has to put themselves in the as-if position of the child in the room and then simulate the shared attention that is created by the interaction between the child and the experimenter. Alternatively, ToM can be studied in an active participant where ToM is said to be used online and shared attention need not be simulated.

Recent imaging studies on normal healthy adults have focused on the ability to "mentalize" by using a wide range of stimuli that represent the intentions, beliefs, and desires of the people involved (for a review, see Gallagher and Frith 2003). Studies of ToM have identified a brain signature consisting of the anterior paracingulate or medial prefrontal cortex (mPFC), superior temporal sulcus (STS), and the temporal poles. The mPFC is hypothesized to represent mental states decoupled from reality, whereas the STS is hypothesized

to help process a causal relationship between visual motion/action and the intended goals of another person (see Frith and Frith 1999); the temporal poles
are thought to draw on encodings of past experience to "simulate" another
person's experience (see Harris 1992). One possible interpretation of these activations is that the STS and temporal poles help us simulate another person's
experience and interpret their actions within the context of their current choice,
which is then decoupled from reality in the mPFC to provide an abstract encoding of the intentions of another person. Most likely, these regions evolved
as an integral part of human brain processing to allow one person to share (and
to a larger extent understand) another person's strategy.

Jason Mitchell has recently conducted a series of studies on mentalizing
which suggest a functional segregation between judging mental states of similar and dissimilar others (Mitchell et al. 2005a, b, 2006). A part of the mPFC
gets recruited when participants make either self-judgments or judgments
about people whom they perceive as being similar on the basis of appearance
or political attitudes. By contrast, a more dorsal part of the mPFC—close to
the activations found in previous mentalizing studies cited above—reveal enhanced activation when judging mental states of people perceived as dissimilar
to oneself. This suggests that we may use two different strategies when inferring another person's mental states: (a) we can simulate the other on the basis
of knowledge we have about ourselves or (b) we can infer mental states of the
other on the basis of more abstract knowledge that we have acquired about the
world. The latter may also involve knowledge about stereotypes and opens
the interesting question of whether judging another person's mental state may
be biased in two different ways, depending on whether we perceive them as
similar or dissimilar: An "egocentric bias," the propensity to understand other
people's states in terms of one's own, may easily occur if we simulate others
on the basis of our self, ignoring possible differences between self and others.
Misattribution may, however, also occur when judging other people's mental
states on the basis of stereotyped and categorical knowledge underestimating
the similarity between the other and us. An interesting twist for future research
in this domain would be to explore whether brain data can be used to predict
differential decisions in social exchange with others, based on whether ventral
or dorsal mPFC is activated reflecting an unconscious perception of people as
being similar or dissimilar to ourselves.

Empathizing

In addition to the ability to understand mental states such as beliefs, intentions,
and thoughts of others, humans can also empathize with others (i.e., share and
understand their feelings and emotions). Humans can feel empathy for other
people in a wide variety of contexts: for basic emotions and sensations (e.g.,
anger, fear, sadness, joy, pain, and lust) as well as for more complex emotions
(e.g., guilt, embarrassment, and love). The idea that neural systems enable

people to share others' states has recently been expanded to include the ability to share their feelings and sensations (Preston and de Waal 2002; de Vignemont and Singer 2006; Decety and Jackson 2004; Decety and Lamm 2006).

Even though there are perhaps nearly as many definitions of empathy as people working on the topic, we provide here a definition of empathy inspired by neuroscientific approaches on empathy (for details, see de Vignemont and Singer 2006):

> We empathize with others when we have an affective state that is isomorphic to another's person's affective state, elicited by the observation or imagination of another person's affective state, and accompanied by the awareness that one knows that the other person is the source of one's own affective state.

The latter requirement is important to differentiate empathy from emotional contagion, which also includes affect sharing but does not require a self–other distinction. Consider, for example, the scenario of babies who begin to cry because other babies in the vicinity are crying. This occurs long before infants develop a sense of a self that is separate from others. In cognitive perspective taking or mentalizing, by contrast, we do not share affects but rather more abstract, propositional states with others, such as intentions or beliefs. Finally, empathy differs from sympathy or compassion in that it refers to sharing a similar affect with the other person but lacks the other related motivation associated with the wish to alleviate the others suffering. In principle, very empathic people may share other people's negative affect in order to know how to let them suffer even more. Alternatively, too much empathy may lead to personal distress, which in turn leads to a withdrawal from the suffering person instead of engaging in helping behavior. In general, however, empathy is suggested to be the first step in a chain that begins with affect sharing and which leads to an understanding of the feelings of others, which in turns motivates other related concerns and helping behavior. In that way, empathy and prosocial decision making are closely linked.

Recently, social neuroscience has started to uncover the mechanism that allows a person to be aware of what it feels like for another individual to be in pain, touched or disgusted in the absence of any stimulation to the body. Overall, results have revealed that common neural responses are elicited when (a) pictures are observed that depict disgusted faces or disgusting odors are smelled directly (Wicker et al. 2003); (b) videos are viewed that show people trying pleasant or unpleasant tastes, or similar tastes are experienced directly (Jabbi et al. 2007); and (c) a person is touched or when someone else is observed to be touched in a video (Keysers et al. 2004). Most of the studies in the domain of empathic brain responses, however, have been conducted in the domain of pain. For example, Singer et al. (2004) recruited couples who were in love with each other and assessed their empathy "*in vivo*" by assessing brain activity in the female partner while painful stimulation was applied either to her own or to her partner's right hand via electrodes attached to the back of the hand. The male partner was seated next to the MRI scanner and a mirror system allowed the female to see both her partner's as well as her own hands lying on a tilted board in front of her. Flashes of different colors on a big screen behind the board pointed either to her hand or that of her partner, indicating which of them would receive the painful stimulation and which would be subject to the non-painful stimulation. This procedure enabled pain-related brain activation to be measured when pain was applied to the scanned subject (the so-called "pain matrix") or to her partner (empathy for pain). The results suggest that the parts of the "pain matrix" were also activated when empathizing with the pain of others. Thus, bilateral anterior insula (AI), the rostral anterior cingulate cortex (ACC), brainstem, and cerebellum were activated when subjects either received pain or a signal that a loved one experienced pain. These areas are involved in the processing of the affective component of pain (i.e., how unpleasant the subjectively felt pain is). Thus, both the experience of pain to oneself and the knowledge that a loved partner experiences pain activates the same affective pain circuits, suggesting that if a loved partner suffers pain, our brains also make us suffer from this pain. Activation in this network could also be observed when an unknown but likable person was observed to suffer pain (Singer et al. 2006) or when a person was merely exposed to videos showing body parts in potentially painful situations (Jackson et al. 2005, 2006), painful facial expressions (Lamm et al. 2007), or needles pricking into hands (Morrison et al. 2004; for a review see de Vignemont and Singer 2006). Overall, findings of shared circuitries underlying sensation and feelings in oneself and observation of similar sensations and feelings in others suggest that we use neuronal representations reflecting our own emotional responses to understand how it feels for others to be in a similar state. Further, they suggest that our ability to empathize may have evolved from a system which represents our own internal feeling states and allows us to predict the affective outcomes of an event for ourselves as well as for other people (e.g., Singer et al. 2004).

These neuroscientific findings seem to be in agreement with earlier action–perception models of motor behavior and imitation, as well as with their extension to the domain of empathy (Preston and de Waal 2002; Gallese 2003). Preston and de Waal (2002), for example, proposed a neuroscientific model of empathy, suggesting that observation or imagination of another person in a particular emotional state activates automatically a representation of that state in the observer with its associated autonomic and somatic responses. In this case, the term "automatic" refers to a process that does not require conscious and effortful processing, but which can nevertheless be inhibited or controlled. Indeed, in most of the above studies, empathic brain responses were observed even though subjects were not even told the goal of the study but were merely instructed to watch passively the scene or movies. Are empathic brain responses really automatic, and do we really always empathize automatically with others when exposed to their emotional states?

To prove automaticity of empathic brain responses, we would require studies showing such responses in the absence of awareness of the empathy-inducing stimulus. Similar to earlier studies in the domain of emotional face perception, which show amygdala responses to faces with fearful expressions when presented subliminally (i.e., without the subjects being consciously aware of the stimulus being presented), we would need to present our subjects displays of people suffering without our subject being aware of seeing those suffering. Despite the fact that such an experiment is difficult to conduct, it is also questionable whether we would then still measure empathic responses. Most people would probably agree that empathy is a conscious experience and that people are aware of what they feel when empathizing with others (for similar arguments, see de Vignemont and Singer 2006).

Recently, de Vignemont and Singer (2006) have proposed an alternative model in which they suggest that empathy is actually not merely the automatic consequence of the passive observation of emotional cues in others, but rather is subject to contextual appraisal and modulation. For example, Singer et al. (2006) found evidence for the modulation of such empathic brain responses as a function of the perceived fairness of another person. Male and female volunteers first played repeated sequential Prisoner Dilemma games with two confederates: one confederate played fairly while the other played unfairly. Empathy-related activation in ACC and AI were observed for both genders when the fair, likable player was in pain. Men, but not women, showed an absence of such empathic activity when an unfair player was perceived to be in pain. On average, an increase in areas associated with reward (nucleus accumbens) was observed in men, which was positively correlated with the expressed desire for revenge assessed after the study by questionnaires. These results suggest that, at least in men, a desire of revenge won over an empathic motivation when someone, who in their view deserved to be punished, was observed suffering. Similarly, Lamm et al. (2007) showed that subjects elicited less empathic responses in pain-related areas when the subjects knew that the pain inflicted to the other was justified to invoke a cure. Even though these findings suggest a modulation of empathic brain responses based on appraisal of the situation, it still remains open whether these empathic brain responses are first elicited and then suppressed, or whether contextual appraisal occurs first and its outcome decides whether an empathic response will or will not be elicited. Due to the poor time resolution of fMRI, answers to these questions will have to be sought, for example, through the use of EEG or MEG.

Studying Brain Signatures in Economic Games

The three games described below all involve two persons in a social interaction. In each game, one person decides first; we will call this person DM1. The person affected by DM1's decision is called DM2. In the second and third games, DM2 will then have an opportunity to make a decision which, in turn, affects DM1. (Note that DM stands for decision maker and serves as a neutral term for describing the roles of the two players in the game.) We also include a brief description of some of the relevant experiments on decision making in these games. However, for a more complete review, the reader is referred to Camerer (2003) and Houser and McCabe (2008).

A valuable model of a person's strategy for brain imaging is the finite state machine, which determines a person's next move based on his or her current state. A state can include a person's information, motivational goals, and affective state. In the finite state case, person 1 has a ToM of person 2 if person 1 infers both the state in which person 2 is as well as the state to which person 2 desires to achieve. In the false beliefs task, state includes the false information the child has (i.e., the toy is in the right-hand cupboard) as well as the motivational goal of the child (i.e., get the toy). An important question is how simple or complex a person's state may be. For example, an overly pessimistic child might reenter the room believing that he will be tricked, perhaps because this has happened to him in the past. In such a case, the child reentering the room would go to the left-hand cupboard, assuming he had been tricked and presupposing a normal brain; given the appropriate information, one can infer that this would be the child's strategy.

Here, we propose the following definition of ToM in two-person extensive form games. One player has an online ToM of another player if, and only if:

1. person 1 and 2 have shared attention over a mutual, and salient, terminal node of the game (goal state);
2. a person chooses a branch that leads to the goal state, it is taken as evidence of both shared attention over that state as well as that person's desire to reach the goal state;
3. the accumulation of evidence of shared attention over a desired goal state increases the likelihood that a player will try to reach that state.

As players move toward a desired goal state, this is treated as evidence to each other that they both desire to reach the goal state, and this evidence makes them more likely to try to reach this state as they continue to move.

Several recent studies involved the brain imaging of subjects while they played strategic games with another partner outside the scanner room (e.g., McCabe et al. 2001; Gallagher et al. 2002; Rilling et al. 2004). The first two studies examined the brain areas involved when a subject plays against an intentional actor (i.e., another person) as compared to playing against a computer. All of these studies have repeatedly demonstrated the involvement of the medial prefrontal lobe. The mPFC, however, is not only involved when mentalizing about the thoughts, intentions, or beliefs of others, but also when people attend to their own states.

The Dictator Game

In the dictator game, DM1 is given (or in some cases earns) an amount of money, M. DM1 is then asked to decide how much M, if any, they wish to send to an anonymous stranger, DM2. How much will DM1 give DM2? The results for four variations in the dictator game are shown in Figure 5.2. Figures 5.2a and 5.2b are typical of a number of experiments (see Hoffman et al. 1996b) where the experimenter gives the money to DM1 and controls for the ability to observe what DM1 does. Data in Figure 5.2a shows how much DM1 gives when he is aware that he is being observed. While a significant mode occurs when zero money is sent, money is often given to DM2, but the amount varies considerably. Figure 5.2b illustrates the results when the experimenter gives DM1 the money, but does not watch what DM1 does. Much less is sent, which suggests that being observed by the experimenter influences how DM1 will act toward DM2. Figures 5.2c and 5.2d show how much DM1 gives DM2 when DM1 earns the money, instead of simply being given the money by the experimenter (Cherry et al. 2002). In Figure 5.2c the experimenter again observes DM1, but now far less money is sent. In Figure 5.2d the experimenter does not observe DM1.

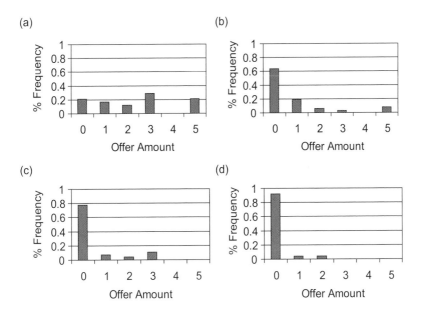

Figure 5.2 Results from four dictator games are shown where decision maker 1 (DM1) is given the opportunity to send some money to DM2. Each subfigure shows the percentage of DM1s who sent $0 up to $5 in $1 increments. In (a) and (b), DM1s were given $10, while in (c) and (d) DM1s earned $10 by taking a quiz. In (a) and (c) the experimenter observed how much each DM1 sent to DM2, while in (b) and (d) the experimenter did not observe the individual identities of the DM1s.

One explanation of these results is that self-interested responses in the dictator game (i.e., to keep all the money) are at least weakly regulated by a social "equity" norm, which implicitly states that the distribution of rewards should be proportional to the effort of participants. Dictators who give more may believe that the other participant was entitled to some of the money. The two treatments show how social regulation may be reduced in favor of self-interest either through anonymity, which weakens compliance, or through earning the money, which increases entitlement.

The Ultimatum Game

In the ultimatum game, DM1 and DM2 must decide jointly how to split an amount of money, M. DM1 moves first by making a nonnegative offer (m1, m2) that sums up to M. DM2 looks at the offer and decides to accept or reject. If the offer is rejected, both players get zero; if the offer is accepted, DM1 gets m1 and DM2 gets m2. What will DM1 offer? The results for four variations of the one-shot ultimatum game are shown in Figure 5.3. Figure 5.3a shows the typical percentage of M offered to DM2 and the percentage of offers rejected (see Hoffman et al. 1996a). However, when DM1 has earned the right in a contest to make the proposal offers become more self-serving, as shown in Figure 5.3b. Notice in Figures 5.3a and 5.3b that there are very few rejections (solid black bars), suggesting that DM2s more or less agree with the offers they are getting. Xiao and Houser (2005) modify the ultimatum game to increase the likelihood of rejections as shown when 10% or 20% of M is offered to DM2 in Figure 5.3c. They then go on to show that when DM2s are allowed to express their anger, they are more likely then to accept an "unfair" offer. Compare the 20% offers rejected in Figure 5.3c to the rejection rates in Figure 5.3d.

To understand this data it helps to consider the following thought experiment. As you are walking along, you see a dollar bill (or similar unit of currency of your home country). Do you pick it up? If you respond affirmatively, then you are willing to exert some energy to make a dollar compared to not having the dollar. So why would not DM1 think that a dollar will be an acceptable offer to DM2? The answer must be that social context matters. When we compare the distribution of offers in Figure 5.3a to the distribution of amounts sent in Figure 5.3b, we see a relative large effect in making DM2 an active participant who can influence the mutual outcome by accepting or rejecting the offer. This suggests that in the ultimatum game, DM1 must have a ToM of DM2.

In their neuroimaging experiments of the ultimatum game, Sanfey et al. (2006) find, in the repeat single play of the ultimatum game with different fictional counterparts, that a DM2 subject not only tends to reject unfair offers of 8–2 or even 9–1, but that this rejection also activates the insula, suggesting that DM2 is in a negative affective state at the time. Furthermore, the larger the insula BOLD response, the more likely DM2 is to reject an unfair offer. Sanfey et al. also find BOLD responses in the ACC and dorsal lateral prefrontal cortex

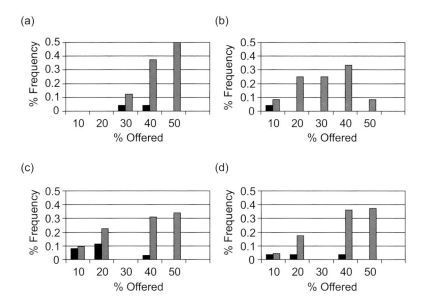

Figure 5.3   Results from four ultimatum games are shown where decision maker 1 (DM1) makes an offer to DM2 on how to split an amount of money, which DM2 can either accept or reject. Each subfigure shows the percentage of DM1s who offered 10–50% of the money to DM2 in 10% increments (gray bars). Solid black bars indicate the relative number of times the offer was rejected. (a) Results are shown from a typical one-shot game with a modal offer of 50% and very few rejections. (b) Offers shift in favor of DM1 when DM1 has earned the right in a contest to be first mover. (c) Increased rejection rates on low offers are shown in a modified ultimatum game designed to produce higher rejection rates. Note that when DM2 can express his anger over a low offer, he is more likely to accept the offer.

(DLPFC) as well as in ToM areas, such as the mPFC and STS (see Rilling et al. 2004). Subsequent experiments by Knoch et al. (2006), using TMS to disrupt the DLPFC while people were playing the ultimatum game, show that this increases the likelihood of accepting unfair offers. These results suggest that the DLPFC may play an important downstream role in overwriting prepotent action tendencies; that is, in the context of an ultimatum game, DLPFC would usually help to reject unfair offers in controlling the tendency to accept any offer even if the offer was unfair.

Figures 5.3c and 5.3d suggest that emotional processing can be inhibited in two different ways. An interesting research issue concerns whether or not the "earned right" treatment causes early inhibition of the emotional response through an early appraisal system, whereas the "expression" treatment causes late inhibition of emotional response through a late appraisal system. Also, do social norms, such as equity, exist in part to provide greater consistency between early and late appraisal systems?

The Investment/Trust Game

In the investment/trust game, DM1 and DM2 are each given an amount of money, M. DM1 must decide how much of M, if any, to send to DM2. Call this decision K. Both DM1 and DM2 are told, before DM1 makes a decision, that the amount sent to DM2 will be tripled to 3K. DM2 must then decide how much money to send back to DM1. What will DM1 send? What will DM2 send back? Figure 5.4 shows four results for the investment/trust game introduced by Berg et al. (1995). In a one-shot investment/trust game (Figure 5.4a), DM1s send on average about half of their money ($5 out of $10) with a great deal of variance (everything from $0–10 is sent). In return, about half of the DM2s reciprocate by returning at least as much as was originally sent back, but the rest of the DM2s defect on DM1s trust.

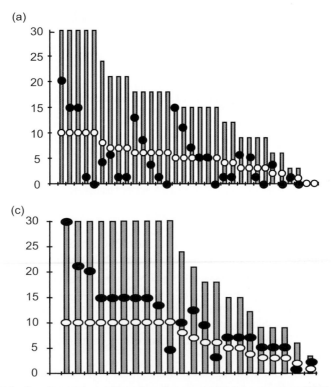

Figure 5.4 Results are shown from three investment/trust games where DM1 decides how much of $10 to send to DM2. Whatever is sent to DM2 is tripled; thereafter DM2 must decide how much of the tripled amount to return to DM1. Open circles indicate the amount sent (data has been ordered by this variable) by DM1. Gray bars represent the tripled amounts. Black circles show the amount that DM2 returned. (a) Typical results are shown: about half of the DM2s reciprocated DM1s trust by returning at least as much as the DM1s sent and about half defecting on the trust.

When we compare Figure 5.4a to Figure 5.2a, we see that social context matters here as well. In the investment/trust game, DM2s are essentially in the same role as DM1s in the dictator game, with one notable exception: The money that DM2s return in the investment/trust game is a direct consequence of DM1's choice to send money. We can thus interpret DM2's reciprocal be-havior as basically paying back a social obligation that was created when DM1 sent the money originally. This social obligation can be increased with social information, as shown in the greater trustworthiness of DM2s in Figure 5.4b. In this treatment, DM1s and DM2s are given the results from the experiment shown in Figure 5.4a. What is interesting is that social obligation, and not self-interest, seems to be the salient information extracted from this record.

Social obligation can also lead to strategic responses in repeat interactions of the investment/trust game. In Figure 5.4c and 5.4d, we show the results

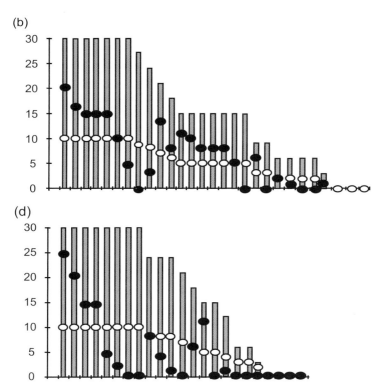

Figure 5.4 (continued) (b) Reciprocity increases when subjects are shown what DM1s and DM2s did in a previous one-shot investment game. The effects of reputation building in a two-period investment game with the same partner are shown in (c) and (d). In period one (c), almost all of the DM2s reciprocate; in the second and final period, much of this reciprocity disappears (d).

when the investment/trust game is played twice with the same partner in the same role. In the first play (Figure 5.4c), DM2s are much more likely to reciprocate the social obligation created by DM1. However, in the second play, many of the same DM2s fail to reciprocate the second social obligation. Why is this the case? One possible interpretation is that repeated play invites more strategic intentions, and part of the game is to realize that this has happened. An interesting effect of the repeated play is that DM2s are much more likely to split the 3K and return 50%. This does not occur in one-shot games (Figure 5.4a, b), suggesting that equal split is, in fact, part of the strategy being used to convince DM1s that they are playing with a cooperative counterpart.

In neuroimaging experiments of the investment/trust game, McCabe et al. (2001) showed a significant increase in anterior paracingulate and DLPFC when subjects in the scanner tried to cooperate with a human versus a computer counterpart outside of the scanner. They interpret these results as suggesting that ToM is essential to the establishment of a trust relationship where subjects must maintain prefrontal control over their desire to defect. In a subsequent experiment, King-Casas et al. (2005) showed that the neural correlate of the intention to increase trust could be modeled directly as a reinforcement-learning signal in the caudate of DM2's brain in a repeated trust interaction with DM1. Finally, Krueger et al. (2007) find evidence for two different neural pathways for two different types of trusting behavior by DM1s. In their experiment, DM1 and DM2 played repeatedly but DM2 faced varying amounts of temptation (by varying payoffs in the game) to defect on DM1. Some subjects showed early activation in the anterior paracingulate (ToM region) followed by later activation in the septal region of the brain (rich in oxytocin receptors for the hormone oxytocin known to increase social approach and trusting behavior in humans; see Kosfeld et al. 2005.) These neural activations were consistent with an unconditional trust strategy where DM1s placed their trust in DM2 without concern for the size of the temptation facing DM2. Other subjects showed no early activation in anterior paracingulate and no subsequent septal activation, but they did show a late activation in the anterior paracingulate consistent with the need to develop a ToM of the temptations their partner faced as DM2. These subjects also showed significantly greater activation in the ventral tegmental area consistent with the need for dopamine for contingent reward learning.

Integrating Empathy and Theory-of-Mind with Game Playing

How can we integrate our knowledge of brain signatures with the way in which people play games? This broader question can be subdivided into two more easily researchable questions: Can we design experiments to study when and how people integrate empathy and ToM? Can we design experiments to study how people use this integrated system to inform their own decisions better?

Singer (2006) answers the first question by proposing a thought experiment, integrating both the cognitive (ToM) and emotional (empathy) perception of pain. Consider her earlier research on the perception of pain in others and the additional task of evaluating how unpleasant pain is to a person who is introduced to process pain very differently from a typical person, where pain is perceived to be enjoyable rather than unpleasant. In such a case, empathic simulation would not lead to an adequate result but has to be inhibited and replaced by more cognitive perspective taking (ToM) in order to conclude that the person suffering pain is probably feeling reward rather than pain. In most cases, however, both systems will cooperate together when inferring the states of another person. An interesting open issue concerns what, if any, new binding sites will emerge to coordinate and/or integrate these two processing streams.

A similar thought experiment to see how these two systems affect decision making is as follows: Person 1 is put into two ultimatum games, acting as DM1 and DM2, respectively. As DM1, person 1 is asked to make a proposal to DM2. As DM2, person 2 receives an identical proposal from a different DM1 and is asked to respond. Person 1 is then asked to evaluate how unhappy DM2 was with their proposal after which they see DM2's response to their proposal.

In this second thought experiment, a critical feature would seem to be how a subject uses empathy and ToM to predict what the other player will do. In principle, if we play the same game often enough with the same person, we can learn to predict what they will do simply from what they have done in the past. This is, in fact, the basis of fictitious play (also called naive Bayesian learning, or reinforcement learning.) However, such learning requires very little empathy or ToM.

Conclusions

Identifying the brain signatures that occur when individuals make decisions in game contexts and in accordance with theories of functional adaptation is necessary but not sufficient for integrating the three levels of research that are needed to understand human social behavior better. These three levels are: (a) the ultimate causes of behavior produced by genetic evolution; (b) the proximal causes of behavior produced by the underlying neuronal mechanism; and, (c) the institutional causes of behavior produced by institutional/organizational governance and processing rules, herein the rules of the game. Sufficiency requires that we build a computational model with equilibrating conditions that can integrate all three levels and demonstrate the two-way influence of genes, neuronal machinery, and the rules of the game on one another.

Existing research suggests some constraints that our models will have to satisfy: context dependency, individual heterogeneity of strategic response (including diversity at the genetic level), flexibility (or the ability to adapt to changing circumstances), and ecological efficiency (producing maximum return at minimal cost) given material, informational, and societal constraints. At the same time, many open questions remain that may change these constraints: the degree of modularity in the brain, how coordination occurs within the brain, the extent to which the same area of cortex may be involved in functionally different cortical computations, and the relative plasticity of neuronal function.

References

Berg J., J. Dickhaut, and K. McCabe. 1995. Trust, reciprocity and social history. *Games Econ. Behav.* **10**:122–142.

Camerer, C. 2003. Behavioral Game Theory: Experiments in Strategic Interaction. Princeton, NJ: Princeton Univ. Press.

Cherry, T., P. Frykblom, and J. Shogren. 2002. Hardnose the dictator. *Am. Econ. Rev.* **92(4)**:1218–1221.

Decety, J., and P. L. Jackson. 2004. The functional architecture of human empathy. *Behav. Cogn. Neurosci. Rev.* **3(2)**:71–100.

Decety, J., and C. Lamm 2006. Human empathy through the lens of social neuroscience. *Sci. World. J.* **6**:1146–1164.

de Vignemont, F., and T. Singer. 2006. The empathic brain: How, when and why? *Trends Cogn. Sci.* **10(10)**:435–441.

Frith, C. D., and U. Frith. 1999. Interacting minds: A biological basis. *Science* **286(5445)**:1692–1695.

Frith, C. D., and U. Frith. 2003. The neural basis of mentalizing. *Neuron* **50**:531–534.

Gallagher, H. L., and C. D. Frith. 2003. Functional imaging of "theory of mind." *Trends Cogn. Sci.* **7(2)**:77–83.

Gallagher, H. L., A. I. Jack, A. Roepstorff, and C. D. Frith. 2002. Imaging the intentional stance in a competitive game. *NeuroImage* **16(3)**:814–821.

Gallese, V. 2003.The roots of empathy. The shared manifold hypothesis and the neural basis of intersubjectivity. *Psychopath.* **36**:171–180.

Harris, P. L. 1992. From simulation to folk psychology: The case for development. *Mind Lang.* **7**:120–144.

Hoffman, E., K. McCabe, K. Shachat, and V. Smith. 1996a. Preferences, property rights, and anonymity in bargaining games. *Games Econ. Behav.* **7**:346–380.

Hoffman, E., K. McCabe, and V. Smith. 1996b. Social distance and other-regarding behavior in dictator games. *Am. Econ. Rev.* **86(3)**:653–660.

Houser, D., and K. McCabe. 2008. Experimental neuroeconomics and non-cooperative games. In: Neuroeconomics: Decision Making and the Brain, ed. P. Glimcher, C. Camerer, E. Fehr, and R. Poldrack. New York: Academic Press, in press.

Jabbi, M., M. Swart, and C. Keysers. 2007. Empathy for positive and negative emotions in the gustatory cortex. *NeuroImage* **34(4)**:1744–1753.

Jackson P. L., A. N. Meltzoff, and J. Decety. 2005. How do we perceive the pain of others? A window into the neural processes involved in empathy. *NeuroImage* **24**:771–779.

Jackson, P. L., P. Rainville, and J. Decety. 2006. To what extent do we share the pain of others? Insight from the neural bases of pain empathy. *Pain* **125**:5–9.

Keysers, C., B. Wicker, V. Gazzola, J. L. Anton, L. Fogassi et al. 2004. A touching sight: SII/PV activation during the observation and experience of touch. *Neuron* **42**:335–346.

King-Casas, B., D. Tomlin, C. Anen, C. Camerer, S. Quartz et al. 2005. Getting to know you: Reputation and trust in a two-person economic exchange. *Science* **308**:78–83.

Knoch, D., A. Pascual-Leone, K. Meyer, V. Treyer, and E. Fehr. 2006. Diminishing reciprocal fairness by disrupting the right prefrontal cortex. *Science* **314(5800)**:829–832.

Kosfeld M., M. Henrichs, P. Zak, U. Fishbacher, and E. Fehr. 2005. Oxytocin increases trust in humans. *Nature* **435**:673–676.

Krueger, F., K. McCabe, J. Moll, N. Kriegeskorte, R. Zahn et al. 2007. Neural correlates of trust. *Proc. Natl. Acad. Sci.,* early edition, December.

Lamm, C., C. D. Batson, and J. Decety. 2007. The neural substrate of human empathy: Effects of perspective-taking and cognitive appraisal. *J. Cogn. Neurosci.* **19(1)**:42–58.

McCabe, K., D. Houser, L. Ryan, V. Smith, and T. Trouard. 2001. A functional imaging study of cooperation in two-person reciprocal exchange. *Proc. Natl. Acad. Sci.* **98**:11,832–11,835.

McCabe, K., S. Rassenti, and V. Smith. 1996. Game theory and reciprocity in some extensive form experimental games. *Proc. Natl. Acad. Sci*. **93**:13,421–13,428.

McCabe, K., M. Rigdon, and V. Smith. 2003. Positive reciprocity and intentions in trust games. *J. Econ. Behav. Org.* **52**:267–275.

Mitchell, J. P., M M. Fason, C. N. Macrae, and M. R. Banaji. 2005a. Thinking about people: The neural substrates of social cognition. In: Social Neuroscience: People Thinking about People, ed. J. T. Cacioppo, P. S. Visser, and C. L. Pickett, pp. 63–81. Cambridge, MA: MIT Press.

Mitchell, J. P., C. N. Macrae, and M. R. Banaji. 2005b. Forming impressions of people versus inanimate objects: Social-cognitive processing in the medial prefrontal cortex. *NeuroImage* **26**:251–257.

Mitchell, J. P., Macrae, C. N., and Banaji, M. R. 2006. Dissociable medial prefrontal contributions to judgments of similar and dissimilar others. *Neuron* **50**:655–663.

Morrison, I., D. Lloyd, G. di Pellegrino, and N. Robets. 2004. Vicarious responses to pain in anterior cingulate cortex: Is empathy a multisensory issue? *Cogn. Affec. Behav. Neurosci.* **4**:270–278.

O'Doherty, J., H. Critchley, R. Deichmann, and R. J. Dolan. 2003. Dissociating valence of outcome from behavioral control in human orbital and ventral prefrontal cortices. *J. Neurosci.* **23**:7931–7939.

O'Reilly, R. C., T. S. Braver, and J. D. Cohen. 1999. A biologically based computational model of working memory. In: Models of Working Memory: Mechanisms of Active Maintenance and Executive Control, ed. A Miyake and P. Shah, pp. 375–411. New York: Cambridge Univ. Press.

Povinelli, D. J., and J. M. Bering. 2002. The mentality of apes revisited. *Curr. Dir. Psychol. Sci.* **11**:115–119.

Preston, S. D., and F. B. M. de Waal. 2002. Empathy: Its ultimate and proximate bases. *Behav. Brain Sci.* **25**:1–72.

Rilling, J. K., A. G. Sanfey, J. A. Aronson, L.E. Nystrom, and J. D. Cohen. 2004. The neural correlates of theory of mind within interpersonal interactions. *NeuroImage* **22(4)**:1694–1703.

Sanfey, A. G., G. Loewenstein, S. M. McClure, and J. D. Cohen. 2006. Neuroeconomics: Cross-currents in research on decision-making. *Trends Cogn. Sci.* **10**:108–116.

Schultz, W., P. Dayan, and P. R. Montague. 1997. A neural substrate of prediction and reward. *Science* **275**:1593–1599.

Singer, T. 2006. The neuronal basis and ontogeny of empathy and mind reading: Review of literature and implications for future research. *Neurosci. Biobehav. Rev.* **30(6)**:855–863.

Singer, T., B. Seymour, J. O'Doherty, H. Kaube, R. J. Dolan, and C. D. Frith. 2004. Empathy for pain involves the affective but not sensory components of pain. *Science* **303(5661)**:1157–1162.

Singer, T., B. Seymour, J. P. O'Doherty, K. E. Stephan, R. J. Dolan, and C. D. Frith. 2006. Empathic neural responses are modulated by the perceived fairness of others. *Nature* **439(7075)**:466–469.

Wicker, B., C. Keysers, J. Plailly, J.-P. Royet, V. Gallese et al. 2003. Both of us disgusted in *my* insula: The common neural basis of seeing and feeling disgust. *Neuron* **40(3)**:655–664.

Xiao, E., and D. Houser. 2005. Emotion expression in human punishment behavior. *Proc. Natl. Acad. Sci.* **102(20)**:7398–7401.

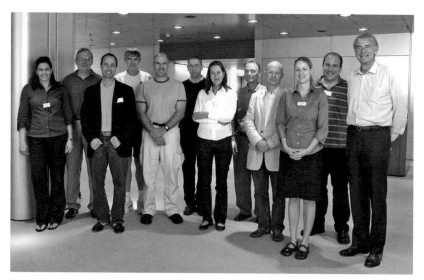

Left to right: Elizabeth Phelps, Kevin McCabe, Michael Shadlen, Roger Ratcliff, Michael Platt, Peter Dayan, Fredericke Wiedemann, Randolf Menzel, Stanislas Dehaene, Hilke Plassmann, Gordon Pipa, Wolf Singer

6

Neuronal Correlates of Decision Making

Michael Platt, Rapporteur

Peter Dayan, Stanislas Dehaene, Kevin McCabe,
Randolf Menzel, Elizabeth Phelps, Hilke Plassmann,
Roger Ratcliff, Michael Shadlen, and Wolf Singer

Abstract

Decision making involves selection from sets of options based on current evidence
about the state of the world and estimates of the value or utility of different outcomes.
The neural correlates of evidence assessment that guide simple perceptual judgments
are now well understood, and we argue that this process can serve as a simple model for
organizing behavioral and neural correlates of decision making in more complex contexts, including those that involve economic transactions, social interaction, emotional
stimulation, and conscious awareness. Bridging the methodological and theoretical gaps
between simple and more complicated decision problems remains a fundamental, but in
our view soluble, challenge for understanding the neurobiology of decision making.

Introduction

Over the past ten years, neurobiologists have made significant advances in the
understanding of the neural correlates of decision making. Given the nature
of this problem, it is perhaps not surprising that the most significant progress
has been achieved in understanding the neuronal mechanisms underlying perceptual decision making, in which there is a satisfying match between computational models of behavior and the response properties of single neurons in
cortical areas traditionally associated with sensorimotor processing. Building
on this work, we have begun to achieve an understanding of the contribution
of valuation to this process as well as the neural systems that contribute to
learning and applying value to decisions. The extension of this work to social

interaction, the role of emotions in coloring or modulating the decision process, and the contributions of conscious and nonconscious processes to decision making remain deeply important yet relatively immature fields of inquiry. We predict that important insights can be gained by comparing the principles governing decision processing in diverse animals, like humans and honeybees, which highlight divergent neural architecture. In our report, we outline current understanding of these issues, highlight significant controversies, and pose questions to stimulate new avenues for research.

What Is a Decision?

Before delving into the neuronal correlates of decision making, let us define what we mean by a decision: A decision is a commitment to a choice or course of action selected from more than one option. We start by considering *perceptual* decision making, which involves committing to one of a number of propositions about an aspect of the state of the outside world. Such commitment is meant to imply a conversion from an uncommitted state, in which evidence and other factors are considered in relation to all the alternatives, to a state in which one of the alternatives is chosen. Later we will discuss more general decisions, which are typically more divorced from propositions about the state of the world. Viewed as a process, a decision has a beginning and an end, and it evolves over time. Commitment implies termination of the decision process, but it does not imply that a decision cannot be superseded or reversed.

Often, a decision results in an action. If that action is immediate, then the process reveals its time of termination. If there is no explicit action, or if the action is delayed, then there is still a termination, but there is no (obvious) behavioral manifestation. There is good evidence that a single mechanism accounts for termination and choice selection; that is, both when and what is decided (reviewed in Gold and Shadlen 2007). A commitment need not result in an action (immediate or planned) but can instead lead to a choice of strategy or choice to make a new decision about something else or a commitment to implement a complex rule or program (e.g., if told "S1," reply "A1"; else if told "S2", reply "A2"; else wait). It is useful to expand the concept of "choice of action" to incorporate this broader class of decision outcomes.

The key elements of a perceptual decision among N alternatives include:

1. *Identification of alternatives.* These are commonly regarded as hypotheses or beliefs about the world. They are ultimately true or false, although this may not be revealed to the decision maker, and are denoted $h_1, h_2, \ldots$

2. *Identification of actions*: For perceptual decisions, in the general sense developed above, the actions define the states associated with commitment to each of the alternatives: $H_1, H_2,...$ [1]

3. *Evidence* is an item of information that has bearing on the alternatives: $P(e_i|h_j)$. Evidence can originate from a variety of sources and can arrive as a stream in time or all at once.

4. *Priors* are knowledge about the likelihood of each of the alternatives, absent any evidence; that is, the probability $P(h_i)$ that each of the alternatives is true, before receipt of any evidence.

5. *Value and utilities* are the consequences of a decision associated with the possible outcomes: $u(H_i, h_j)$. Notice that the outcomes include both the actual state of the world and the action of the decision maker. Utilities are based on values and costs, are influenced by motivational and emotional factors, and may be accumulated across sequential choices to define the utility or value of a strategy.

6. *Decision variable* is a number (or vector of numbers) that combines the preceding terms. An operation on the decision variable establishes the outcome of the decision.

7. *Decision rule* is often a criterion of the decision variable or a bound to accumulated evidence.

8. *Objectives and goals* are desired consequences of making decisions. They are usually stated in terms of values, utility, and time.

9. *Policy and strategy* are operations on control factors (e.g., criteria, decision variable, utility) that influence the decision process to obtain objectives and goals.

Many decisions are not described as choices among discrete alternatives but involve instead an estimate of a quantity or a parameter. For example, instead of deciding whether motion is left, right, up, or down, an observer might be asked to judge its actual direction of movement. It is an open question how and whether the mechanisms of decisions among discrete alternatives can be applied to this problem. In statistical contexts, hypothesis testing and parameter estimation are types of inference. Commitment implies termination of the decision process, but it does not imply that a decision cannot be superseded or reversed.

An alternative perspective that is common in statistical treatments is to separate the hypotheses and actions a little more distinctly. In this case, choices are not treated purely as commitment to hypotheses, but rather as independent

---

[1] It is important to respect the distinction between hypotheses and actions. *P(h)* refers to the probability that a state of the world holds. It also represents the degree of belief in that state. *P(H)* refers to the probability that the decision maker will choose a particular outcome. It is not a term that is commonly used, but it could be if the mapping between hypothesis and action were complicated.

entities in their own right. Further, the state of the world is often considered as being well known, in which case it is only the utilities that are important for determining choices. This encourages a firm functional (though not necessarily an algorithmic or implementational) separation between compiling information about the posterior distribution over the states of world based on the evidence, $P(h_i|e)$, and the choice of action as maximizing the expected short- or long-run utility averaging over this posterior. Later, we consider cases in which the state of the world is considered as being well known, where it is only the utilities that are important for determining choices.

Drift-diffusion Models of Perceptual Decision Making

The neuronal correlates of perceptual decision making have been explored extensively in association cortical areas that intervene between sensory processing and motor affordance (Gold and Shadlen 2007; Sugrue et al. 2004; Smith and Ratcliff 2004; Glimcher 2003; Romo and Salinas 2003). These studies have revealed a number of important features of the decision process. Specifically, the decision process unfolds in time as the output system is continuously fed sensory information that supports a particular motor affordance. For example, the lateral intraparietal area (LIP) contributes to the selection of a target for an orienting movement of the eyes. Neurons in this area continuously query sensory areas for information supporting a particular orienting movement. The value or utility of a particular orienting saccade influences this temporally extended process (Platt and Glimcher 1999; Sugrue et al. 2004).

The temporal unfolding of activity in neurons in the LIP (Shadlen and Newsome 2001; Roitman and Shadlen 2002; Huk and Shadlen 2005) as well as other areas, such as the frontal eye fields (Roesch and Olson 2003; Ding and Hikosaka 2006), the dorsolateral prefrontal cortex (Kim and Shadlen 1999; Heekeren et al. 2004), premotor cortex (Romo et al. 2004), and superior colliculus (Horwitz and Newsome 2001), has been argued to represent a decision variable. Furthermore, the decision variable has been argued to resemble diffusion to boundary models developed to explain choice and reaction time data in psychophysical studies (Ratcliff 1978; Ratcliff et al. 2003). In these models, the decision variable has a starting point, a drift rate or rate of accumulation, and a terminal boundary representing the end of the decision process. According to this view, neurons represent a decision variable that integrates sensory information favoring a particular oculomotor response until the boundary is crossed, after which a movement is initiated. Remarkably, models of this sort can explain a large fraction of the variance in both choice and reaction time based on the spike rates of neurons in many of these areas (Mazurek et al. 2003; Ratcliff et al. 2003).

Complementing the prediction of behavioral data from neuronal activity, computational modeling has also demonstrated that it is possible to fit behavioral data with a diffusion class model and predict neuronal firing rates (Ratcliff et al. 2003). Specifically, in a simple brightness discrimination task, a dual diffusion model was fit to behavioral data, accuracy, and correct and error reaction time distributions. Then, position in the process was assumed to represent firing rate, and functions predicting firing rate were able to match most of the main features of the observed firing rate data quantitatively. This correspondence between behavioral models and neurophysiological data are startling, to say the least, given the history of compartmentalization in much of science.

The consilience of the psychophysical model and neurophysiological data thus represents a major success in understanding the neurobiology of decision making. This model has been extended to the neuronal correlates of somatosensory guided decisions (Romo and Salinas 2003), behavioral and imaging data from human subjects performing numerical judgment tasks (Dehaene 2007; Sigman and Dehaene 2005) and object classification tasks (Heekeren et al. 2004). Moreover, similar processes seem likely to underlie decisions about a choice of strategy so the model is not limited to overt actions. For instance, in a dual-task setting, where subjects have to perform quickly, in the order they prefer, a visual numerical judgment and an auditory tone judgment, choosing which of two tasks to perform first adds a stage to the response time which can be modeled as involving a noisy accumulation of evidence up to a threshold (Sigman and Dehaene 2006). It might even be possible to extend these ideas to more complex real-life decisions, as when children select which algorithm (e.g., memory retrieval, explicit calculation, shortcut) to apply to an arithmetic problem, a high-level decision that has been modeled as a differential weighing of evidence for the efficiency of the various alternatives (Siegler 1988).

The model also has the attractive feature that confidence in the decision could, in principle, be estimated from the length of time needed to commit to a response or information encapsulated in integrators that fail to reach the boundary for commitment. We note, however, that thus far computational modeling of psychophysical data does not support the idea that observers use elapsed time as an estimate of uncertainty.

Despite these advances, significant controversies remain. Do all decisions evolve in time? Although it would appear that every decision takes time, it remains unclear as to how the decision process unfolds when there is no relevant sensory information to guide choice. Further, can the model account for decisions extended across long periods of time and involving multiple sources of information, such as choosing whether or not to buy a car? Likewise, decision making at the institutional level may not always involve the extended transmission of evidence. Conversely, legal decision making often involves backward contingency of evidence that alters the decision process.

A second set of questions focuses on whether decisions of this type are more appropriately modeled using nonlinear system dynamics (cf. Wang 2002; Wong and Wang 2006; Machens et al. 2005). These questions notwithstanding, the perceptual model of decision making extended in time represents a set of formal, quantitative principles for organizing neurophysiological (and perhaps neuroimaging) evidence gathered in other decision-making contexts, including those that unfold over long periods of time, emotional situations, and social interaction.

The Origins of Variability in Decision Making

Psychological Models

One important feature of decision models in psychology is that they assume different sources of noise during processing. There is noise within the decision process, noise in the evidence entering the process from trial to trial, and noise in the decision criteria (or starting point of the process, which is to a large degree equivalent). We would like to emphasize two main points: First, these sources of noise are discriminable in the models. Simulated data can be generated from the model with different values of these noise parameters and these can be recovered. Second, these sources of noise are necessary to fit behavioral data. A diffusion process with equal boundaries predicts that reaction times on correct and error trials are identical. For example, variability in evidence (drift rate) from trial to trial leads to errors slower than correct responses and variability in decision criteria from trial to trial gives fast errors.

Noise and Randomness in Decision Making

Most decisions of interest from a psychological, economic, or evolutionary point of view appear stochastic. In part, this is because evidence and/or valuation does not uniquely guarantee only one optimal choice. Moreover, the neuronal correlates of the assumed decision variable can only be revealed when there is incomplete agreement between information and choice. For these reasons, psychological and neurobiological research has focused on decisions based on evidence and/or valuation that tends to favor, but does not determine, one choice. In these situations, knowledge of the variables influencing choice appears to govern the probability of an outcome without guaranteeing it. Thus, the actual choice appears to be random.

There are two qualitatively different classes of mechanisms which could give rise to probabilistic behavior (Shadlen et al., this volume; Luce and Suppes 1965). The difference between these two mechanisms is whether the noise is in the assessment of evidence and utilities (first stage) or in the application of the decision rule (second stage). If it is in the first stage, then the decision arises deterministically based on the sign of a noisy decision variable relative to a criterion. In this case, variability arises because the representation of evidence is intrinsically noisy (Shadlen and Newsome 1994, 1998). This model is similar to the random utility model of Manski (1977), which assumes that the decision rule is applied deterministically. This model implies that individual preferences or utilities will not always be the same under identical conditions because of measurement error and random variation in the assessment of preference or utility. Utilities are thus conceptualized as random variables.

If the noise is in the second stage, the decision process uses errorless representations of the utility of options to compute a probability of choice and realizes it in an explicitly random act, equivalent to flipping a weighted coin (Glimcher 2005). This model is similar to the constant utility theory of Luce (1959), which states that choice is a probabilistic function of preferences or utilities (Luce 1959). Thus, accordingly, utilities can be deduced from the relative frequency with which an individual chooses various alternatives under identical conditions.

These two models of probabilistic behavior cannot be distinguished behaviorally. An animal that chooses "right" on 71% of trials could be choosing "right" every time the value of a normally distributed variable with $\mu = \sigma = 1$ exceeds 0, or it could be doing so by flipping a weighted coin on each trial ($p = 0.71$). For well-studied perceptual decisions, the first idea has strong support (see Gold and Shadlen 2007). Enthusiasm for the deliberate random act derives mainly from theoretical claims that randomness confers survival advantage in predator–prey situations and competitive games (Glimcher 2005; Maynard Smith 1982).

Neuronal Noise and Decision Making

In perceptual decisions, variability in choice and response time can be traced to the variable activity of neurons in the cortex (for a review, see Parker and Newsome 1998; Mazurek and Shadlen 2003). Recordings from the neurons that represent evidence and the neurons that represent the decision variable show trial-to-trial variation in spike rates which explains (a) the behavioral sensitivity overall, (b) errors on single trials, and (c) some of the variance in reaction time. This implies strongly that although, in principle, behavioral variability could have a variety of causes—including the representation of states that are simply unknown to the experimenter or irrelevant to the task at hand—the brain is unable to eliminate these causes. It is affected by variability in the way that conforms to the noise in the engineering sense, and this leads to mistakes.

What is the source of the neural noise? This is an immense topic beyond the scope of our report. We note, however, that there is clear and compelling empirical evidence that cortical neurons discharge irregularly (Shadlen and Newsome 1994, 1998). This implies that every quantity that the neocortex represents—be it evidence, a decision variable, or a representation of elapsed time—is corrupted in some sense by response variability, and thus includes both signal and noise. Although noise may be an intrinsic feature of the biophysical properties and synaptic connections of cortical neurons, this does not exclude the possibility that intrinsic neuronal noise has been exploited by evolution to promote behavioral variability or flexibility, which can have obvious survival advantages (Glimcher 2005).

Value-based Decision Making

As noted, decisions involve selecting among possibilities based partly on their value or utility. We can define the value of a *state* as the expected long-run summed reward, discounted by the delay to its receipt, starting from that state; the value of an *action* at a state (sometimes called a Q value) can be defined as the expected long-run summed reward starting from initiating that particular action when in that state, again discounted by delay. From a formal perspective, it is appropriate to consider net rewards after costs are taken into account, although the neural realization of costs and punishments is less clear than that for rewards.

As mentioned, much of the work on perceptual decision making has focused on uncertainty about the state of the world and the decision variables that accumulate sensory information favoring one state over another. In contrast, the tradition of studies investigating complex, long-run values has tended to assume that states are well known, thus placing the emphasis squarely on the utilities. This tradition is the focus of our discussion for the remainder of this section. However, two important caveats point to the future merging of these approaches: First, although the state of the subject in the world may be known, the rules of the world (e.g., what transitions between states are occasioned by which actions) are not. In this case, subjects face an exploration–exploitation dilemma associated with their uncertainty about the nature of the environment. Although not generally couched in such terms, this implies that there exist some higher-order decision variables that control the course of exploration. Second, value-based decision making still requires a physical realization of competition among the options. This likely involves the same sort of mechanisms as discussed for perceptual decision making, and it may be possible to endow the variables coded by neural firing rates in the competing populations with some form of decision variable semantics.

Value Systems

Consideration of the psychological and neural data suggests that value thus defined is not a unitary concept: there are different ways of defining and calculating value, and there are different ways of using values to control decisions. These different notions of value also appear to map onto somewhat distinct neural systems. Available data suggest the existence of four different systems for computing and representing value, although there is by no means consensus that this is the only scheme that can adequately encapsulate all available data:

1. The first value system is the *native value system*. Native values are influenced by motivational states (e.g., hunger, thirst) and (probably) mood. Thus, native values may differ from true, real-world values. This system has been described as the "liking" system (Berridge and Robinson 2003) and is most likely mediated by the primary taste system, hypothalamus, and periaqueductal gray region of the brainstem and can be modulated by opioids and benzodiazepines.

2. The second value system is the *forward model system*. This system learns a full tree of states, actions, transitions, and outcomes, and it infers values by extensive search of this tree. Since the forward model's evaluation of the outcomes it encounters during this search appears to be sensitive to motivational state, it is goal directed. This model of value is computationally hard to compute and is probably the best candidate to be considered as an explicit value system. The neural systems associated with outcome evaluation in the forward model remain a subject of debate, but may be related to physiological evaluation mechanisms (discussed further below). The inference process appears to involve the dorsolateral prefrontal cortex as well as the dorsomedial striatum and places a heavy burden on working memory.

3. The *cached value system* represents the learned value of a state or an action, which is typically independent of motivational state or changes in the environment. Thus, the cached value system is inflexible and cannot generalize to different motivational states or contexts. The normal form of learning uses dopamine to report an appetitive prediction error, with values being represented in the amygdala and possibly the ventral striatum. It has been speculated that serotonin calculates cached values for aversive outcomes (Daw et al. 2002).

4. The fourth value system computes the *long-run expected value*, which putatively acts as an opportunity cost of inaction and controls the vigor of responding. This value system is important for determining when to act and may be linked to tonic dopamine levels (Niv et al. 2006).

Value-based Control Systems

These four value systems contribute in a variety of ways to four different systems controlling decision making:

1. *Goal-directed control* follows from state-action values computed by the forward model. Since choices are based on extensive search of all states, actions, and outcomes, goal-directed decision making provides a sophisticated, but computationally expensive, control system.

2. *Habitual control* operates on cached state-action values. Because cached values are insensitive to motivational state, habit-based control is inflexible.

Habitual control depends strongly on the dorsolateral striatum and is influenced by the neuromodulators, dopamine, and serotonin.

These two control systems are conventionally assumed to compete through a softmax function (essentially rolling dice) according to their relative uncertainties, although the mechanisms that compute uncertainty remain unclear. Competition within each system could possibly be implemented instead by a diffusion-to-bound mechanism, similar to the one proposed to account for perceptual decision making (Shadlen et al., this volume; Gold and Shadlen 2007). The long-run expected value influences action latency.

3. The *episodic controller* can best be viewed as a replacement for the forward model because it is more accurate in very early learning. This system simply recommends repeating any action or sequence of actions that was successful in the past, a strategy that can be shown to be optimal (i.e., to have minimal uncertainty) in some particular circumstances. The hippocampus likely plays a key role in episodic control.

4. The *Pavlovian controller* specifies actions regardless of their instrumental suitability. This control system consists of intrinsic, instinctive mechanisms that have been programmed by evolution due to their routine efficacy. Pavlovian control includes spontaneous approach and avoidance behaviors in the light of value-based predictions of reward, and thus leads to behavioral phenomena such as autoshaping, negative automaintenance, and Pavlovian-instrumental transfer. Preparatory appetitive and aversive effects appear to depend on the ventral striatum, whereas more consummatory defensive and aggressive Pavlovian responses appear to depend on the dorsal periaqueductal gray region of the brainstem.

These four value systems and associated decision control systems can account for a wide array of observations following specific manipulations (e.g., such as incentive devaluation) as well as damage to specific brain areas (e.g., the dorsolateral striatum), and these promote particular behavioral responses. There are, however, other conceptualizations of value and control systems that might equally account for these observations. This caveat becomes clear when we consider precisely how a single decision evolves in time within and across these systems. Specifically, how can evidence for these four systems be reconciled with neurophysiological observations of integration with respect to time in perceptual decision making? Do the resultant values computed in each of these four systems contribute to the decision variable apparently computed in cortical areas mediating sensorimotor processing? If so, how do they influence the decision variables? It is not yet clear precisely how competition between decisions is instantiated (i.e., whether decision variables are parsimoniously seen as being involved) and what influence uncertainty has on states (as in perceptual decision making). For instance, there is evidence for value-related bias of the decision variable (Platt and Glimcher 1999; Sugrue et al. 2004;

Klein et al., in prep.) as well as motivationally induced changes in the rate of integration (Bendiksby and Platt 2006) of neurons in the LIP. Certainly, the mechanisms underlying value-related influences on the decision variable, as well as precisely where value-related signals enter the decision process, remain to be explicated fully, thus providing a fruitful avenue for future research.

The Role of Emotion in Decision Making

Value and Emotion

As discussed above, the concept of value is fundamental to current models of decision making. When considering the impact of emotion on decision making, one might begin by considering the relation between value and emotion.

Current models do not limit emotion to a subjective feeling. There is no question that many of us make choices when we do not have strong feelings. One does not need to have a strong subjective experience to invoke an emotional process (LeDoux 1996). The distinction between feeling and emotion is prominent in current models of emotion, but it is less familiar to those from other disciplines and can thus result in some confusion.

What distinguishes value from emotion? The answer to this depends on how we understand the purpose and limits of emotion. It is has been argued by some that emotion is a *relevance detector* in that it allows us to determine what is or is not important in a given situation, in order to generate an adaptive response (Cosmides and Tooby 2000). In this broad framework, we can clearly see the intersection of emotion and value. Although emotion may encompass more than value, value is a fundamental component of emotion. However, others have argued that systems that mediate emotion as well as those that do not both contribute to the calculation of value (Cohen 2005). Accordingly, emotion and value are clearly related, but remain distinct. This latter view is more prominent in current models of decision making.

What Is Emotion?

Prior to considering the role of emotion in decision making, it is necessary to define precisely what we mean by the term "emotion." Emotion is often discussed as a unitary concept in the decision-making literature, but there are clearly a number of components that should be differentiated if we are to understand the range of means by which it might impact our choices. How to best characterize the components or dimensions of emotion has been widely debated by psychologists and philosophers, and there is no clear agreement. As a working framework, we will refer to Scherer's (2000) model of emotion.

In Scherer's model, *emotion* refers to synchronized responses, which may include physiological activation, motor expression, subjective feeling, and action tendencies, that are triggered by internal or external events and which are of significance to the organism. *Mood* reflects a more diffuse, long-lasting, and likely less intense state and is characterized primarily by a change in subjective feeling. *Attitudes* are relatively enduring, affectively colored beliefs, preferences, and predispositions toward objects or persons. *Personality traits* are emotionally laden, stable dispositions, and behavioral tendencies typical for a person.

These four distinctions represent classes of states one might include under the term "emotion." Within each class, one might further differentiate specific types of responses or states, such as fear, happiness, sadness, or social emotions (e.g., guilt). Another common distinction in emotion research is to characterize reactions or states with dimensions, such as valence (i.e., positive or negative) and arousal (intensity). As this framework makes clear, the term "emotion" is often used to represent a class of processes, each of which might have a unique impact on decision making.

Current Models of Emotion and Decision Making

Dual Selves Models

One of the main ways that the impact of emotion on decision making has been characterized is to view emotion and cognition as two alternative means by which we can arrive at a choice. The notion that we can make choices with either our heart (emotion) or our head (reason) was first proposed in early philosophical writings, and this distinction persists to this day in common language use, legal reasoning, as well as scientific investigations. A primary contention of this dual selves approach is that emotion and reason compete with one another when arriving at a decision.

As the popularity of the dual selves model suggests, there is clearly some intuitive appeal in viewing decision making this way. However, there are also numerous problems which lead us to suggest that the model is simply too simplistic, as well as unrealistic, to capture the role of emotion in decision making.

For example, one function of emotion is to allow us to interact adaptively with our environment, thus avoiding situations that are dangerous or threatening and moving us toward choices that are likely to increase evolutionary fitness. Emotion plays an important role in the assignment of value. In this way, emotion is a critical component of models of decision making.

Another primary difficulty with the dual selves model is that it suggests a unitary role for emotion in decision making. As discussed below, there are several means by which different components of emotion can influence decisions, and no single characterization will suffice. Although one might argue that under some circumstances an emotional reaction might interfere with one's ability to reason about a decision, there are also several other ways that emotion might influence decisions. How cues from emotional reactions and states are integrated into the "rational" decision-making process has yet to be fully understood. There is, however, abundant evidence to suggest that the relation between emotion and reason in decision making is not simply competitive.

Somatic Marker Hypothesis

One model for emotion's role in decision making that has received considerable attention is the somatic marker hypothesis (Damasio 1996). Damasio and his collaborator Antoine Bechara suggest that emotion can provide a heuristic for decision making by associating physiological bodily reactions, called somatic markers, with specific choices or options (Bechara and Damasio 2005). When faced with a decision, the somatic marker allows one to assess the potential emotional consequences of a possible option without having to use reason. In this way, emotion provides a shortcut for fast, intuitive decisions and does not depend on deliberative assessment or awareness of potential outcomes. It is suggested that the ventral medial prefrontal cortex and the insular cortex play critical roles in representing somatic markers.

Although it is likely that physiological emotional reactions—and their learned associations with objects, persons, or potential outcomes—play an important role in decision making, there are several aspects of the somatic marker hypothesis that have not been supported by the data.

One problem relates to how the physiological response is mapped onto a particular choice. In the initial Bechara gambling task (Bechara et al. 1994), it was proposed that when considering a possible option, an increased physiological response (i.e., somatic marker) causes one to move away from that option (which is riskier and, ultimately, less rewarding) toward another that does not invoke as strong an emotional response. However, simply changing the order or outcomes of the possible options has been shown to lead to the opposite result; that is, a stronger physiological response for the preferred option (Tomb et al. 2002). In other words, somatic markers do not predict the appropriate action.

In addition, a dissociation between the physiological response and choice has been demonstrated in a number of studies. Patients who do not have a normal representation of bodily states perform normally on the Iowa gambling task used in the initial Bechara studies (Bechara et al. 1994). In addition, lesion evidence in rats suggests that the neural circuits mediating the physiological response to a conditioned fear stimulus are partially distinct from those mediating the decision to avoid the conditioned stimulus (Amorapanth et al. 2000).

Components of Emotion and Decisions

In spite of difficulties with some of the strong claims of the somatic marker hypothesis, one of the advances of this approach is that it considers the independent contribution of a specific component of emotion: the physiological response. This component approach has been extended in recent work by Lerner and colleagues (Lerner and Keltner 2001).

There is evidence, for example, that distinct emotional reactions, each of which leads to a similar physiological response and bodily state, can have the opposite effects on decision making. Despite years of investigation, researchers have been unable to detect clear differences in the physiological responses that characterize discrete emotional states, such as anger and fear. For this reason, and others, emotion researchers have suggested that an appraisal of the situation is an important component of the subjective qualities of an emotional response. Lerner and Keltner (2001) suggest that anger and fear, which elicit a similar physiological profile, can have opposite effects on the assessment of risk in decision making. Anger, along with happiness, results in less risk aversion, whereas fear leads to increased risk aversion. This effect was observed both when assessing anger and fear as personality traits and when experimentally manipulating mood. Lerner and Keltner (2001) suggest that this reflects differences in the cognitive sense of certainty and control between anger and fear. An alternative interpretation is that anger and fear promote different action tendencies (i.e., approach and avoid). In either case, it is clear that the physiological state alone cannot determine emotion's influence on the assessment of risk. In a related series of studies, Lerner and Lowenstein (2003) demonstrated that the induction of a sad or disgusted mood differentially influences the endowment effect, with a sad mood essentially reversing the endowment effect and a disgusted mood simply eliminating it.

Proposed Framework for Future Investigations of Emotion and Decision Making

As the studies by Lerner and colleagues cited above demonstrate, examination of the components of emotion reveals a range of effects on decision making, including opposite patterns depending on the specific emotional state. To date, much of the research on emotion and decision making has been rather imprecise in defining the specific aspects of emotion that are important. Given the range of processes and functions encompassed by the term emotion, future research on the neural mechanisms of emotion and decision making would benefit from a more precise characterization and assessment of emotion and its impact on specific aspects of decision making.

In addition, it is clear that decision making can also impact emotion. For instance, one can choose to engage in a cognitive strategy to regulate one's emotional state (i.e., the glass is half full). This choice may not only influence emotional reactions, but also subsequent decisions made while in this state. In addition, choosing an option can represent an investment in that option, which in turn can change its perceived value. Through processes such as cognitive dissonance, social psychologists have identified a range of means by which our choices will impact our attitudes and subsequent decisions. Clarifying the complex interactions of emotion and decision making, and the relation to value, is an important challenge for the future.

Finally, we suggest that an initial approach to understanding the mechanisms of emotion and decision making might be to link specific components of emotion to aspects of existing models of decision making. For instance, we suggest that specific emotional states and reactions elicit action tendencies, such as fear and withdrawal or anger and approach. In the context of the particular model of value-based decision making discussed above, these action tendencies are likely reflected in the motivational state in the native value system and forward model system (Dayan, this volume). Similarly, one might incorporate the impact of physiological arousal in the assessment of outcomes in this model or take advantage of a detailed description of emotion to further characterize components of the value-based model, such as behavioral vigor or the Pavlovian controller.

We have provided examples from only one model, but it is the approach that we wish to emphasize here. Although there are components of the mechanisms of emotion that are clearly distinct from those of decision making, there are likely several levels of integration. By emphasizing the integration of models of emotion and decision making in future research, we can avoid the implications of the intuitively appealing, but inaccurate, dual selves models which have dominated both the layperson's perceptions and research on emotion and decision making.

Conscious and Subliminal Decision Making

Defining and Measuring Conscious and Unconscious Processing

Descriptions of valuation and decision-making systems at the functional and neurophysiological levels often remain agnostic about whether these processes occur at a conscious or nonconscious level. To address this, we must find minimally different conditions in which availability of conscious information varies, measure the extent to which information is processed consciously and nonconsciously, and provide a means for measuring the influence of these processes on valuation and decision making (Dehaene, this volume).

There are, in fact, many ways to study the conscious/nonconscious contrast (e.g., blindsight, forgetting, hemi-neglect, masking, attentional blink). Typically, one compares two conditions that are as minimally different as possible, yet promote either conscious or nonconscious processing; for instance, a word followed by a mask (Kouider and Dehaene 2007). Asserting whether processing is or is not conscious, however, can be difficult. The key feature of conscious processing is the subjective awareness of an event. This is usually assessed by reportability; that is, the ability to give a verbal or nonverbal report or "commentary" on the event. However, when a subject is unable to report, there is no universal agreement that this indicates a lack of subjective awareness.

Nonetheless, reportability seems to be an excellent index of a major transition occurring in the availability of information for many tasks. For example, masking tasks require subjects to perform a discrimination as well as provide a verbal report about a stimulus followed by a mask. The delays between stimulus and mask determine reportability as well as discrimination performance on this task. Although subjects often perform better than chance when the stimulus remains subliminal, objective performance measures and subjective reportability share a similar threshold: a value of the delay beyond which stimulus information is available for discrimination, report, or, in fact, essentially any task (Del Cul et al. 2007).

Influence of Conscious and Subliminal Processing on Decision Making

Neurobiological evidence suggests that nonconscious events can influence the decision processes that integrate evidence favoring a particular motor response, as outlined above. For example, subliminal priming can evoke biased activation in motor structures associated with the behavioral report (Dehaene et al. 1998). Furthermore, changes in reaction time associated with subliminal processing can be explained by partial accumulation of evidence provided by the prime (e.g., Vorberg et al. 2003). These observations suggest that the temporal accumulation of sensory evidence can operate without conscious processing. Importantly, this can occur at a fairly high level of processing since subliminal primes can be processed in terms of their semantic content (Dehaene et al. 1998) or motivational value (Pessiglione et al. 2007). Recently, subliminal cues have even been found to influence executive-level processing such as task switching (Lau and Passingham 2007).

Despite the importance of nonconscious processing for decision making, items or events that enter awareness can differentially influence the decision process. Numerous differences between subliminal and conscious-level processing have been proposed (Dehaene and Naccache 2001). Subliminal primes typically have only a minimal subthreshold influence on behavior, altering task-related choices by a few tens of milliseconds and error rates by a few percent. This is compatible with the hypothesis that many if not all of the brain's evidence accumulation systems can begin to operate nonconsciously; however, it also suggests that crossing the threshold for a full-blown decision is often, if not always, associated with conscious-level processing. Usually, subliminal primes have a short-lived influence on decision processes that does not continue beyond a few hundreds of milliseconds; this suggests that active maintenance of information is somehow tightly correlated with conscious-level processing. Finally, there is evidence that some inferential and/or executive processes depend on conscious-level reflection. For example, if in a conflict task the prime conflicts with the target on a majority of trials, such that subjects can exploit prime information to anticipate an *opposite* target, this information can only influence the decision process when the prime is consciously perceived (Merikle and Joordens 1997). Conscious-level processing seems needed when the decision involves non-automatized changes in high-level processes; for instance, the strategic changes that adapt decision parameters such as the decision threshold from one trial to the next as a function of perceived task difficulty (the Gratton effect; see Kunde 2003).

Neural Systems Supporting Conscious and Nonconscious Processing

These observations raise the question of the neurobiological substrate of conscious and nonconscious processing. There is some evidence that conscious processing involves large-scale interactions between diverse brain areas, which may be evident in synchronized electrophysiological responses detectable on the scalp using EEG. Experiments exploiting the phenomenon of binocular rivalry suggest that access to conscious processing is associated with enhanced synchronization of neuronal responses (Fries et al. 1997, 2002; Tononi et al. 1998). This notion has received further support by the demonstration that the earliest electrographic correlate distinguishing conscious from nonconscious processing is a transient increase of precise phase synchronization of oscillatory activity in the gamma frequency range across a widely distributed network of cortical areas. This transient phase locking occurs around 180 ms after stimulus presentation and appears to be the trigger event gating the access of signals to the work space of consciousness (Singer 2007; Melloni et al. 2007). The subsequent transfer and maintenance of consciously processed information to working memory is accompanied by sustained oscillatory activity in the theta frequency range, again involving a widespread network of cortical areas, and by enhanced gamma oscillations during recall (Melloni et al. 2007). Dorsolateral prefrontal cortex is thought by many to be a key node for conscious processing and is frequently activated or found synchronized with posterior areas in fMRI contrasts of conscious/nonconscious processing. Intriguingly, electrophysiological markers for conscious processing take approximately 200 ms to develop and are therefore not evident in ERP components, such as the N170 (Del Cul et al. 2007; Sergent et al. 2005), but consciously processed stimuli lead to an enhanced P300 component which is considered as a correlate of the transfer of information to working memory (Melloni et al. 2007). Later, ERP components can be directly related to reportability using temporal accumulation models. Subliminal stimuli may fail to create enough cascading activation to activate large-scale circuits in an effective, coherent manner, and thus their effects on the decision process may be weaker and restricted to a small set of task-related processes.

An important open issue concerns the relation of these observations to top-down attentional control, which evokes similar patterns of neural activity. Attention and conscious processing are expected to share some features, since awareness requires selection of some events or stimuli over others. In this context, it is noteworthy that focused attention does not only lead to enhanced responses to the selected stimuli but also to an anticipatory entrainment of neuronal populations into coherent gamma oscillations (Fries et al. 2001). Despite this covariance, the neural mechanisms underlying attention and consciousness are separable.

Outstanding Questions Regarding Conscious and Nonconscious Processing

One question that we pondered was whether consciousness as a process might be construed or modeled as a nonconscious decision process to engage or report (Shadlen and Kiani 2007). Such an analogy might help to explain the apparent consistency between discrimination performance and reportability on a trial by trial basis observed in human subjects. This observation suggests that the representation of evidence and its accumulation are intact, whereas the policy that guides and implements decision termination is faulty. If conscious processing reflects an integration process for access to report, then one would predict that reportability and discrimination performance curves should be related by a criterion shift. This model could thus help to provide a description of a mechanism that can be linked to the neural correlates of conscious processing. Additional ideas suggest the importance of working memory in conscious processing. For example, working memory storage is more efficient for consciously perceived stimuli than those that remain subliminal.

One important question is to what degree such conscious processing, and its influence on decision making, is confined to humans. Addressing this question requires developing behavioral techniques that encourage subjective reportability in animals. This has been achieved in studies of binocular rivalry (Logothetis and Schall 1989) as well as blindsight (Cowey and Stoerig 1991). Such evidence supports the notion that some animals may process information both consciously and nonconsciously, but it remains to be determined whether there are quantitative differences between species or whether these differences might be qualitative.

Another relevant question relates to how we can provide a neurobiological understanding of the qualia of consciousness. There may be signatures in behavior, such as confidence ratings, that are measures of qualia. Formal models may permit us to determine whether qualia and reportability represent distinct aspects of the mechanisms associated with conscious processing.

A final question relates to the interfering effects of consciousness on decision making. In general, nonconscious processing is inefficient; in subliminal priming, for example, only a small subthreshold amount of information is available to bias decisions. However, certain tasks, such as swinging a baseball bat or searching for the name of the author of a paper from 1967, may be better performed without conscious awareness. Indeed, we may consciously banish such tasks to unconscious processing to solve them more efficiently. Understanding such nonconscious incubation phenomena and how they eventually lead to "aha" moments seems particularly important for understanding creativity and insight. When people engage in explicit, verbal reflection, this interferes with finding a solution by insight but does not interfere with solving logical problems using analytic techniques. Moreover, explicit, deliberative processing seems particularly disruptive for aesthetic judgments. Such observations suggest that conscious and nonconscious processes can be complementary and must be actively integrated, yet how these processes differ (what are the powers and limits of nonconscious processing) and what the neural mechanisms underlying these processes are remain to be explored. Further, just how these processes are related to habitual systems underlying valuation and decision making remains to be determined.

Accounting for Individual Differences in Decision Making: Sources of Heterogeneity in the Decision Process

An important, but unresolved, question is how we can account for differences in decision making between individuals, age groups, neurological conditions, and behavioral contexts. Perceptual and economics-based models provide two different but complementary approaches to address this issue.

Perceptual and Cognitive Decision Making

At the simplest level, differences in perceptual decision making can be usefully studied using the diffusion-to-bound model described above. This approach has been applied to individual and group differences in a range of experimental tasks, including numerosity discrimination, letter discrimination, brightness discrimination, recognition memory, and lexical decision. In all tasks except letter discrimination, the evidence extracted from stimuli is the same when performed by college students or 60–75 year olds (Ratcliff et al. 2006). In contrast, letter discrimination with masking shows a decrease in evidence accumulation with age because older adults progressively lose higher spatial frequency vision. There is a modest slowing of nondecision components with aging, but the main source of longer reaction times is the application of a more conservative decision criterion. In some discrimination tasks, model parameters change systematically with age during childhood (i.e., nondecision components speed up and decision criteria are reduced), whereas for other tasks there is a dramatic increase in drift rates by age 9 or 10. There is a range of drift-diffusion model parameters expressed in the neurologically intact young adult population.

This style of analysis can also be applied to behavioral changes associated with neurological disorders. For example, in lexical decision tasks, patients with aphasia show drift rates in the normal range, but their decision criteria is impaired relative to neurologically intact individuals. This suggests that the representation of evidence and its accumulation are intact, whereas the policy that guides and implements decision termination is faulty. Because similar models have been successfully applied to studies of the neuronal correlates of decision making, this approach shows great promise of directly linking individual differences in decision components to the underlying neurobiology.

Social and Economic Decision Making

Traditionally, economists have explained heterogeneity in observed behavior either through differences in preferences, differences in information sets, or the selection of different equilibrium strategies. Neuroscience can help document and further explain the sources of these differences, for example, by revealing the variances in information-processing strategies, computational capacity, or valuation systems. This will be enhanced by directly linking these variances to quantifiable components of the decision architecture revealed in neurophysiological studies.

One possible explanation for variance may be due to the heterogeneity of preferences or valuations in the brain. For example, in the gambling task depicted in Figure 6.1, person 1 must choose a or b, against Nature, N. In standard theory, we can talk about $U(10)$, $U(15)$, and $U(0)$ as the subjective utility of the monetary outcomes 0, 10, and 15. Assume Nature is governed by the following random process: play left with probability p and play right with probability $1 - p$. This can then be solved using an expected utility calculation:

$$U(10) = p^* \ U(15) + (1 - p \ ^*) \ U(0),$$

where $U' > 0$, $U'' < 0$, and p^* is chosen to give the equality. One reason people may show different patterns of choice in this situation (i.e., have different p^*) is because their preferences, U, may be different. Supporting this notion, parametric brain activation correlates of different preferences have been reported in the parietal cortex of people playing a gambling task (Huettel et al. 2006). Although the reasons why people might hold different utility function remains to be determined fully, it seems likely that genetic background, developmental trajectory, and context reactivity contribute to differences in the neural architecture that supports valuation, emotional responses, evidence accumulation, and the decision threshold setting mechanisms outlined above.

A second reason people make different decisions may be because they process information differently. In the voluntary trust game (Figure 6.2) by McCabe and Smith (2000), player 1 moves left 50% of the time. In response, player 2 moves right (reciprocated) 75% of the time in one-shot play. This occurs more frequently than predicted by the Nash equilibrium of player 1 always moving left and player 2 always moving right. For those players moving left, their estimated q must have been less than q^*, and for those moving right, their estimated q must have been greater than q^*.

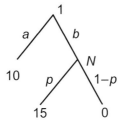

Figure 6.1 Gambling task: Choose *a* or *b* against Nature (*N*).

It is difficult to imagine that this strong reciprocity is simply the result of differences in risk aversion, but instead seems more likely to be due to social factors. For example, player 1 (who played right) may have thought that this would create a social obligation for player 2 to move left—a notion supported by behavioral observations in the involuntary trust game (Figure 6.3; McCabe et al. 2001). When player 1 is forced to move right and player 2 could not see player 1's foregone opportunity cost, player 2 was twice as likely to play right when compared to player 2's behavior in the voluntary trust game. Furthermore, McCabe et al. (2001) found that cooperators showed significantly greater activation in the anterior paracingulate cortex when playing other humans than when playing against a computer. This area has been found to be active in numerous fMRI experiments examining theory-of-mind (Gallagher and Frith 2003), suggesting social contexts and interactions promote approach behavior, engage reward systems in the brain, and encourage empathy and social reasoning.

A third reason people vary in their decisions could be due to the use of different strategies in playing the game. Krueger et al. (in preparation) look at repeat play of the voluntary trust game played by the same partners who alternated roles between player 1 and player 2. Consistent with earlier behavioral findings, they find that players can be divided into two types: unconditional and conditional cooperators. Intriguingly, these two types of cooperators exhibit different neural signatures in the brain. Thus, individual differences in decision making may arise from differences in strategy identified with distinct patterns of neural activity.

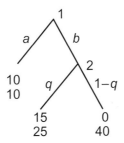

Figure 6.2 Trust game: Choose a or b against person 2.

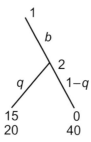

Figure 6.3 Involuntary trust game: Choose *a* or *b* against person 2.

The economic approach to understanding the heterogeneity of decisions made by different people or promoted by different contexts provides a tantalizing hint at the complexity underlying real-world social decisions. Despite the attractiveness of this approach, however, considerable questions remain unanswered. This reflects, in part, the relative maturity of neuroeconomics relative to the neurobiology of perceptual decision making. Importantly, although it is relatively easy to describe the equilibrium point in a game formally, it seems much harder to map this number onto underlying neurobiology. What would an equilibrium look like at the neurophysiological level? In social situations, there is an explosion of degrees of freedom that all must, ultimately, be reduced to a single quantity, the decision variable, in order to inform choice. How could an equilibrium be instantiated in a decision variable that is integrated over time to a threshold for commitment?

Extending Neuronal Models of Decision Making to Long Temporal Scales

It seems unlikely that simple accumulation models will be able to be extended to long timescales, such as decisions over hours or days. Over intermediate timescales, a model such as Busemeyer's decision field theory may apply (Busemeyer and Townsend 1993, 1995). For example, in buying a car, one may pay attention to different features of the stimulus (e.g., gas mileage, color, power). Decision field theory assumes that these features drive a single decision process—at each time step, one of the features drives the process towards one or the other possible options. Over tens of seconds or a few minutes, this seems a reasonable candidate that connects well to established models of perceptual decision making and to our current understanding of the neurophysiology in which the decision process is embodied.

However, in tasks that require minutes, hours, or days, (e.g., planning out a chess move, deciding whether to go to a conference, and so on), a decision will almost certainly involve multiple steps which take some information computed as intermediate products that are required by later stages for the final decision or choice. In addition, intermediate results will have to be stored and retrieved when the decision process is interrupted, for example, by boisterous children, work, or the television. Because the timescale can be long, behavior will depend on the combinations of the various stages of processing and not so much on the individual steps. Of course, in the range of a few seconds, behavior will be determined by the distribution of the individual decisions; however, when decision times are tens of seconds or longer, the organization of stages will then dominate. Connecting long timescale decision processes to the underlying neurobiology will require both reasoned computational modeling and improved understanding of the neural processes that permit information to be accumulated, stored, evaluated, and connected over long delays.

Evolution of Neural Architectures for Decision Making

As large-brained primates we often neglect the fact that quite complex decision making can be accomplished by much smaller and differently organized nervous systems. There is an enormous richness and complexity of behavior that appears to occur without any conscious processing. In fact, one might argue that such behaviors are better than conscious; that is, they are highly efficient, infallible, fast, and exquisitely adapted to a local environment. Although many of these behaviors reflect the ineluctable releasing of a motor pattern by a sign stimulus, many more behaviors appear to rely on flexible processes quite similar to those guiding behavior in humans and other vertebrates. These observations raise the important question of whether similar computational rules underlie the decision process when it is embodied in dramatically different nervous systems.

This complexity is demonstrated aptly by the behavior of the honeybee (Menzel et al. 2007). These diminutive volant insects use the well-known waggle dance to communicate navigational information to others in the hive. The dance can convey the location of nectar, pollen, resin, water, or a new nest site. How other bees interpret these signals varies with the vigor of the dance as well as each bee's current motivational state. Furthermore, the honeybee appears to interpret different destinations as options that can be weighed in terms of evidence bearing on their likelihood or their current value. When a foraging bee that has been trained to visit a feeding station is unexpectedly displaced, it displays search components in the direction of both the hive and the feeder, and ultimately chooses one or the other (Menzel et al. 2005). This behavior can be interpreted as each individual bee differentially investing in each of the possible options, before selecting one and committing to that action. Even more astonishing, bees appear to compute social decisions, in a process akin to voting, to choose a new nest site when swarming (Lindauer 1955).

Presently, we know little about how these processes are encoded in the honeybee brain. The bee brain includes an analog of the vertebrate dopamine system, the octopamine system, which apparently serves a similar role in value learning (Menzel and Giurfa 2001). How this valuation system might influence valuation and decision processes carried out elsewhere in the bee brain remains to be studied. One clue to the design of the neural architecture supporting value-based decisions in both vertebrates and invertebrates is that neuromodulatory systems such as dopamine and octopamine project widely and appear to broadcast a message related to values and emotions of a single class (e.g., appetitive, aversive; Schultz and Dickinson 2000). Similar principles characterize the serotonergic, cholinergic, and norepinephrine systems, which appear to promote changes in the value of different options or behavioral strategies. In this scheme, the message computed by any individual neuron may change with respect to the weighting of inputs and channeling of outputs by altering modulatory states. Future progress in understanding the principles governing decision making and how the decision process is embodied in large networks of neurons in humans and other vertebrates will profit from an understanding of how decision making is accomplished by a limited number of highly specialized neurons in the invertebrate nervous system (Menzel and Giurfa 2006). In particular, one may ask whether the computational role of individual neurons embedded in their anatomical and functional network may change with modulatory states and expected outcomes.

Extending Neuronal Models of Decision Making to Legal Issues and Group Processes

Can an understanding of the neurobiology of decision making have clear implications for decision making at the group or institutional level?

Institutions are humanly devised formal (rules, laws, constitutions) or informal (norms of behavior, conventions, and self imposed codes of conduct) constraints that govern the behavior of two or more individuals (North 1990). These constraints define the incentive structure of societies and, specifically, economies. Institutions are a central concern for law, which serves as the formal regime for political rule making and enforcement. In general, understanding the neurobiology of decision making could be important for understanding how institutions have evolved over time (see McElreath et al., this volume), as well as how institutions impact human decision making (e.g., judge and jury decision making) and behavior (see Lubell et al., this volume). At the present time, it is not possible to state whether neurobiology can ultimately help us reach a better understanding of institutional decision making. However, in the following sections, we explore current neuroscientific data and their potential impacts on institutional decision making.

Evolution and Formulation of Institutions and Neural Models of Decision Making

Although institutions may be deliberately and intentionally formulated by people, the evolution and function of institutions might be better understood as emergent phenomena. In other words, institutions evolve and operate in a fashion that cannot be predicted from the decisions made by any single individual. If institutions are truly emergent, this raises the important questions of what we can learn from neurobiological or behavioral studies in animals to explain how institutions have evolved (see McElreath et al., this volume) and whether neurobiology can inform the formulation of rules by political and legal institutions to promote desired social behavior.

These questions have begun to be addressed explicitly in the realm of public policy. As we have discussed in this report, motivation and emotion contribute in important ways to decision making; thus, understanding how the cognitive control of motivation and emotion is implemented in the brain might provide important insights for institutional decision making. If, for example, a society wishes to regulate a particular form of undesirable behavior, knowledge of the neural mechanisms underlying cognitive control may provide important insights in developing legal rules to achieve this goal. Ochsner and Gross (2005), for example, have proposed that cognitive control of emotional states requires both attentional selection of information and cognitive modulation of emotional processes; that is, processes which appear to be implemented by distinct neural systems. To the extent that this model provides an accurate description of the neurobiology of cognitive control, different types of legal rules might be developed to engage these different systems differentially in order to attain desirable goals. In a similar vein, Bernheim and Rangel (2004) recently applied current understanding of the neurobiology of addiction to the formulation of better economic policies on addictive substances. These models suggest that neurobiological understanding, when thoughtfully applied, may positively inform public policy making.

Legal Decision Making and Neural Models of Decision Making

Understanding the neuronal correlates of decision making may also impact how we address the problem of determining culpability and setting standards of punishment in the legal system. Clearly, people's actions (i.e., the outcome of their decisions) are determined by processes that occur in their brains. This obvious fact raises the troubling question of whether we are responsible for our actions, and it has clear implications for attributing agency and assigning punishment.

The problem can be illustrated by the difference in culpability one would ascribe to a defendant who impulsively acts out his aggression against another person due to a large brain tumor in the medial prefrontal cortex. In this case, most people would not hold the defendant responsible for his actions. Contrast this situation with a defendant who commits the same act due to a nonobvious change in neural circuitry as a result of environmental or physiological deficits that arose during development, subliminal brain injury, or genetic factors. Whether this defendant should be treated any differently under the law than the defendant with the obvious brain tumor is a highly contentious and hotly debated issue. Yet, as evidence accumulates favoring the idea that brain states reflect the interaction of genes and environmental influences during development, which means they are thus out of the control of the individual, this legal problem will become thornier indeed. Witness the interaction between the expression of different genetic variants involved in neuromodulatory function (e.g., monoamine oxidase A, serotonin transporter gene), developmental stress, and likelihood of being incarcerated for violence (Caspi et al. 2002).

It is perhaps worth considering the various goals of the legal system in this regard. If the goal is to mitigate the risk of recidivism, then scientific evidence supporting a clear relationship between broken connections among genes, brains, and appropriate action should play an important role in the legal process. If the goal of the legal system is, however, to determine moral agency and thus culpability for antisocial behaviors (perhaps to deter such behaviors in the society) absent of preventing future illegal behavior, then the utility of neuroscientific evidence becomes less clear. Current models of perceptual- and value-based decision making may help guide the assessment of neuroscientific evidence favoring a link between genes, development, brain states, and action. Yet even as neuroscience begins to explain the mental capacities that underlie agency, motivation, and initiative—and hence responsibility and free will—it does not explain away these phenomena. Insights from neurobiology may *augment* the discussion of such legal concepts as negligence, but it should not override traditional approaches.

Conclusions

Neurobiologists now understand, in great detail, how simple decisions are made by individual neurons and groups of neurons in several well-defined experimental contexts. This understanding has proceeded from the simultaneous application of formal computational models to both behavior and the activity patterns of individual neurons. This achievement was unthinkable fifty years ago, and thus we should feel optimistic that even more progress will be made over the next half century. Despite this optimism, significant challenges remain. Most importantly, a wide gulf remains between the simple decisions typically studied in the laboratory and the complex decisions made in the real world. Bridging this gap will require concerted integration across multiple disciplines and levels of analysis. This has already begun in the fields of neuroscience, psychology, and economics, but only a brave few have crossed the chasms separating these fields from anthropology, evolutionary biology, political science, and the law. Equally important to dispel natural fears of a brave new world of biological determinism and moral ambiguity, our boldness in crossing these boundaries must be bolstered by the quality of our science and the care with which our conclusions are communicated to the wider community.

References

Amorapanth, P., J. E. LeDoux, and K. Nadar. 2000. Different lateral amygdala outputs mediate reactions and actions elicited by a fear-arousing stimulus. *Nature Neurosci.* **3(1)**:74–79.

Bechara, A., and A. R. Damasio. 2005. The Somatic Marker Hypothesis: A Neural Theory of Economic Decision. *Games Econ. Behav.* **52**: 336–372.

Bechara, A., A. R. Damasio, H. Damasio, and S. W. Anderson. 1994. Insensitivity to future consequences following damage to human prefrontal cortex. *Cognition* **50**:7–15.

Bendiksby, M. S. and M. L. Platt 2006. Neural correlates of reward and attention in macaque area LIP. *Neuropsychologia* **44(12)**:2411–2420.

Bernheim, B. D., and A. Rangel. 2004. Addiction and cue-triggered decision processes. *Am. Econ. Rev.* **94(5)**:1558-1590.

Berridge, K. C., and T. E. Robinson. 2003. Parsing reward. *Trends Neurosci.* **26(9)**:407–513.

Busemeyer, J., and J. Townsend. 1995. Decision field theory. In: Mind as Motion, ed. R. Port and T. van Gelder. Cambridge, MA: MIT Press.

Busemeyer, J. R., and J. T. Townsend. 1993. Decision field theory: A dynamic-cognitive approach to decision making in an uncertain environment. *Psychol. Rev.* **100(3)**:432–459.

Caspi, A., J. McClay, T. E. Moffitt, et al. 2002. Role of genotype in the cycle of violence in maltreated children. *Science* **297(5582)**:851–854.

Cohen, J. D. 2005. The vulcanization of the human brain: A neural perspective on interactions between cognition and emotion. *J. Econ. Persp.* **4**:3–24.

Cosmides, L., and J. Tooby. 2000. Evolutionary psychology and the emotions. In: Handbook of Emotions (2nd ed.), ed. M. Lewis and J. M. Haviland-Jones, pp. 91–115. New York: Guliford.

Cowey, A. and P. Stoerig. 1991. The neurobiology of blindsight. *Trends Neurosci.* **14(4)**:140–145.

Damasio, A. R. 1996. The somatic marker hypothesis and the possible functions of the prefrontal cortex. *Phil. Trans. Roy. Soc. Lond. B* **351(1346)**:1413–1420.

Daw, N. D., S. Kakde, and P. Dayan. 2002. Opponent interactions between serotonin and dopamine. *Neural Networks* **15(4-6)**:603–616.

Dehaene, S. 2007. Symbols and quantities in parietal cortex: Elements of a mathematical theory of number representation and manipulation. In: Attention and Performance XXII. Sensorimotor Foundations of Higher Cognition, ed. P. Haggard and Y. Rossetti. Cambridge, MA.: Harvard Univ. Press, in press

Dehaene, S. and L. Naccache 2001. Towards a cognitive neuroscience of consciousness: Basic evidence and a workspace framework. *Cognition* **79**:1–37.

Dehaene, S., L. Naccache, G. H. Le Clec, et al. 1998. Imaging unconscious semantic priming. *Nature* **395**:597–600.

Del Cul, A., S. Baillet, and S. Dehaene. 2007. Brain dynamics underlying the non-linear threshold for access to consciousness. *PLoS Biol.*, in press.

Ding, L., and O. Hikosaka. 2006. Comparison of reward modulation in the frontal eye field and caudate of the macaque. *J. Neurosci.* **26(25)**:6695–6703.

Fries, P., J. H. Reynolds, A. E. Rorie, and R. Desimone. 2001. Modulation of oscillatory neuronal synchronization by selective visual attention. *Science* 291:1560–1563.

Fries, P., P. R. Roelfsema, A. K. Engel, P. König, P., and W. Singer. 1997. Synchronization of oscillatory responses in visual cortex correlates with perception in interocular rivalry. *Proc. Natl. Acad. Sci.* 94:12,699–12,704.

Fries, P., J. H. Schröder, P. R. Roelfsema, W. Singer, and A. K. Engel. 2002. Oscillatory neuronal synchronization in primary visual cortex as a correlate of stimulus selection. *J. Neurosci.* **22(9)**:3739–3754.

Gallagher, H. L., and C. D. Frith. 2003. Functional imaging of "theory of mind." *Trends Cogn. Sci.* **7(2)**:77–83.

Glimcher, P. W. 2003. The neurobiology of visual saccadic decision making. *Ann. Rev. Neurosci.* **26**:133–179.

Glimcher, P. W. 2005. Indeterminacy in Brain and Behavior. *Ann. Rev. Psychol.* **56**:25–56.

Gold, J. I., and M. N. Shadlen. 2007. The neural basis of decision making. *Ann. Rev. Neurosci.* **30**:535–574.

Heekeren, H. R., S. Marrett, P. A. Bandettini, and L. G. Ungerleider. 2004. A general mechanism for perceptual decision making in the human brain. *Nature* **431**:859–862.

Horwitz, G. D., and W. T. Newsome. 2001. Target selection for saccadic eye movements: Prelude activity in the superior colliculus during a direction-discrimination task. *J. Neurophysiol.* **86**:2543–2558.

Huettel, S. A., C. J. Stowe, E. M. Gordon, B. T. Warner, and M. L. Platt. 2006. Neural signatures of economic preferences for risk and ambiguity. *Neuron* 49:765–775.

Huk, A. C., and M. N. Shadlen. 2005. Neural activity in macaque parietal cortex reflects temporal integration of visual motion signals during perceptual decision making. *J. Neurosci.* 25:10,420–10,436.

Kim, J.-N., and M. N. Shadlen. 1999. Neural correlates of a decision in the dorsolateral prefrontal cortex of the macaque. *Nature Neurosci.* **2(2)**:176–185.

Kouider, S., and S. Dehaene. 2007. Levels of processing during non-conscious perception: A critical review of visual masking. *Phil. Trans. R. Soc. Lond. B* **362(1481)**:857–875.

Kunde, W. 2003. Sequential modulations of stimulus-response correspondence effects depend on awareness of response conflict. *Psychon. Bull. Rev.* **10(1)**:198–205.

Lau, H. C., and R. E. Passingham. 2007. Unconscious activation of the cognitive control system in the human prefrontal cortex. *J. Neurosci.* **27(21)**:5805–5811.

LeDoux, J. E. 1996. The Emotional Brain. New York: Simon and Schuster.

Lerner, J.S., and D. Keltner. 2001. Fear, anger, and risk. *J. Pers. Soc. Psychol.* **81**:146–159.

Lowenstein, G. A., and J. S. Lerner. 2003. The role of affect in decision making. In: Handbook of Affective Sciences, ed. R. J. Davidson, K. R. Scherer, and H. H. Goldsmith. Oxford: Oxford Univ. Press.

Lindauer, M. 1955. Schwarmbienen auf Wohnungssuche. *Physiol.* 37:263–324.

Logothetis, N. K., and J. D. Schall. 1989. Neuronal correlates of subjective visual perception. *Science* **45(4919)**:761–763.

Luce, R. D. 1959. Individual Choice Behavior: A Theoretical Analysis. New York: Wiley.

Luce, R. D., and P. Suppes. 1965. Preference, utility, and subjective probability. In: Handbook of Mathematical Psychology, vol. 3. ed. R. Luce, R. Bush, and E. Galanter, New York: Wiley.

Machens, C. K., R. Romo, and C. D. Brody. 2005. Flexible control of mutual inhibition: A neural model of two-interval discrimination. *Science* **307(5712)**:1121–1124.

Manski, C. 1977. The Structure of Random Utility Models. *Theory and Decision* **8**:229–254.

Maynard Smith, J. 1982. Evolution and the Theory of Games. Cambridge: Cambridge Univ. Press.

Mazurek M. E., J. D. Roitman, J. Ditterich, and M. N. Shadlen. 2003. A role for neural integrators in perceptual decision making. *Cerebral Cortex* **13**:1257–1269.

McCabe, K., and V. L. Smith. 2000. A two person trust game played by naïve and sophisticated subjects. Proc. Natl. Acad. Sci. **(97)7**:3777–3781.

McCabe, K., D. Houser, L. Ryan, V. Smith, and T. Trouard. 2001. A functional imaging study of cooperation in two-person reciprocal exchange. Proc. Natl. Acad. Sci. **98**:11,832–11,835.

Melloni, L., C. Molina, M. Pena, D. Torres, W. Singer, and E. Rodriguez. 2007. Synchronization of neural activity across cortical areas correlates with conscious perception. *J. Neurosci.* **27(11)**:2858–2865.

Menzel, R., B. Brembs, and M. Giurfa. 2007. Cognition in invertebrates. In: Evolution of Nervous Systems, vol. II: Evolution of Nervous Systems in Invertebrates, ed. J. H.Kaas, chapter 1.26, pp. 403–422. Oxford: Academic Press.

Menzel, R., and Giurfa, M. 2001. Cognitive architecture of a mini-brain: The honeybee. *Trends Cogn. Sci.* **5**:62–71.

Menzel, R., and Giurfa, M. 2006. Dimensions of cognition in an insect, the honeybee. *Behav. Cogn. Neurosci. Rev.* **5**:24–40.

Menzel, R., U. Greggers, A. Smith, S. Berger, R. Brandt et al. 2005. Honey bees navigate according to a map-like spatial memory. *Proc. Natl. Acad. Sci.* **102(8)**:3040–3045.

Merikle, P. M., and S. Joordens. 1997. Parallels between perception without attention and perception without awareness. *Conscious Cogn.* **6(2–3)**:219–236.

Niv, Y., N. D. Daw, D. Joel, and P. Dayan. 2006. Tonic dopamine: Opportunity costs and the control of response vigor. *Psychopharm.* **191(3)**:507–520.

North, D. C. 1990. A Transaction cost theory of politics. Washington, St. Louis: School of Business and Political Economy, Papers 144.

Ochsner, K. N., and J. J. Gross. 2005. The cognitive control of emotion. *Trends Cogn. Sci.* **9(5)**:242–249.

Parker, A. J., and W. T. Newsome. 1998. Sense and the single neuron: Probing the physiology of perception. *Ann. Rev. Neurosci.* **21**:227–277.

Pessiglione, M., L. Schmidt, B. Draganski, et al. 2007. How the brain translates money into force: A neuroimaging study of subliminal motivation. *Science* **316(5826)**:904–906.

Platt, M. L., and P. W. Glimcher. 1999. Neural correlates of decision variables in parietal cortex. *Nature* **400(6741)**:233–238.

Ratcliff, R. 1978. A theory of memory retrieval. *Psychol. Rev.* **85**:59–108.

Ratcliff, R., A. Cherian, and M. Segraves. 2003. A comparison of macaque behavior and superior colliculus neuronal activity to predictions from models of two-choice decisions. *J. Neurophysiol.* **90(3)**:1392–1407.

Ratcliff, R., A. Thapar, and G. McKoon. 2006. Aging and individual differences in rapid two-choice decisions. *Psychon. Bull. Rev.* **13(4)**:626–635.

Roesch, M. R., and C. R. Olson. 2003. Impact of expected reward on neuronal activity in prefrontal cortex, frontal and supplementary eye fields and premotor cortex. *J. Neurophysiol.* **90(3)**:1766–1789.

Roitman, J. D., and M. N. Shadlen. 2002. Response of neurons in the lateral intraparietal area during a combined visual discrimination reaction time task. *J. Neurosci.* **22(21)**:9475–9489.

Romo, R., A. Hernández, and A. Zainos. 2004. Neuronal correlates of a perceptual decision in ventral premotor cortex. *Neuron* **41(1)**:165–173.

Romo, R., and E. Salinas. 2003. Flutter discrimination: Neural codes, perception, memory and decision making. *Nature Rev. Neurosci.* **4**:203–218.

Scherer, K. R. 2000. Psychological models of emotion. In: The Neuropsychology of Emotion, ed. J. C. Borod, pp. 137–163. New York: Oxford Univ. Press.

Schultz, W., and A. Dickinson. 2000. Neuronal coding of prediction errors. *Ann. Rev. Neurosci.* **23**:473–500.

Sergent, C., S. Baillet, and S. Dehaene. 2005. Timing of the brain events underlying access to consciousness during the attentional blink. *Nature Neurosci.* **8(10)**:1391–1400.

Shadlen, M. N., and R. Kiani. 2007. Neurology: An awakening. *Nature* **448**:539–540.

Shadlen, M. N., and W. T. Newsome. 1994. Noise, neural codes and cortical organization. *Curr. Opin. Neurobiol.* **4**:569–579.

Shadlen, M. N., and W. T. Newsome. 1998. The variable discharge of cortical neurons: Implications for connectivity, computation and information coding. *J. Neurosci.* **18**:3870–3896.

Shadlen, M. N., and W. T. Newsome. 2001. Neural basis of a perceptual decision in the parietal cortex (area LIP) of the rhesus monkey. *J. Neurophysiol.* **86**:1916–1936.

Siegler, R. S. 1988. Strategy choice procedures and the development of multiplication skill. *J. Exp. Psychol.: Gen.* **117(3)**:258–275.

Sigman, M., and S. Dehaene. 2005. Parsing a cognitive task: A characterization of the mind's bottleneck. *PLoS Biol* **3(2)**:e37 doi:10.1371.

Sigman, M., and S. Dehaene. 2006. Dynamics of the central bottleneck: Dual-task and task uncertainty. *PLoS Biol* **4(7)**:e220 doi:10.1371.

Singer, W. 2007. Large-scale temporal coordination of cortical activity as a prerequisite for conscious experience. In: The Blackwell Companion to Consciousness, ed. M. Velmans and S. Schneider, pp. 605–615. Oxford: Blackwell.

Smith, P. L., and R. Ratcliff. 2004. Psychology and neurobiology of simple decisions. *Trends Neurosci.* **27**:161-168.

Sugrue, L. P., G. S. Corrado, and W. T. Newsome. 2004. Matching behavior and the representation of value in the parietal cortex. *Science* **304(5678)**:1782–1787.

Tononi, G., R. Srinivasan, D. P. Russell, and G. M. Edelman. 1998. Investigating neural correlates of conscious perception by frequency-tagged neuromagnetic responses. *Proc. Natl. Acad. Sci.* **95**:3198–3203.

Tomb, I., M. Hauser, P. Deldin, and A. Caramazza. 2002. Do somatic markers mediate decisions on the gambling task? *Nature Neurosci.* **5(11)**:1103–1104.

Vorberg, D., U. Mattler, A. Heinecke, et al. 2003. Different time courses for visual perception and action priming. *Proc. Natl. Acad. Sci.* **100(10)**:6275–6280.

Wang, X. J. 2002. Probabilistic decision making by slow reverberation in cortical circuits. *Neuron* **36(5)**:955–968.

Wong, K. F., and X. J. Wang. 2006. A recurrent network mechanism of time integration in perceptual decisions. *J. Neurosci.* **26(4)**:1314–1328.

7

The Evolution of Implicit and Explicit Decision Making

Robert Kurzban

Department of Psychology, University of Pennsylvania,
Philadelphia PA 19104, U.S.A.

ABSTRACT

In the history of psychology, the relative attention paid to implicit versus explicit processes has fluctuated dramatically. Since the time of the structuralist school of thought, when the methodological commitment to introspection left little room for implicit processes, the pendulum has swung in the opposite direction. The rise of cognitive science has seen a steady, even inexorable rise in the importance attached to implicit processes. Here it will be argued that, evolutionarily, implicit cognitive processes antedate explicit processes, which might be phylogenetically quite recent. Two questions are distinguished. First, why did explicit *kinds* of mechanisms evolve? The answer to this question is very difficult, and possibly intractable without a compelling theory of consciousness, which at this point seems to be at best debatable and at worst absent in psychological thinking. Second, why did the *particular systems, which seem to be (or, perhaps, happen to be) explicit*, evolve? In other words, what are the functions of particular explicit systems? The answer to this question directs attention to the possible functions of explicit systems. It is suggested that the answers to these questions might be found in the answers to questions about the functions of (natural) language, social learning, and strategic social interaction.

Distinguishing Implicit and Explicit Cognition

Though debate continues about the best way to articulate the distinction between "implicit" and "explicit" computations (see, e.g., Keysers et al., this volume), there are themes sufficiently common among commentators to sketch the locus of the difference. Cognitive procedures are said to be "explicit" when they are associated with "awareness," "consciousness," or, somewhat less precisely, a sense of "control" of the procedure (see Dienes and Perner, 1999, and associated commentaries), and these terms will be used somewhat interchangeably here. Procedures are implicit when they are not associated with any of these and will be referred to here as "unconscious" or "outside of awareness."

Examples at the extremes are perhaps most illustrative. The formation of a visual image requires a great deal of processing, including identifying lines, shapes, and objects in the visual field. These low-level visual computations are executed without awareness, consciousness, control, or attention. People are aware of a visual scene but unaware of the complex operations that constructed it. Neither aware of these low-level processes nor conscious of the computations performed, it is difficult to imagine "choosing" to see no edges or changing the algorithm by which edges are detected. A similar and often-used example is grammaticality judgments in one's native tongue. People are often able to judge *that* a sentence is ungrammatical while being unaware and unable to articulate *why* it is or *which* rule has been violated (Pinker 1994).

At the other end might be experiences such as playing chess, in which there is a strong phenomenological sense of directing one's attention to the task, considering possible moves (and one's opponent's countermoves), and entertaining hypothetical trajectories of play. Importantly, during one's reflection on one's move, if one were asked to report about the process, it would be reasonable to expect that the player could, with reasonable accuracy, report their thoughts: "I am considering castling, queen side, which has the strategic advantage of protecting my king and the tactical advantage of protecting my queen's pawn, which is currently threatened."

This continuum is not meant to imply that there is no dynamic element. Some processes, for example, might begin at one end of the spectrum and, through learning, finish at the other. The case of motor learning, such as the mastery of a musical instrument, would be one such example (Keysers et al., this volume).

I begin with a brief review of the historical development of this distinction, ending with a discussion of the current state of the art. In particular, the functions of implicit and explicit cognitive systems are discussed, with a focus on what inferences one can draw once one knows whether a given system is operating implicitly or explicitly. Starting from this foundation, it is possible to begin to address the potentially difficult question about the evolution of these two different kinds of computational systems, which in turn leads to two different questions. The first, which is potentially counterintuitive, is why explicit cognition evolved at all. To foreshadow, the answer to this question will be disappointing, as it will be argued that current understanding does not afford any tidy answers to this question. The second question is why specific explicit systems evolved, looking at the functions of systems that are known (or at least thought) to be involved in explicit decision making. After discussing some possible (kinds of) answers to the second question, I conclude with some suggestions about which questions will prove fruitful in subsequent investigations of the evolution of implicit and explicit decision making. Here the emphasis is on articulating the functions of explicit decision-making systems, with an eye toward discerning commonalities among them in an effort to explain why these systems—but not others—are associated with attention, awareness, and "consciousness" (for a lucid discussion of these distinctions at the neurophysiological level, see Dehaene et al. 2006).

An Explicit History

The history of the role of implicit mental processes in science can be thought of as a journey with two peaks. It begins, appropriately enough, in the floor of a valley, with implicit processes having little or no role. The work of Wundt and the structuralist school, to a first approximation, took conscious (explicit) processes to be the topic of study of psychology. The emphasis on introspection as a method carried the clear implication that whatever it was that was the object of study, it was something to which one could, in principle, have conscious access. Though somewhat different in flavor, William James (1890) had a similar confidence that consciousness was the proper study of the psychologist.

The emergence of interest in nonconscious processes in the beginning of the twentieth century can be multiply attributed to, but is most famously associated with, the works of Freud. According to Freud, individuals are not (currently) conscious of any number of things. These included pedestrian elements (e.g., names and events not currently relevant to the individual) but also, and more importantly for Freud, "primitive" thoughts and desires repressed and kept out of conscious thought by the suite of defense mechanisms familiar to students of psychoanalysis (e.g., projection, sublimation).

Broadly concurrent with Freudianism, though with arguably a longer half-life (at least outside the clinic), the rise of Behaviorism led to the decline of the unconscious in the scientific study of psychology. Because (classical) behaviorism, in the tradition of John Watson, was skeptical of the utility of studying the activity in organisms' brains, both conscious processes and unconscious processes tended not to be the subject of theorizing. Research in this tradition has, of course, undergone considerable change (e.g., Rescorla 1990).

From this valley, the so-called "cognitive revolution" elevated unconscious processes to heights even greater than under Freudianism. The view of the mind as a computer—taking in (sensory) information, operating on it, and generating (behavioral) output—put both explicit and implicit processes in play. Cognitive science not only made the workings of the brain a legitimate topic of study, but provided a language—that of computation—to talk about it.

The relative importance placed on the two types of processes has, perhaps unsurprisingly, been the source of considerable disagreement and dramatic change over time in the psychological community. To give a sense of the trajectory of the weight accorded to nonconscious processes, in an important milestone in the study of implicit processes, Kihlstrom (1987, p. 1445) claimed that, at the time he was writing, "many psychologists...have been reluctant to admit that nonconscious mental structures and processes are psychologically important" but concluded by emphasizing the potentially critical role played by the "cognitive unconscious."

The increasingly important role accorded to nonconscious processes has been boosted by many seminal studies and papers. One of these was Nisbett and Wilson's (1977) review of people's ability to report on aspects of the processes underlying their decision making. Among other research discussed was a field study in which people were asked to choose which of four identical pairs of panty hose they liked best. The right-most pair was most frequently selected, but the people making the choice never indicated that the position was the causal antecedent of their choice, citing instead some feature of the panty hose. Nisbett and Wilson concluded from this, and a wealth of other data accumulated, that "...there may be little or no direct introspective access to higher order cognitive processes" (Nisbett and Wilson 1977, p. 231).

A second paper, published at about the same time, investigated "split brain" patients whose corpus collosum, which connects the two hemispheres, had been severed (Gazzaniga and LeDoux 1978). Because of the way that the sensory system is wired, each hemisphere could be provided with different information. In this case, a chicken claw was shown to the left hemisphere, which controls speaking, while a wintry scene was presented to the right hemisphere. When faced with an array of objects and asked to point to one related to what they observed, the patients' left hand pointed to a shovel, which is logical given the image presented to the right hemisphere (which controls the left hand). For present purposes, the crucial finding is that when asked to explain the reason for the choices, the patient reported that the shovel is related to what was seen because it was for cleaning up after the chickens (Gazzaniga and LeDoux 1978). This illustrates that people are quite willing to tell a narrative to explain their actions even when this narrative cannot possibly be the causal locus of their behavior (e.g., Gazzaniga 1998). Of course, this is a patient population, but it mirrors Nisbett and Wilson's (1977) findings above, and thus can be expected to occur in nonpatient populations as well (Hirstein 2005).

Finally, Libet et al. (1983) asked participants to perform a simple motor movement—a flick of the wrist—at a moment of their choosing. Using a clever experimental design, the researchers were able to look at the temporal relationship between the neural activity that occurred as the act was initiated and the participant's awareness that they wished to initiate the movement. As Libet (1999, p. 49) later said: "In the traditional view of conscious will and free will, one would expect conscious will to appear before, or at the onset, of RP" (or readiness potential, i.e., the electrical activity in the brain that indicates the initiation of the activity). Leaving aside for the moment the seemingly dualist notion that a mental act ("conscious will") could occur *before* associated neural activity, the finding was that subjective awareness followed the onset of the electrical activity initiating the event by roughly 400 milliseconds. Again in Libet's (1999, p. 50) terms, the "brain initiates [the] voluntary act unconsciously." (For further discussion, see Glimcher, this volume.)

Modern Views

These classic experiments and others have changed the modern conception of the role of implicit, unconscious processes. From their humble origins as beneath the notice of the founders of modern psychology, they have come to loom larger than even Freud would have had them. This change is perhaps best illustrated by Timothy Wilson's (2002) recent book, in which he calls attention to estimates of the information that impinges on the senses that are on the order of millions per second, while estimates of conscious processing suggest that capacity is roughly 40 per second. In the domain of reasoning, of focal interest here, it has been suggested that the vast majority is performed by implicit processes (Oaksford and Chater 2001, p. 356).

Taken together with evidence that information obtained from the world can have important effects about which people cannot report, this leaves open the possibility that early accounts of consciousness got it nearly exactly backwards, and that far from being the focus of psychology, conscious processes might be not only the tip of the iceberg, but in fact a very, very small tip, with implicit processing responsible for the overwhelming majority of computation. This view makes it important to look in more detail at what is known about each of these kinds of cognition.

Explicit and Implicit Processes

Properties and Functions of Explicit and Implicit Processes

The distinction between explicit and implicit systems has come under a number of labels and is often considered to be a subspecies of so-called "dual process" models. Some researchers, for example, have preferred to use the somewhat neutral appellation of system 1 (akin to implicit) and system 2 (akin to explicit) (Stanovich and West 2000). Independent of the terminology, there is relatively broad (though not complete) agreement about the properties of these two systems. This field represents a vast research enterprise, and thus the overview presented here should be considered an approximation of current thinking, as views and terms differ across disciplines and researchers.

Very generally, the implicit system is taken to be evolutionarily older, automatic and fast in operation, and divided into multiple, distinguishable subsystems which operate in parallel. These systems are broadly understood to be domain specific, having relatively narrow functions, and include at least a large fraction of the sensory systems. They are sometimes considered to be relatively "inflexible," an entailment of their automatic operation.

In contrast, the explicit system is evolutionarily more recent, perhaps "uniquely human" (Evans 2003, p. 454). It is often referred to as more "unitary" than the implicit system, subject to conscious (or volitional) control, capable of responding to instructions in natural language, and operating in a more serial fashion. Many researchers link the explicit system to particular cognitive systems such as working memory, which is taken to operate serially, with a particular capacity, integrating information from multiple sources; this in part contributes to the claim that the explicit system tends to be slower in operation than the implicit system but capable of more abstract representations. Anatomically, these systems are believed to reside in the evolutionarily more recent areas of the brain.

These properties can be understood in the context of the putative functions of these different systems. Acting quickly and in parallel, the implicit system allows fast response to the immediate environment by taking in information, sorting its relevance, and organizing potential adaptive responses. The explicit system, in contrast, integrates slowly but more meticulously information to generate conclusions and plans. The functional relationship between these two systems is also a subject of debate. One prominent possibility is that the explicit system, at least in part, can inhibit the implicit systems to facilitate accuracy at the expense of speed.

What Can Be Concluded from the Implicit/Explicit Distinction?

Before discussing the evolution of implicit and explicit systems, it is worth clarifying what *logical inferences* can be drawn about computational systems, when one knows that a particular system is implicit or explicit. For example, does the fact that, on present understanding, explicit systems tend to integrate information or compute more "globally" imply that any system with this feature or function will necessarily be explicit? In other words, given the empirical observations about the operations of systems that are explicit, what can we, as a matter of logical deduction, broadly conclude about such systems?

The answer is: unfortunately, not very much. First, the puzzling claim by Libet above suggests the necessity of a brief digression into physicalism, the rejection of dualism (Bloom 2004). That is, as essentially every cognitive scientist would agree (explicitly, if not implicitly), the mind is just the body, and cognition is just what the mind does. Therefore, if there are two kinds of computation—implicit and explicit—without knowing what makes a computation unable, in principle, to be one type or the other, one cannot say why a particular computation (or computational system) could not, in principle, be the other way round. For example, the claim that the explicit system is good at integrating new knowledge does not mean that an implicit system could not be designed to do the same thing, or that a system designed as such could not be implicit. Without knowing the link between this distinction and computation, neither inference is possible.

Consider for a moment Libet's (1999) musing that the execution of conscious will could come *before* computation is ruled out by this view. Any computation, whether it happens to have the property of awareness or consciousness, must be implemented physically in the brain. The notion of conscious will preceding neural activity seems to be precluded by monism. Nothing about explicitness or control or awareness licenses any departure, at all, from physicalism.

Thus, while the properties and functions of explicit and implicit processes can broadly be distinguished empirically as a result of work such as that reviewed above, these results do not carry any logical entailment in either direction. Knowing that a particular process is implicit, for example, does not guarantee that it will have the features associated with other implicit processes. It does not even guarantee in any meaningful sense that the process in question had to have the property in question. We cannot know, from the current state of knowledge, whether any given computation is, in principle, implicit or explicit. In similar fashion, we cannot know that there are limits on what explicit or implicit processes can include. In short, there seems no principled reason to allow us to think that because a certain computation has a particular property (or lacks a particular property) that it can therefore only be an implicit process.

Examples are illustrative. Consider the phenomenon of "blindsight" (e.g., Weiskrantz 1986), in which a person who reports that they have no visual experience is able to accomplish tasks that clearly require visual representations, such as pointing to objects (that they deny being able to see). This is a potentially important example that informs speculation about the possible functions of awareness. Such cases clearly show that conscious awareness of the visual field (or, at least, the ability to talk about what one sees) is not necessary for the performance of tasks that require visual information. These are not limited to physical tasks. There is evidence of emotional blindsight, in which patients report being unable to perceive faces but show evidence of processing information about emotional facial expressions (Pegna et al. 2005).

A number of other interesting and entertaining examples have recently been made part of the public awareness with the success of Malcom Gladwell's 2005 book, *Blink*, which recounts cases in which processes of which people are unaware guide their judgments and decisions. In the opening story, various experts are able to report that an ancient statue did not look right, though they were unable to articulate the source of their (as it turns out, correct) judgment. As with the many similar cases discussed by Gladwell, people's implicit judgments, often involving the integration of a large amount of information drawn from previous experience and from the world, yield correct judgments and decisions in the absence, apparently, of awareness of the underlying computations underlying them. This is not to say, of course, that such processes are always superior, as even the examples from *Blink* illustrate: quick intuitive judgments can also lead the decision maker astray.

Questions about the Evolution of Explicit Cognition

Evolutionary History of Implicit Cognition

Depending on one's views on the construal of what constitutes explicit processes or explicit representations, the phylogenetic origin of explicit cognition is either recent or thoroughly unknowable.

If explicitness is equated with "awareness," "consciousness," or qualia, then it is clear that explicitness is unknowable. As many have pointed out, behavior does not fossilize; clearly, neither does qualia. Indeed, the problem is much worse than that. There is little guidance for knowing what other organisms have explicit representations because, to take one well-known example, we simply cannot know what it is like to be a bat (Nagel 1974).

However, if we limit our discussion to computational systems that have the *properties associated with explicit* processing, then it seems reasonable to make some guesses. Looking at such properties, it would appear that evolutionarily ancient decision making must have been implicit. At the very least, we can suppose that organisms without nervous systems did not have the capacity for explicit representation as they did not have the capacity for representation. Many plants will "decide"—to anthropomorphize—to turn toward the sun, but it must be assumed that this is accomplished without "attention," "qualia," or "control."

What about creatures with nervous systems? Consider the high school biology labs' favorite primitive organism: the planarium (*Dugesia tigrina*), a small flatworm with light-sensitive areas that guide the organism's movement. The "decision" to move away from light is likely to be a result of implicit decision making. The system in question has many features associated with implicit decision making: acting quickly, presumably without awareness, and certainly not subject to conscious control. It is impossible to be certain, but a counter-claim seems hard to credit.

Indeed, one could take, and some have taken, a strong position on this. It could be that explicit representation is evolutionarily very novel indeed. Where one draws the line would seem to be a matter of speculation (or possibly semantics), but some view explicit processes as uniquely in the domain of humans. One can debate when these processes evolved, and then the date of various kinds of representations might be very recent, on the order of hundreds or even tens of thousands of years (Mithen 1996).

Such a view resonates with the claim that evolutionarily recent systems tend to be the home of explicit representations (Platt et al., this volume). This view, if one takes it seriously, also predicts that because the brain is by far composed of structures that date back much further than the last few hundred thousand years, then *nearly all cognitive processes are implicit*. That is, if only evolutionarily novel systems are explicit, and evolutionarily novel systems comprise only a small fraction of the computational systems of the brain, then this conclusion is inescapable.

This (speculative) conclusion leads naturally to a central question. If it is true that the vast and overwhelming number of organisms has been doing just fine with only implicit representations, and that the bulk of human computational abilities are implicit rather than explicit, then why did explicit representational systems evolve at all?

Evolutionary Function of Explicit Cognition – Two Questions

Two questions surround the function of explicit cognition and ought to be kept distinct. Their separation is important because not only might they well have very different answers, they might even differ in whether or not they can be answered or, at least, can be answered given the current state of knowledge. (For an alternate view of some of the issues raised in this section, see Stevens, this volume.)

The first question is: Why did explicit *kinds* of mechanisms evolve? That is, what does the fact that a representation is explicit add to their function? The answer depends, of course, on what precisely one takes explicit representation to mean. This, in itself, is difficult enough, given disagreements on the topic. It is even more difficult if one factors in certain views of explicitness. For example, if explicitness is tied to consciousness, then the answer to the question of the evolved function of explicitness is connected to the answer of the evolved function of consciousness. This is, of course, no small task.

Even if one takes a different view of explicitness, one is still left with describing how *whatever it is that explicit representation is contributes to the function of the computation*. To give a sense in which this question might be answerable, consider the identity of explicitness with something like a cognitive representation whose meaning is some proposition (Dienes and Perner 1999). In such a case, it might be possible to describe computational advantages to explicit representations.

Consider one, but by no means the only, version of this possibility. Suppose we take the opposite of explicit in this sense to be implicit in the sense that the information is embodied in a set of representations, but is not represented as a proposition in some particular format. For example, given the implicit representations about broad facts about a word—such as "moon"—until the reader processes this sentence, it is unlikely that the proposition "there are no penguins on the moon" was represented in propositional form.

If a representation is some proposition in some format, rather than a set of representations that implicitly carry the implication of the proposition, then one can imagine that certain computations could be performed on the explicit proposition that could not be performed otherwise. For example, it might be computationally easier to negate an explicitly represented proposition and generate the explicit negative of the proposition than negate a proposition that is represented only implicitly. By maintaining—or constructing—representations in explicit format, operations can be performed on them that could not otherwise be done.

In similar fashion, explicit representations considered in this way might have an obvious connection to language. It seems plausible that it is easier to verbalize explicit representations than implicit ones. Indeed, the ability to verbalize has occasionally been taken to be the defining characteristic of explicit knowledge, and this idea is at the root of the well-known distinction some draw between declarative and procedural knowledge.

The second question one can ask requires less of a commitment to what one means by explicit representation and can be posed as follows: Why did the particular systems, which seem to be (or, perhaps, happen to be) explicit, evolve? In other words, what are the functions of the systems that are (or, again, just happen to be) explicit?

The advantage to asking the question in this way is twofold. First, to the extent that consciousness (in the phenomenological sense) is related to explicitness, the problem of what plausible function phenomenology might have is finessed. Second, to the extent that people agree on processes that are explicit, *independent of the definition of explicitness*, we can agree on the systems whose functions are worth investigating in this context.

Potential Answers about the Evolution of Explicit Cognition

The most clear-cut cases of explicit cognition involve processes in which the properties that people associate with the phenomenon are all present. This would be cases in which individuals report conscious awareness and talk about using natural language. In order to say "I see Cinderella's Castle," one must presumably be aware of the experience of seeing the castle, have a representation that it is oneself that is having the experience, be able to formulate the proposition, and be able to represent the proposition in natural language. Without these elements, it is hard to see how the utterance might occur. In short, episodic representations refer to events that are experienced (Tulving 1983).

Episodic memory allows one to report, through natural language, on events that one has experienced and distinguished from two other kinds of representations: semantic and procedural. Without engaging in a deep discussion of the surrounding literature and debates on this topic, it is possible to review briefly these forms of memory. Semantic knowledge or memory can be conveniently thought of as a database of information in propositional or other form. The fact that roses are red is an example of semantic knowledge. Procedural knowledge or memory refers to representations of skills or patterns of behavior. A usual example is tying one's shoes. The information about how this is done must be in the heads of those who tie shoes, but few can articulate how they do it. In this sense, in contrast to episodic memory, procedural memory is implicit.

Language

To the extent that explicit representations are bound up with language, it is natural to infer that explicit representations are tied to communication. The literature on natural human language is vast (e.g., Pinker 1994) and cannot be summarized here. However, one broad generalization seems reasonably consensual among researchers: Natural language is for communicating or transferring representations from one individual to another individual (Pinker 1994). So, it is possible that explicit representational capacities evolved in the service of language, which in turn evolved in the service of whatever it is that the ability to communicate does. Since there is more than sufficient debate on the latter, I will not venture a guess or even list the numerous possibilities. There seems little doubt that language is useful and that it evolved by natural selection to transfer information from one person to another (Pinker and Bloom 1990). Thus, without entering this debate let us nonetheless look at one particular function that language serves: social learning.

Social Learning

Many organisms acquire information from the world during the process of development. In humans, ontogenetic information acquisition is taken to an extreme. Humans acquire substantial information from other people, rather than through interaction with other elements of the environment. There are, of course, reliably developing intuitive domains of knowledge, such as folk physics and folk biology, which acquire information in a way that mirrors what one might expect in other organisms; that is, through the normal daily interaction with the physical world (Hirschfeld and Gelman 1994).

Still, a great deal of information is transmitted from the brain of one individual to the brain of another individual through the use of language. This is not, to be sure, a "direct" process (Sperber and Wilson 1986). Representations are generally converted to linguistic form, decoded by the listener, and re-encoded into the proper representational format.

There is little doubt that natural language makes the transmission of information much easier. Two examples make this clear. First, consider the game of charades: Stripped of the ability to use (spoken) language, conveying even single words, let along abstract ideas, is a time-consuming and difficult (if enjoyable) process. Second, consider putative examples of social learning in nonhumans: Even among chimpanzees, our phylogenetically close relatives, social learning without language is a difficult process. Social transmission of one of their most famous behaviors—termite fishing—is not a simple process by which one chimp observes another and thereby discovers the secret. What is socially acquired seems to be that there is a relationship between a fishing stick and getting termite meals. The use of the stick to accomplish the task is a time-consuming process of individual learning, involving various experiments with the stick and termite mounds (Myowa-Yamakoshi and Matsuzawa 1999).

Humans communicate a great deal of information from person to person. Language acquisition itself—the specific meaning of words—is a clear-cut example. Without information from social others, language learning would not be possible. Social knowledge acquisition extends, of course, well beyond language. People acquire information about behavioral conventions, moral norms and laws, and technical information about tools and their use, to name just a few examples (Kurzban 2007). This has resulted in potentially enormous benefits.

Individual learning through interacting with the environment entails potentially large costs. These include the opportunity costs associated with the time spent acquiring the information, the possibility that one will learn the wrong information, any potential dangers of individual learning, such as mistakes in trial and error learning, and so on. Social learning, while it carries its own potential costs, has many advantages. One can have the benefit of *accumulated* knowledge, one can learn quickly, and one can learn things that are simply not able to be learned, ontogenetically, from the environment (Boyd and Richerson 1985; Boyd and Richerson, this volume; McElreath et al., this volume).

In short, for a species such as ours, in which there is a vast amount of information that must be obligatorily acquired ontogenetically, social learning is tremendously important. In addition, to the extent that explicit representations facilitate the social transfer of information, it is easy to see a connection between explicit representation and social learning. In other words, perhaps explicit representational formats have been selected before, during, or subsequent to the evolution of language to enable individuals to teach—and learn—ontogenetically valuable information, such as norms, morals, and tool use.

This is not to say that all social learning is explicit. Indeed, any number of experiments show many different kinds of contexts for which the implicit system is superior to the explicit system, artificial grammars being perhaps among the best-studied examples (Cleeremans et al. 1998). Along the same lines, the important effects of learning by imitation, without either language or explicit pedagogy, have been the object of investigation for some time (e.g., Bandura et al. 1961). It might well be that some forms of social learning are actually better suited to behavioral imitation than explicit verbal instruction.

In any case, it seems at least possible that the unique human capacity for language and the vast reliance on social learning in humans is not a coincidence, and that the former functions in service of the latter, and explicit representations function in the service of natural language.

Strategic Social Interaction

A related possibility derives from another distinctly human characteristic: humans are, zoologically speaking, spectacularly social. Humans engage in a tremendous number and variety of interactions with other humans. These include many prosocial behaviors that extend beyond kin, beyond reciprocal dyads, and into large-scale group-based behaviors, including group-level co-operation, a phenomenon that has attracted a massive amount of attention from theorists in the natural and social sciences.

Because social life is complex, it involves many different kinds of interactions in which the payoffs to different kinds of behaviors vary widely. Some interactions mirror coordination games, in which everyone is better off doing the same sort of thing. Driving on one side of the road is a commonly used example. Other games are mixed-motive games, such as the well-known Prisoner's Dilemma, in which, in the one-shot version, each player is best off following their economic self-interest even though both would be better off if they chose the more altruistic option. Since this has been discussed in depth elsewhere (e.g., Axelrod 1984), further discussion is omitted here. The focal point is that people play many different types of games, with differentiable strategic configurations (DeScioli and Kurzban 2007).

In addition, and most crucially, *these games are all played over time*. As is well known by even casual students of game theory, adding a dynamic element to strategic play has profound implications for optimal play (Axelrod 1984). To take but one example, adding repeated play to mixed-motive interactions means that under many conditions there are an arbitrarily large number of equilibria.

This is important in the present context because we should expect human evolved psychology to embody equilibrium solutions to repeatedly faced game theoretical problems. Further, many strategies are history-dependent. Consider again the Prisoner's Dilemma game and "Tit-for-Tat." Tit-for-Tat requires some representation (whether explicit or implicit) of what a particular individual did in the context of a particular game (the previous Prisoner's Dilemma interaction). One computational system that looks well designed to accomplish this particular task is the poster child of explicit representation: episodic memory.

Representing who did what to you on previous "moves" of social games is of potentially enormous adaptive value for an organism involved in many different repeated games with many different strategic structures (e.g., Cosmides and Tooby 1992). Because others are likely to use similar representations in their interactions with oneself, it follows that an organism involved in complex social interactions with many other organisms would be well served by maintaining a representation *of one's own strategic actions*. To anticipate others' future moves, one might need to represent one's own previous moves, given that others are likely to condition their behavior on one's own previous behavior.

This is not to say that semantic information is not useful in the context of strategic dynamics. Knowing who is in one's kin group—and specifically relatedness information—as well as information about coalitions and alliances can be useful in predicting behavior. Instead, the argument here—many versions of which have been made before (e.g., Dennett 1996)—is that explicit representation might be tied in some important way to the representation of oneself as the agent. That is, explicitness emerges as a result of the representation undertaken by an individual to depict something about the world.

To clarify, there are two related ideas, both of which might hint at the origins of explicit information. First is the notion that one must represent, in strategic settings, what others know and *that you know what others know*, and so on (Schelling 1960). It could be that this sort of recursive representation is special in some way, and, in particular, special in its relationship with consciousness (Hofstader 1999). The second is the notion that representation of oneself as the owner of strategic knowledge is the key element. Both of these ideas have featured prominently in discussions of explicit representations.

Continuing further along this general line of reasoning, it has recently been suggested that socially strategic information is stored in an explicit representational system, the "social cognitive interface" (Kurzban and Aktipis 2007). Drawing on modern interpretations of modularity (Barrett and Kurzban 2006), the suggestion is that there is a "pool" of information that might be advantageous to retain for strategic purposes, even if this information is not necessarily the most accurate representation about what is true (which can be stored elsewhere, for nonsocial purposes). Thus, for example, this representational system might retain positive views about the individual which are difficult for others to verify, but might be communicated and consumed by listeners. The social cognitive interface acts as a press secretary, carefully controlling the flow of information, striking the optimal balance between plausibility and casting oneself in a positive light. According to this view, explicit representations are part of the socially strategic repertoire, but are viewed as a set of semi-isolated systems rather than a broader class of computational systems.

Consider the recent explosion of research using the implicit association task (Greenwald et al. 1998), which reveals, as the name implies, implicit associations. Findings that suggest people have negative associations with certain groups, while explicitly denying such associations (which is the socially desirable response), gives the flavor of the value of such a system. It might be functional to use information about social categories to make inferences, while at the same time denying that one is engaged in any such process for reasons of social desirability. If one is not able to talk (explicitly) about these (implicit) associations, this might be all to the good in terms of strategic self-presentation.

Conclusion

The Relationship between Evolution and Function

Beginning with the notion that cognition was, phylogentically, essentially all implicit, the key to understanding explicit decision making is to comprehend why explicit representational systems evolved. This, in turn, requires an understanding of the *function* that explicitness has; that is, what functions can be executed with explicit representations that cannot be executed with implicit representations?

This question is hobbled by several important obstacles. First is the very basic question of what is meant by explicitness. The diversity of views in the scientific literature makes answering functional questions difficult because of the lack of agreement about the phenomenon in question. Related to this issue, explicitness is often defined with respect to qualities or properties that are themselves not well understood. To the extent that explicitness is related to concepts such as "consciousness," "intention," and "attention" (Schacter 1987), uncertainty surrounding these terms precludes a rigorous treatment of explicitness. The notions of "automaticity" and "control" are similarly problematic, as they are notoriously slippery concepts (see Keysers et al., this volume).

Second, substantial research has shown that implicit representational systems (i.e., systems that are widely acknowledged to be implicit) seem to be extremely powerful and diverse in their functions. To the extent that implicit systems can discharge many different functions, one is left to wonder what work is left for explicit representational systems.

In this case, as argued above, the best we might be able to do is look at computational systems that are broadly, consensually agreed to be "explicit" and investigate the functions of these systems. Although this approach is somewhat oblique, it is appealing because of the problems with the more direct approach alluded to above. It might be that understanding the functions that explicit systems have will allow us to infer the function of explicitness in representation.

Perhaps the best example of explicitness can be found in processes that people report that they are aware of and are able to describe through linguistic means. The link between explicitness and communication, which is a deeply social enterprise, hints that explicit representations might function to facilitate social tasks. This might include social learning, in general, or social strategic maneuvering. These might be productive avenues of future research.

This approach has the potentially valuable effect of ruling out certain putative functions of explicit representations. For example, in his discussion of conscious representations, Wilson (2002) points to long-term computation as one of the signal features of conscious cognition. However, it is not at all clear that consciousness or explicitness is needed for computations in association with long-term planning. The animal literature is replete with cases of organisms behaving in such a way so as to defer, for example, present consumption to improve their long-term prospects. Caching in birds and hoarding in rodents are good examples.

Similarly, it is not clear that explicit representational systems are more functionally suited to any particular sort of learning. As indicated above, numerous examples have shown that awareness, consciousness, or the ability to articulate the rule in question is not necessary for acquisition of complex rules. Information integration fits into the same category. There seems to be no principled reason why implicit systems cannot integrate large amounts and different kinds of information. Perhaps this will turn out to be the case, but it does not seem obvious that it necessarily is.

This analysis, of course, has a potentially important implication for the focal issue of the present volume, "Better than Conscious?" (see Engel, this volume.) If the foregoing framing is correct, then the answer to this question, as with so many in psychology, is: It depends. Some, but not all, decision-making processes might very well be more likely to generate "correct" or "adaptive" decisions when conscious computations are dominant, but other decision-making processes might yield better results when only implicit processes guide the decision. Domains such as discounting, moral reasoning, and aesthetic judgments (Keysers et al., this volume; Hastie, this volume) provide examples that favor one direction or the other.

By extension, the issue of when unconscious or subconscious procedures are "better than conscious" might need to be replaced with a set of questions that could be glossed as: "Better than conscious *for what*?" If implicit processes guide good decision making in some cases, but not all, then the question of the added—or diminished—value of explicit systems in decision making will have to be evaluated on a case-by-case basis. This is discouraging news in terms of developing an overarching theory, but is possibly the most productive route for additional research.

Where to Go

Clearly, progress on the evolution of explicit decision making will hinge critically on our ability to define precisely what is meant by explicit representations. To the extent that there is a divergence of views of what is to be explained, the correct functional explanation will be handicapped.

If researchers can agree, however, on a set of processes that are mutually recognized as explicit, then a good strategy might be to identify the features of these processes and look for commonalities. These commonalities might help to triangulate on function.

Finally, it is worth closing with a commonsense observation. "Explicit," in the lay sense, refers to the idea that something is expressed, in language, rather than implied. Taken seriously, this leads us to look for the function of explicitness in the (computational) value of formatting a representation in (some kind of) language (or representational format), though not necessarily natural language. A representation that is made explicit in, say, some particular format in the language of thought (Fodor 1975) can, presumably, take part in any computational process that accepts representations in that format as an input. The value of explicitness, then, lies in the surrounding computational systems of the explicit representation. If we knew a lot about important elements of human decision making, and the kinds of representations they took as input, we should be able to make inferences about when representing the relevant information explicitly in this representational format would make good, functional sense.

References

Axelrod, R. 1984. The Evolution of Cooperation. New York: Basic Books.

Bandura, A., D. Ross, and A. Ross. 1961. Transmission of aggression through imitation of aggressive models. *J. Abnorm. Soc. Psychol.* **63**:575–582.

Barrett, H. C., and R. Kurzban. 2006. Modularity in cognition: Framing the debate. *Psychol. Rev.* **113**:628–647.

Bloom, P. 2004. Descartes' Baby: How the Science of Child Development Explains What Makes Us Human. New York: Basic Books.

Boyd, R., and P. J. Richerson. 1985. Culture and the Evolutionary Process. Chicago: Univ. Chicago Press.

Cleeremans, A., A. Destrebecqz, and M. Boyer. 1998. Implicit learning: News from the front. *Trends Cogn. Sci.* **2**:406–416.

Cosmides, L., and J. Tooby. 1992. Cognitive adaptations for social exchange. In: The Adapted Mind: Evolutionary Psychology and the Generation of Culture, ed. J. Barkow, L. Cosmides, and J. Tooby, pp. 163–228. New York: Oxford Univ. Press.

Dehaene, S., J. P. Changeux, L. Naccache et al. 2006. Conscious, preconscious, and subliminal processing: A testable taxonomy. *Trends Cogn. Sci.* **10**:204–211.

Dennett, D. 1996. Kinds of Minds. New York: Basic Books.

DeScioli, P., and R. Kurzban. 2007. The games people play. In: Evolution of Mind: Fundamental Questions and Controversies, ed. S. Gangestad and J. Simpson, pp. 130–136. New York: Guilford Press.

Dienes, Z., and J. Perner. 1999. A theory of implicit and explicit knowledge. *Behav. Brain Sci.* **22:**735–755.

Evans, J. 2003. In two minds: Dual-process accounts of reasoning. *Trends Cogn. Sci.* **7**:454–459.

Fodor, J. A. 1975. The Language of Thought. Cambridge, MA: Harvard Univ. Press.

Gazzaniga, M. S. 1998. The Mind's Past. New York: Basic Books.

Gazzaniga, M. S., and J. E. Ledoux. 1978. The Integrated Mind. Dordrecht: Kluwer Acad. Publ.

Gladwell, M. 2005. Blink: The Power of Thinking without Thinking. New York: Little, Brown and Co.

Greenwald, A. G., D. E. McGhee, and J. L. K. Schwartz. 1998. Measuring individual differences in implicit cognition: The implicit association test. *J. Pers. Soc. Psychol.* **74**:1464–1480.

Hirschfeld, L., and S. Gelman. 1994. Mapping the Mind: Domain Specificity in Cognition and Culture. New York: Cambridge Univ. Press.

Hirstein, W. 2005. Brain Fiction: Self-Deception and the Riddle of Confabulation. Cambridge, MA: MIT Press.

Hofstadter, D. 1999. Gödel, Escher, and Bach: An Eternal Golden Braid. New York: Basic Books.

James, W. 1890. The Principles of Psychology. New York: Henry Holt and Company.

Kihlstrom, J. F. 1987. The cognitive unconscious. *Science* **237**:1445–1452.

Kurzban, R. 2007. Representational epidemiology: Skepticism and gullibility. In: Evolution of Mind: Fundamental Questions and Controversies, ed. S. Gangestad and J. Simpson, pp. 357–362. New York: Guilford Press.

Kurzban, R., and C. A. Aktipis. 2007. Modularity and the social mind: Why social psychologists should be less self-ish. *Pers. Soc. Psychol. Rev.* **11**:131–149.

Libet, B. 1999. Do we have free will? *J. Consc. Stud.* **6(8–9)**:47–57.

R. Kurzban

Libet, B., C. A. Gleason, E. W. Wright, and D. K. Pearl. 1983. Time of conscious intention to act in relation to onset of cerebral activity (readiness potential): The unconscious initiation of a freely voluntary act. *Brain* **106**:623–642.

Mithen, S. 1996. The Prehistory of the Mind. London: Thames and Hudson.

Myowa-Yamakoshi, M., and T. Matsuzawa. 1999. Factors influencing imitation of manipulatory actions in chimpanzees (*Pan troglodytes*). *J. Comp. Psychol.* **113**:128–136.

Nagel, T. 1974. What is it like to be a bat? *Phil. Rev.* **4**:435–450.

Nisbett, R. E., and T. D. Wilson. 1977. Telling more than we can know: Verbal reports on mental processes. *Psychol. Rev.* **84**:231–259.

Oaksford, M., and N. Chater. 2001. The probabilistic approach to human reasoning. *Trends Cogn. Sci.* **5**:349–357.

Pegna, A. J., A. Khateb, F. Lazeyras, and M. L. Seghier. 2005. Discriminating emotional faces without primary visual cortices involves the right amygdala. *Nature Neurosci.* **8**:24–25.

Pinker, S. 1994. The Language Instinct. New York: William Morrow and Company.

Pinker, S., and P. Bloom. 1990. Natural language and natural selection. *Behav. Brain Sci.* **13**:707–784.

Rescorla, R. A. 1990. The role of information about the response-outcome relationship in instrumental discrimination learning. *J. Exp. Psychol: Anim. Behav. Proc.* **16**:262–270.

Schacter, D. L. 1987. Implicit memory: History and current status. *J. Exp. Psychol.: Learn. Mem. Cogn.* **13**:501–518.

Schelling, T. 1960. The Strategy of Conflict. Cambridge, MA: Harvard Univ. Press.

Sperber, D., and D. Wilson. 1986. Relevance: Communication and Cognition. Oxford: Blackwell.

Stanovich, K. E., and R. F. West. 2000. Individual differences in reasoning: Implications for the rationality debate. *Behav. Brain Sci.* **23**:645–726.

Tulving, E. 1983. Elements of Episodic Memory. Oxford: Clarendon Press.

Weiskrantz, L. 1986. Blindsight: A Case Study and its Implications. Oxford: Oxford Univ. Press.

Wilson, T. D. 2002. Strangers to Ourselves: Discovering the Adaptive Unconscious. Cambridge, MA: Harvard Univ. Press.

8

Passive Parallel Automatic Minimalist Processing

Roger Ratcliff and Gail McKoon

Department of Psychology, Ohio State University, Columbus, OH 43210, U.S.A.

Abstract

Research for which the idea that many basic cognitive processes can be described as fast, parallel, and automatic is reviewed. Memory retrieval/decision processes have often been ignored in the cognitive literature. However, in some cases, computationally complex processes can be replaced with simple passive processes. Cue-dependent retrieval from memory provides a straightforward example of how encoding, memory, and retrieval can interact. Three other examples are reviewed: inference in text processing, compound cue models for priming, and implicit memory. In each case, the research benefits from a focus on retrieval and decision processes. For implicit memory, consideration of these kinds of processes leads to a view of implicit memory different than hypothesizing new specialized memory systems. Finally, how behavioral data from simple decisions and the models that explain the behavior can be related to neuroscience research on neural firing rates are discussed.

Introduction

Our research is relevant to two major topics of this Ernst Strüngmann Forum: (a) the distinction between implicit and explicit memory processes and (b) the diffusion models in psychology and neuroscience that explain simple decision-making processes. In our view, a number of issues in these domains are interconnected by their reliance on cognitive processes that occur quickly, automatically, and passively.

In conjunction with fast automatic passive processes, we suggest that in many cases, active, computationally expensive processes should be replaced by mechanisms that instantiate passive uses of information. We also emphasize that the retrieval of information from memory cannot be understood without consideration of the retrieval context in which memory is tested. In the final section of this paper, we suggest connections between these ideas, behavioral data, and neural processes.

Our view is that relatively simple processes operate on perceptual inputs. The results of these computations are usually integrated with already known information, producing outputs that are added to the database upon which other cognitive processes can operate. This view is similar in many ways to John Anderson's (1990, 1993; Anderson and Lebiere 1998). Both views stress that representations of easily accessible knowledge have large impacts on cognitive processes.

Retrieval and decision processes are important given their usual neglect in comparison with encoding processes. Crucially, it is often possible to model empirical findings such as priming in lexical decision or inferences in reading with retrieval processes instead of encoding processes. To give one example, which will be elaborated on below, in reading, people can produce a large number of answers to questions based on a text. The key question, however, is whether the inferences required to answer the questions were made during reading or at the time the question is asked. It is clear that many plausible inferences are not made during reading. In this respect, our view is similar to Gigerenzer's view of decision making in that minimalism is stressed in the theoretical proposals as compared to other views.

One way to divide up the domains of cognitive processing is to separate perceptual encoding computations that are carried out in parallel and automatically from those that are carried out as strategic processes. Fundamental to the modeling of cognitive phenomena, automatic and strategic processes, and encoding and retrieval processes, must be examined jointly, empirically, and theoretically. The goal is to develop models that explicitly bridge empirical phenomena.

The idea that memory can never be assessed without taking into account the retrieval cues that interact with memory was made central in cognitive psychology 35 years ago by Tulving (1974). Cue-dependent retrieval is an integral component of all current memory models. Recognition and recall of items in memory are understood in a theoretical framework that relates retrieval cues to encoding and memory representations.

We discuss a number of cognition phenomena. Their common theme is that sometimes complicated assumptions about representations or processes can be replaced by simpler mechanisms that depend on quickly accessible, context-relevant information and provide a base for the operation of higher-level processes.

Cue-dependent Retrieval

One of the key tenets of cue-dependent retrieval is that it is not possible to draw conclusions about memory without understanding the retrieval environment, including the cues presented at retrieval. Tulving (1972) presented a number of compelling experimental demonstrations which show that memories can be recovered with appropriate cues when, with other cues, even presentation of the studied item itself, retrieval fails. In these experiments, the conclusion from the experiments with suboptimal cues would have been that the information had been lost.

Tulving (1972) suggests a view in which retrieval processes and cues presented at retrieval interact with memory to produce a response. It is this interaction that should be key in understanding how the retrieval environment affects processing. Perhaps the most dramatic example is recognition failure of recallable words (Tulving and Thomson 1973). The experiments had subjects initially read pairs (A-B) of weakly associated words followed by a forced-choice recognition test of the second member of the pairs (B) with distractors similar to the target words. Finally, a cued recall test, in which the first (A) members of the pairs were presented, showed a significant proportion of words recalled that were not recognized in the recognition phase. From examples like these, Tulving argued that memory cannot be understood without understanding how retrieval cues interact with memory. We have taken this view further, as illustrated below, to understand many aspects of inference in text processing and semantic priming in terms of retrieval processes.

Minimal Inference in Text Processing

In the 1970s and 1980s, most text-processing experiments were concerned with whether some particular kind of inference was encoded during reading. If a fish swam under a rock and a turtle was sitting on the rock, does the reader encode that the fish swam under the turtle (Bransford et al. 1972)? If a workman pounds a nail, does the reader understand that he uses a hammer (Corbett and Dosher 1978)? If an actress falls from a 14-story building, does the reader understand that she will most likely die (McKoon and Ratcliff 1986)? Sorting out the results of many such experiments led to an appreciation of what turned out to be a crucial methodological issue. The procedures used in most early experiments did not allow inferences that were generated at the time of reading to be distinguished from inferences that were generated at the time of the test. Suppose, for example, that after studying a list of sentences, subjects were given a list of words and asked to recall the sentence that went with each word. Given the word "hammer," for instance, the sentence to recall might have been, "the workman pounds the nail." Recall of the sentence could occur either because the subject had generated the connection between "hammer" and the "pounds" sentence when the sentence was read or because the subject generated the connection at the time the word "hammer" was given in the recall test. Corbett and Dosher (1978) presented other sentences, such as "the workman pounded the nail with a rock," and found that "hammer" was just as good as a retrieval cue for those sentences, even though it would not have been encoded, thus concluding that the connection was made at retrieval.

In response to this problem, experimenters began to use procedures by which inferences could be attributed unequivocally to processes that occurred during reading (e.g., Corbett and Chang 1983). To make this argument, two theoretical ideas were borrowed from research on memory. The first has just been discussed, namely Tulving's (1974) notion of cue-dependent retrieval: a cue evokes information from memory directly and selectively; that is, it directly evokes memory of those past events of which it was a part. The second was Posner's (1978) separation of fast automatic cognitive processes from slower strategic ones. These two ideas in combination led to the use of speeded, single-word item recognition as a procedure to examine inference processes. In a typical experiment, subjects read several sentences (or longer texts) and then, after some delay, one or more single test words were presented. For each test word, subjects were asked to make a recognition decision; that is, they were asked to decide whether the test word had appeared in the studied sentences and to respond as quickly as possible. It is assumed that the recognition decision is based on cue-dependent retrieval: if the test word and/or its meaning was encoded as part of the studied sentence, then the test word will quickly contact the information encoded from the sentence, allowing a fast positive response to the test word. For example, given the sentence "the workman pounded the nail," the test word "workman" should quickly evoke the information from the sentence, and there should be a fast positive response. If an inference was encoded about the workman pounding with a hammer, then "hammer" as a test word should also quickly evoke the information from the sentence, leading to a fast positive response—a response that would be an error because "hammer" did not actually appear in the sentence (for discussion of slow responses and the use of deadline methods to ensure fast responses, see McKoon and Ratcliff 1989). The important point for interpretation of the results of recognition experiments is that, following Posner, fast responses are assumed to come from automatic processes—processes that are not under the subject's strategic control. Because the processes are not under strategic control, it is further assumed that responses reflect information that was encoded during reading, not information that was constructed by slower strategic processes occurring at the time of the test.

Applying this reasoning, experiments looked at what kinds of information were encoded during reading in procedures in which subjects were given no special goals to encode any particular types of information. One outcome was the conclusion that in the absence of special goals, relatively few of the inferences that had been studied earlier so extensively were actually generated during reading. This conclusion was summarized by the "minimalist hypothesis" (McKoon and Ratcliff 1992a), which states that the only inferences encoded during reading (unless the reader has special goals in reading, e.g., studying for an exam, reading a report to make a decision, etc.), in the absence of special strategies, are those that depend on information that is easily and quickly available from memory and those that are needed to make the text that is being read locally coherent. This conclusion has not been shared by all text-processing researchers, and considerable debate ensued (e.g., Graesser et al. 1994; Graesser and Zwaan 1995; McKoon and Ratcliff 1995b; Singer et al. 1994). Efforts to map out what kinds of nonminimalist inferences are generated during reading, especially those that create causal links between pieces of text information, still continue.

Although the focus on fast, parallel, and passive evocation of information from memory was first reflected in new experimental procedures, a more important consequence has been its reflection in theoretical thinking. This change was part of a broader movement in cognitive psychology. In memory research, the global memory models (Gillund and Shiffrin 1984; Hintzman 1986, 1988; Murdock 1982) accounted for many and various empirical findings with direct access retrieval processes that are global, passive, fast, and automatic, explicit implementations of cue-dependent retrieval. In text processing, part of the minimalist hypothesis (McKoon and Ratcliff 1992a) is that not only a test word but also every word, concept, and proposition in a text evokes information from memory directly, globally, and quickly. Kintsch's (1974) model for the representation of meaning in propositional structures has acquired processes (Kintsch 1988) by which information from long-term memory is made available by fast, passive retrieval processes. A crucial aspect of this focus is that attention is directed at what is evoked from memory by a text rather than only at what inferences need to be generated to understand the text.

Compound Cue Models for Associative Priming

A phenomenon that has received much attention over the recent history of cognitive psychology is priming in lexical decision and recognition. This kind of priming is seen as a speedup in processing for a word that results from processing a related word just before it. For example, in making word/nonword lexical decisions about strings of letters, if a target test word "doctor" is preceded by a related prime word, "nurse," then the "word" response to "doctor" is speeded up by 30 to 50 ms.

The first and most common theoretical interpretation of priming is based on spreading activation: the prime word activates other words related to it in memory, and this advance activation leads to a speedup on the target (McNamara 1992a, 1992b, 1994). This view requires that items be stored as distinct and connected entities in memory, in accord with a commonsense view of processing that has its roots in computer science and implementation on digital computers (e.g., Quillian 1969). This mechanism places a lot of importance on processes that operate at the time the prime is presented. In this respect, the mechanism is similar to a constructionist view of inference making.

It is, however, important to note that there are widely used cognition models for which the representations in memory are distributed. In such representations, activation cannot spread. If items are stored in common overlapping vectors of features, then all that can happen at retrieval is an assessment of the extent to which a cue matches memory.

We have proposed an alternative to spreading activation, a mechanism that is more passive and operates at retrieval. The assumption is that the information with which memory is probed at retrieval is not simply the tested word, but instead a combination of the test word plus prior words (with the prior words weighted less); for example, the other words that are in short-term memory. If two successively presented words share features or associations to information in memory, then the combination will match memory better than two unrelated words.

The cue combination explanation of priming, the compound cue model (Ratcliff and McKoon 1988, 1994, 1995; McKoon and Ratcliff 1992b, 1995a), can be implemented in the global memory models that are current in cognitive psychology. The compound cue model treats priming pairs of words in the same way that the global memory models treat pairs of words. In pair recognition, a pair of words is presented simultaneously and the task is to decide whether both were on the study list. If the two words were studied in a pair together, the degree of match between the test probe and memory is greater than if both words were studied but in different pairs. This mechanism is implemented differently in different global memory models. In a distributed memory model, such as TODAM (Murdock 1982), a pair is stored as a vector convolution. This means the words of a pair are combined and added to a common memory vector. At test, a compound cue model would assume that the memory vector is matched with either the association between the two prime and target words along with the single item, or that the probe is actually a combination of a lot of the test item and a little of the prime. In both cases, the match between the test item combination is better for the two associated words than for unassociated words.

Ratcliff and McKoon used the same mechanism to explain priming, adding some assumptions about how reaction time is derived from degree of match. There has been considerable controversy over whether spreading activation (ACT*, Anderson 1983) or compound cue mechanisms give the best account of priming, with no clear winner (McNamara 1992a, 1992b, 1994). What is clear is that different models of representation fit better with compound cue and spreading activation models. A compound cue mechanism provides a method of probing memory with a combination of cues that allows retrieval to be more focused; that is, more likely to access conjunctions of information, as in the Gillund and Shiffrin (1984) memory model. It also provides a good analogy for how retrieval and inferences might be processed (i.e., by jointly probing memory with information in the question presented at test).

Implicit Memory

Global memory models address what has been called explicit memory. There is, however, another domain of research concerned with the effects of prior study on performance in tasks that does not require recollection of prior study; this has been called implicit memory. Much research on implicit memory has centered on the experimental finding that repetition of a stimulus produces a benefit to performance, even when conscious memory of the prior episode with the stimulus is not required. A key result is the finding that on many tasks, this repetition priming effect is unimpaired in amnesics, even when their explicit memory, as evidenced by recognition or recall tasks, is severely impaired. It has been claimed that this priming is produced by a memory system separate from that which performs explicit memory tasks. Squire (1992), for example, proposed a hierarchy of separate systems, and Schacter and Tulving (1994) produced a taxonomy of multiple memory systems. The problem with such an approach is that it is driven by hypothesis testing; at no point are the difficult theoretical questions posed about how information is represented within each memory system, how processing works within each system, or how processes interact among the different memory systems. Crucially, there is no discussion of how processing works for the tasks in which repetition effects are found.

Consider, for example, what must happen in a multiple memory systems account of priming in word identification. In tasks used to show this phenomenon, a test word is flashed briefly, then masked. Prior presentation of the word increases the probability of correctly identifying it. If the earlier encounter is stored as a new representation in a separate memory system from that used for word identification, then when the test word is presented it must contact this representation, and the representation must become available to the processes that are standardly used for word identification in time to facilitate them. It seems unlikely to us that any reasonable mechanism could be constructed to work this quickly to both identify the test word in the implicit memory system and use the resulting information to aid identification.

Our data provides the basis for a different interpretation of implicit priming effects (Ratcliff and McKoon 1996, 1997). Using experimental procedures for which costs as well as benefits could be examined, we found that the facilitative priming effect for an exact repetition of an item was accompanied by inhibition in processing when an item closely similar to the test item had been presented earlier. We argue that this shows a bias in processing, not the operation of a separate memory system. We further explain bias with a model for word identification (Ratcliff and McKoon 1997), a modification of the logogen model developed by Morton (1969). Schooler et al. (2001) have also proposed a model for bias that does not make use of a separate memory system; their model uses the mechanisms of REM (retrieving effectively from memory; Shiffrin and Steyvers 1997). In both cases, the primary aim of the models was to explain standard processing; priming was only a by-product of the standard processes (Morton 1970). In addition, each model could be used in conjunction with other criterial tests said to identify separate memory systems: dissociations and stochastic independence (see also Ratcliff and McKoon 1996).

Currently, the domains of implicit and explicit memory are related mainly by contrasts: Is this implicit memory or explicit memory? As models for implicit memory were developed, it was hoped that relationships between explicit and implicit memory systems would become apparent (e.g., Schooler et al. 2001) and that theoretical progress would be made. This did not happen. Instead, the field has become stagnant, and researchers who were most active in implicit memory moved away from it such that relatively little empirical or theoretical progress has been made over the last ten years.

Models of the Time Course of Processing

A major topic of this Forum involved decision-making models and how they relate to neural processes. The current class of diffusion models fits behavioral data in two-choice tasks well (accuracy and response time [RT] distributions for correct and error responses). There are several related versions of these models, which differ on the basis of whether evidence is accumulated as a single sum positively or negatively toward a positive or negative decision criterion (Ratcliff 1978) or through separate diffusion processes, each toward its own criterion. The key to the success of these models is that for all of them, the decisions depend on diffusion processes (Ratcliff and Smith 2004).

The Ratcliff diffusion model is a model of the cognitive processes involved in simple two-choice decisions (Ratcliff 1978, 1988, 2006; Ratcliff and Rouder 1998; Ratcliff et al. 1999). It separates the quality of evidence entering the decision from decision criteria and from other, nondecision processes such as stimulus encoding and response execution. The model should only be applied to relatively fast two-choice decisions (mean RTs < 1000–1500 ms) and only to decisions that are a single-stage decision process (as opposed to the multiple-stage processes that might be involved in, e.g., reasoning tasks).

The diffusion model assumes that decisions are made by a noisy process that accumulates information over time from a starting point toward one of two response criteria or boundaries (Figure 8.1a). The starting point is labeled z and the boundaries are labeled a and 0. When one of the boundaries is reached, a response is initiated. The rate of accumulation of information is called the drift rate (v) and is determined by the quality of the information extracted from the stimulus. In an experiment, the value of drift rate, v, would be different for each stimulus condition that varied in difficulty. For recognition memory, for example, drift rate would represent the quality of the match between a test word and memory. A word presented for study three times would have a higher degree of match (i.e., a higher drift rate) than a word presented once. The zero point of drift rate (the drift criterion; Ratcliff 1985, 2002; Ratcliff et al. 1999)

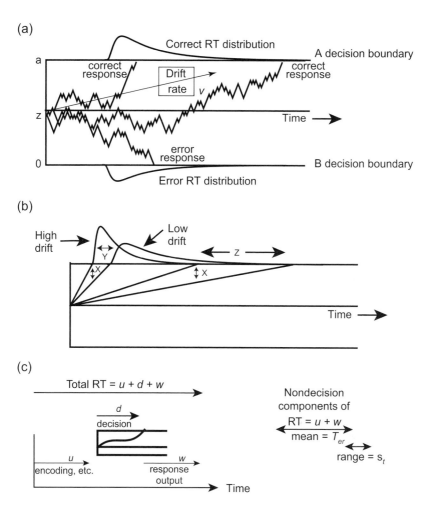

Figure 8.1 An illustration of the diffusion model. (a) The diffusion model with starting point z, boundary separation a, and drift rate v. Three sample paths are shown illustrating variability within the decision process; correct and error RT distributions are illustrated. How distribution shape changes when drift rate changes by an amount X is shown in (b). The fastest responses slow by Y, and the slowest responses slow by Z, leading to a small shift in the forward edge of the distribution and a larger change in the tail, which results in increased skew. The third panel (c) illustrates the components of processing besides the decision process d with the duration of the encoding process u and the duration of processes after the decision process w. These two components are added to give the duration of nondecision components T_{er}. The nondecision component is assumed to have a uniform distribution with range s_t.

divides drift rates into those that have positive values (i.e., mean drift rate toward the A decision boundary in Figure 8.1a) and negative values (mean drift rate toward the B decision boundary).

There is noise ("within trial" variability) in the accumulation of information so that processes with the same mean drift rate (v) do not always terminate at the same time (producing RT distributions) and do not always terminate at the same boundary (producing errors). This is shown by the three processes, all with the same drift rate, in Figure 8.1a.

Empirical RT distributions are positively skewed and in the diffusion model this is naturally predicted by simple geometry. In Figure 8.1b, distributions of fast processes from a high drift rate and slower responses from a lower drift rate are shown. If the higher and lower values of drift rate are reduced by the same amount ("X" in the figure), then the fastest processes are slowed by an amount "Y" and the slowest by a much larger amount, "Z". Our data shows that RT distribution shape is invariant under a number of manipulations (Ratcliff and McKoon 2007), which is exactly what the diffusion model predicts.

Figure 8.1c illustrates component processes assumed by the diffusion model: the decision process with duration d; an encoding process with duration u (this would include memory access in a memory task, lexical access in a lexical decision task, and so on); and a response output process with duration w. When the model is fit to data, u and w are combined into one parameter to encompass all the nondecision components with mean duration T_{er}.

The components of processing are assumed to be variable across trials (Figure 8.2). For example, all words studied three times in a recognition memory task would not have exactly the same drift rate. The across-trial variability in drift rate is assumed to be normally distributed with standard deviation η and the starting point is assumed to be uniformly distributed with range s_z. These two sources of variability have consequences for the relative speeds of correct and error responses, and this will be discussed shortly. One might also expect that the decision criteria would be variable from trial to trial. However, the effects would closely approximate the starting point variability for small to moderate amounts of variability; computationally, only one integration over the starting point is needed instead of two separate integrations over the two criteria.

Error responses are typically slower than correct responses when accuracy is stressed in instructions or in experiments where accuracy is low; errors are usually faster than correct responses when speed is stressed in instructions or when accuracy is high (Luce 1986; Swensson 1972). Early random walk models could not explain these results. For example, if the two boundaries were equidistant from the starting point, the models predicted that correct RTs would be equal to error RTs, a result almost always contradicted by data (e.g., Stone 1960). It has been shown that the combination of across-trial variability in drift rate and across-trial variability in starting point can account for all of the empirically observed patterns of correct and error RTs (Ratcliff et al. 1999; Ratcliff and Rouder 1998): experimental conditions for which error RTs were faster than correct RTs and conditions for which they were slower, even when errors moved from being slower to being faster than correct responses

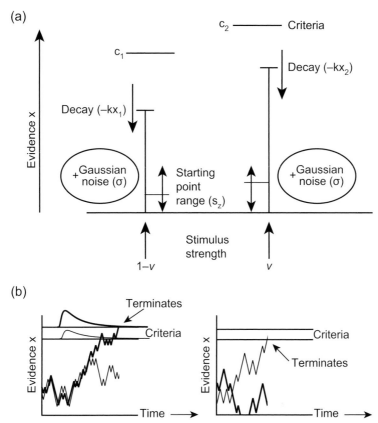

Figure 8.2 The dual diffusion models: (a) two accumulators with accumulation rates $1-v$ and v, within trial Gaussian noise s, decision criteria c_1 and c_2, variability in starting points s_z, and decay k. (b) Sample paths for two pairs of processes: the left panel with the dark process winning and the right with the light process winning.

in a single experiment. A discussion of falsifiability of the model is presented in Ratcliff (2002).

An important feature of the diffusion model with variability across trials in the components of processing is that it allows decision noise to be separated from perceptual or encoding noise (variability in drift rate across trials) and from criterion noise (variability in starting point across trials). The standard signal detection approach collapses these three sources of noise into one. The diffusion model allows these three sources to be extracted from the data and identified uniquely subject to variability in the data (the variability parameters usually have larger standard errors of estimate relative to other parameters; Ratcliff and Tuerlinckx 2002).

A rarely discussed problem is the potentially troubling relationship between accuracy and RT. Accuracy has a scale with limits of zero and 1 while RT has a lower limit of zero and an upper limit of infinity. In addition, the standard deviations in the two measures change differently: the standard deviation in accuracy decreases as accuracy approaches 1, whereas the standard deviation in RT increases as RT slows. In the diffusion model (as well as other sequential sampling models), these relations between accuracy and RT are explained directly. The model accounts for how accuracy and RT scale, relative to each other, and how manipulations of experimental variables affect them differentially. This is a major advance over models that address only one dependent variable: only mean RT or only accuracy.

Applications

The diffusion model has been applied over a wide range of experimental paradigms and in several populations of human (and even animal) subjects. One example is aging and speed of processing. For some time, it has been known that older adults (e.g., 65 to 90 years old) are slower in two-choice tasks than young adults (college students). It was usually assumed that this decrease in performance was the result of a general slowdown in all cognitive processes. However, recent diffusion model analyses of two-choice data from a number of tasks (six experiments with 30 or more subjects in each of three age groups per experiment) show that the slowdown is due almost entirely to the conservativeness of older adults. To avoid errors, they set their decision criteria significantly farther from the starting point of the decision process than young adults. Counter to the previously held view, in most tasks, the quality of the information on which decisions are based (i.e., drift rate) is not significantly worse for the older than the young adults in the tasks we studied (Ratcliff, Thapar, and McKoon 2001, 2003, 2004, 2006, 2007; Ratcliff, Thapar, Gomez, and McKoon 2004; Spaniol et al. 2006; Thapar et al. 2003).

Criterion Setting

An issue that arose during this Forum concerns the processes involved in response feedback and control (see Dayan, this volume). For animal research, this can be explored experimentally. For humans, it is difficult to imagine how a complete theory of criterion setting might be achieved. One problem is that humans can calibrate their responses in a reaction time task on the first trial of an experiment on the basis of verbal instructions alone. For example, if a letter string is presented to a subject and the instruction is to hit one key if it is a word and another key if it is a nonword, subjects can perform this task on the first trial and require no feedback about whether their responses are correct. If they have familiarity with other reaction time tasks, they will be able to start responding quickly and accurately on the very first trial using only the sound waves that carry the verbal instructions. On the many tasks for which there is no feedback about accuracy, reinforcement is not needed for subjects to set criteria. For human subjects, reinforcement and feedback can be used to shape behavior and adjust criteria, but a theory to account for such effects will be incomplete because humans use knowledge in ways that theories cannot as yet explain.

Do Diffusion Processes Reflect Neural Activity?

One way that the connection between diffusion processes and neural activity has been pursued is by simultaneously collecting behavioral data and single-cell recording data. Beginning with Hanes and Schall's pioneering work (1996) and Shadlen and colleagues' efforts to integrate diffusion processes and neural decision making (e.g., Gold and Shadlen 2001), research in this area has advanced rapidly (Ditterich 2006; Huk and Shadlen 2005; Mazurek et al. 2003; Roitman and Shadlen 2002; Schall 2003). Studies using ERP (Philiastides et al. 2006) and fMRI measures (Heekeren et al. 2004) are beginning to appear. The general questions are whether and how the components of processing recovered from behavioral data by the diffusion model or other recent sequential sampling models correspond to the physiological measures.

Research aimed at these questions is illustrated in a recent experiment by Ratcliff, Cherian, and Segraves (2003). Monkeys were trained to discriminate whether the distance between two dots was large or small, indicating their responses by left versus right eye movements. Which response was correct was probabilistic, defined by the history of rewards for correct responses in the experimental sessions. As the monkeys performed the task, data were collected from cells identified as buildup (or prelude) cells in the superior colliculus. The goal was to test whether the decision process and the firing rates (aggregated over individual cells and trials for each cell) were linked such that the closer the diffusion process to a decision boundary, the higher the firing rate of a cell. Ratcliff et al. applied the diffusion model to the behavioral data, fitting the data adequately and obtaining the values of the parameters that best fit the behavioral data. Then, using these parameter values, sample diffusion paths were generated, each path beginning at the starting point of the diffusion process and ending at a response boundary. These paths were averaged and the result was compared to the average of the firing rates, across cells and trials, of the buildup cells. The finding was that the average path closely matched the average neural firing rate. As the average path approached a decision boundary, the average firing rate increased.

In the 2003 experiment, recordings from cells that increased firing for one of the response categories were compared to recordings from cells that increased firing for the other of the response categories (Ratcliff, Cherian, and Segraves 2003). The diffusion model accounted for the difference between the firing rates of the two types of cells, but not for the firing rates of the cells themselves.

To model the two types of cells separately, Ratcliff, Hasegawa et al. (2006) proposed a dual diffusion model. In this model, evidence is accumulated separately for the two response alternatives as in accumulator models (e.g., Usher and McClelland 2001). For each alternative, evidence accumulation is a diffusion process (see Figure 8.2). The amount of evidence at any given point in the process is subject to decay as a function of the amount of evidence in the accumulator. This model fits all the same data as the standard diffusion model, but the advantage of the model is that it predicts the firing rates for the cells that respond in favor of one of the two types of stimuli as well as for the cells that respond in favor of the other type. Ratcliff, Hasegawa et al. (2006) showed that the model provided reasonably good fits to the behavioral data, and they used the best-fitting values of the parameters to generate predicted paths for the two types of cells separately (see also Mazurek et al. 2003). The averages of the predicted paths corresponded closely to the averages of the cells' firing rates.

Discussion

The goal of all the examples above is to think about how a cognitive system might be designed using, to the greatest extent possible, passive, parallel, and automatic processes. The idea is that computations performed passively at encoding or in parallel at retrieval can replace what have been thought to be more active processes or processes operating on new processing systems. This is important in the context of this Forum because it offers a different view of the infrastructure of cognition and provides the basis for initial biases in processing and inferences that are made in processing information.

Acknowledgments

This research was supported by National Institute of Mental Health grant HD MH44640 and National Institute for Deafness and other Communication Disorders grant DC01240.

References

Anderson, J. R. 1983. The Architecture of Cognition. Cambridge: Harvard Univ. Press.
Anderson, J. R. 1990. The Adaptive Character of Thought. Hillsdale, NJ: Lawrence Erlbaum.
Anderson, J. R. 1993. Rules of the Mind. Hillsdale, NJ: Lawrence Erlbaum.
Anderson, J. R., and C. Lebiere. 1998. The Atomic Components of Thought. Mahwah, NJ: Lawrence Erlbaum.
Bransford, J. D., J. R. Barclay, and J. J. Franks. 1972. Sentence memory: A constructive versus interpretive approach. Cogn. Psychol. 3:193–209.

Corbett, A. T., and F. R. Chang. 1983. Pronoun disambiguation: Accessing potential antecedents. *Mem. Cogn.* **11**:283–294.

Corbett, A.T., and B. A. Dosher. 1978. Instrument inferences in sentence encoding. *J. Verb. Learn. Behav.* **17**:479–491.

Ditterich, J. 2006. Computational approaches to visual decision making. In: Percept, Decision, Action: Bridging the Gaps, ed. D. J. Chadwick, M. Diamond, and J. Goode, p. 114. Chichester: Wiley.

Gillund, G., and R. M. Shiffrin. 1984. A retrieval model for both recognition and recall. *Psychol. Rev.* **91**:1–67.

Gold, J. I., and M. N. Shadlen. 2001. Neural computations that underlie decisions about sensory stimuli. *Trends Cogn. Sci.* **5**:10–16.

Graesser, A. C., M. Singer, and T. Trabasso. 1994. Constructing inferences during narrative text comprehension. *Psychol. Rev.* **101**:371–395.

Graesser, A. C., and R. A. Zwaan. 1995. Inference generation and the construction of situation models. In: Discourse Comprehension: Essays in Honor of Walter Kintsch, ed. C. A. Weaver, S. Mannes, and C. R. Fletcher, pp. 117–139. Hillsdale, NJ: Lawrence Erlbaum.

Hanes, D. P., and J. D. Schall. 1996. Neural control of voluntary movement initiation. *Science* **274**:427–430.

Heekeren, H. R., S. Marrett, P. A. Bandettini, and L. G. Ungerleider. 2004. A general mechanism for perceptual decision-making in the human brain. *Nature* **431**:859–862.

Hintzman, D. 1986. "Schema abstraction" in a multiple-trace memory model. *Psychol. Rev.* **93**:411–428.

Hintzman, D. 1988. Judgments of frequency and recognition memory in a multiple-trace memory model. *Psychol. Rev.* **95**:528–551.

Huk, A. C., and M. N. Shadlen. 2005. Neural activity in macaque parietal cortex reflects temporal integration of visual motion signals during perceptual decision making. *J. Neurosci.* **25**:10,420–10,436.

Kintsch, W. 1974. The representation of meaning in memory. Hillsdale, NJ: Lawrence Erlbaum.

Kintsch, W. 1988. The role of knowledge in discourse comprehension: A construction-integration model. *Psychol. Rev.* **95**:163–182.

Luce, R. D. 1986. Response Times. New York: Oxford Univ. Press.

Mazurek, M. E., J. D. Roitman, J. Ditterich, and M. N. Shadlen. 2003. A role for neural integrators in perceptual decision making. *Cerebral Cortex* **13**:1257–1269.

McKoon, G., and R. Ratcliff. 1986. Inferences about predictable events. *J. Exp. Psychol.: Learn. Mem. Cogn.* **12**:82–91.

McKoon, G., and R. Ratcliff. 1989. Inferences about contextually defined categories. *J. Exp. Psychol.: Learn. Mem. Cogn.* **15**:1134–1146.

McKoon, G., and R. Ratcliff. 1992a. Inference during reading. *Psychol. Rev.* **99**:440–466.

McKoon, G., and R. Ratcliff. 1992b. Spreading activation versus compound cue accounts of priming: Mediated priming revisited. *J. Exp. Psychol.: Learn. Mem. Cogn.* **18**:1155–1172.

McKoon, G., and R. Ratcliff. 1995a. Conceptual combinations and relational contexts in free association and in priming in lexical decision. *Psychon. Bull. Rev.* **2**:527–533.

McKoon, G., and R. Ratcliff. 1995b. The minimalist hypothesis: Directions for research. In: Discourse Comprehension: Essays in Honor of Walter Kintsch, ed. C. A. Weaver, S. Mannes, and C. R. Fletcher, pp. 97–116. Hillsdale, NJ: Lawrence Erlbaum.

McNamara, T. P. 1992a. Priming and constraints it places on theories of memory and retrieval. *Psychol. Rev.* **99**:650–662.

McNamara, T. P. 1992b. Theories of priming: I. Associative distance and lag. *J. Exp. Psychol.: Learn. Mem. Cogn.* **18**:1173–1190.

McNamara, T. P. 1994. Theories of priming: II. Types of primes. *J. Exp. Psychol: Learn. Mem. Cogn.* **20**:507–520.

Morton, J. 1969. The interaction of information in word recognition. *Psychol. Rev.* **76**:165–178.

Morton, J. 1970. A functional model for memory. In: Models of Human Memory, ed. D. A. Norman, pp. 203–254. New York: Academic Press.

Murdock, B. B. 1982. A theory for the storage and retrieval of item and associative information. *Psychol. Rev.* **89**:609–626.

Philiastides, M. G., R. Ratcliff, and P. Sajda. 2006. Neural representation of task difficulty and decision making during perceptual categorization: A timing diagram. *J. Neurosci.* **26**:8965–8975.

Posner, M. I. 1978. Chronometric explorations of mind. Hillsdale, NJ: Lawrence Erlbaum.

Quillian, M. R. 1969. The teachable language comprehender. *Comm. ACM* **12**:459–476.

Ratcliff, R. 1978. A theory of memory retrieval. *Psychol. Rev.* **85**:59–108.

Ratcliff, R. 1985. Theoretical interpretations of speed and accuracy of positive and negative responses. *Psychol. Rev.* **92**:212–225.

Ratcliff, R. 1988. Continuous versus discrete information processing: Modeling the accumulation of partial information. *Psychol. Rev.* **95**:238–255.

Ratcliff, R. 2002. A diffusion model account of reaction time and accuracy in a two-choice brightness discrimination task: Fitting real data and failing to fit fake but plausible data. *Psychon. Bull. Rev.* **9**:278–291.

Ratcliff, R. 2006. Modeling response signal and response time data. *Cogn. Psychol.* **53**:195–237.

Ratcliff, R., A. Cherian, and M. Segraves. 2003. A comparison of macaque behavior and superior colliculus neuronal activity to predictions from models of simple two-choice decisions. *J. Neurophys.* **90**:1392–1407.

Ratcliff, R., Y. T. Hasegawa, Y. P. Hasegawa, P. L. Smith, and M. A. Segraves. 2006. A dual diffusion model for behavioral and neural decision making. *J. Neurophys.* **97**:1756–1774.

Ratcliff, R., and G. McKoon. 1988. A retrieval theory of priming in memory. *Psychol. Rev.* **95**:385–408.

Ratcliff, R., and G. McKoon. 1994. Retrieving information from memory: Spreading activation theories versus compound cue theories. *Psychol. Rev.* **101**:177–184.

Ratcliff, R., and G. McKoon. 1995. Sequential effects in lexical decision: Tests of compound cue retrieval theory. *J. Exp. Psychol.: Learn. Mem. Cogn.* **21**:1380–1388.

Ratcliff, R., and G. McKoon. 1996. Biases in implicit memory tasks. *J. Exp. Psychol.: Gen.* **125**:403–421.

Ratcliff, R., and G. McKoon. 1997. A counter model for implicit priming in perceptual word identification. *Psychol. Rev.* **104**:319–343.

Ratcliff, R., and G. McKoon. 2007. The diffusion decision model: Theory and data for two-choice decision tasks. *Neural Comp.*, in press.

Ratcliff, R., and J. N. Rouder. 1998. Modeling response times for two-choice decisions. *Psychol. Sci.* **9**:347–356.

Ratcliff, R., and P. L. Smith. 2004. A comparison of sequential sampling models for two-choice reaction time. *Psychol. Rev.* **111**:333–367.

Ratcliff, R., A. Thapar, P. Gomez, and G. McKoon. 2004. A diffusion model analysis of the effects of aging in the lexical-decision task. *Psychol. Aging* **19**:278–289.

Ratcliff, R., A. Thapar, and G. McKoon. 2001. The effects of aging on reaction time in a signal detection task. *Psychol. Aging* **16**:323–341.

Ratcliff, R., A. Thapar, and G. McKoon. 2003. A diffusion model analysis of the effects of aging on brightness discrimination. *Perc. Psychophys.* **65**:523–535.

Ratcliff, R., A. Thapar, and G. McKoon. 2004. A diffusion model analysis of the effects of aging on recognition memory. *J. Mem. Lang.* **50**:408–424.

Ratcliff, R., A. Thapar, and G. McKoon. 2006. Aging and individual differences in rapid two-choice decisions. *Psychon. Bull. Rev.* **13**:626–635.

Ratcliff, R., A. Thapar, and G. McKoon. 2007. Applying the diffusion model to data from 75–85 year old subjects in 5 experimental tasks. *Psychol. Aging* **22**:56–66.

Ratcliff, R., and F. Tuerlinckx. 2002. Estimating the parameters of the diffusion model: Approaches to dealing with contaminant reaction times and parameter variability. *Psychon. Bull. Rev.* **9**:438–481.

Ratcliff, R., T. Van Zandt, and G. McKoon. 1999. Connectionist and diffusion models of reaction time. *Psychol. Rev.* **106**:261–300.

Roitman, J. D., and M. N. Shadlen. 2002. Response of neurons in the lateral interparietal area during a combined visual discrimination reaction time task. *J. Neurosci.* **22**:9475–9489.

Schacter, D. L., and E. Tulving. 1994. What are the memory systems of 1994? In: Memory Systems, ed. D. L. Schacter and E. Tulving, pp. 1–38. Cambridge, MA: MIT Press.

Schall, J. D. 2003. Neural correlates of decision processes: Neural and mental chronometry. *Curr. Opin. Neurobiol.* **13**:182–186.

Schooler, L., R. M Shiffrin, and J. G. W. Raaijmakers. 2001. A model for implicit effects in perceptual identification. *Psychol. Rev.* **108**:257–272.

Shiffrin, R. M., and M. Steyvers, M. 1997. A model for recognition memory: REM: Retrieving effectively from memory. *Psychon. Bull. Rev.* **4**:145–166.

Singer, M., A. C. Graesser, and T. Trabasso. 1994. Minimal or global inference in comprehension. *J. Mem. Lang.* **33**:421–441.

Spaniol, J., D. J. Madden, and A. Voss. 2006. A diffusion model analysis of adult age differences in episodic and semantic long-term memory retrieval. *J. Exp. Psychol.: Learn. Mem. Cogn.* **32**:101–117.

Squire, L. R. 1992. Memory and the hippocampus: A synthesis from findings with rats, monkeys, and humans. *Psychol. Rev.* **99**:195–231.

Stone, M. 1960. Models for choice reaction time. *Psychometrika* **25**:251–260.

Swensson, R. G. 1972. The elusive tradeoff: Speed versus accuracy in visual discrimination tasks. *Perc. Psychophys.* **12**:16–32.

Thapar, A., R. Ratcliff, and G. McKoon. 2003. A diffusion model analysis of the effects of aging on letter discrimination. *Psychol. Aging* **18**:415–429.

Tulving, E. 1972. Episodic and semantic memory. In: Organization and Memory, ed. E. Tulving and W. Donaldson, pp. 381–403. New York: Academic Press.

Tulving, E. 1974. Cue-dependent forgetting. *Am. Sci.* **62**:74–82.

Tulving, E., and D. M. Thomson. 1973. Encoding specificity and retrieval processes in episodic memory. *Psychol. Rev.* **80**:352–373.

Usher, M., and J. L. McClelland. 2001. The time course of perceptual choice: The leaky, competing accumulator model. *Psychol. Rev.* **108**:550–592.

9

How Culture and Brain Mechanisms Interact in Decision Making

Merlin Donald

Department of Cognitive Science, Case Western Reserve
University, Cleveland, OH 44106–7068, U.S.A.

Abstract

Decision making is a very private thing, individualized and personal. Yet it has a cultural dimension. The human brain does not acquire language, symbolic skills, or any form of symbolic cognition without the pedagogical guidance of culture and, as a result, most decisions made in modern society engage learned algorithms of thought that are imported from culture.

Mathematical thought is a good example of this: it is cultural in origin, and highly dependent on notations and habits invented over many generations. Its algorithms were created culturally, by means of a slow, deliberate process of creation and refinement. Thus, the algorithms that determine many mathematically based decisions reside, over the long run, in culture. The brains of the individuals making the decisions are, in most particular instances, temporary "carriers" of cultural algorithms, vehicles for applying them in a particular time and place. In principle, this conclusion applies to many examples, such as chess-playing, social judgment, business decisions, the composition of poetry, and so on.

Culturally transmitted algorithms can be learned and made so automatic that they can be executed by the brain without much conscious supervision. Unconscious or "intuitive" decisions are often the best, and many successful decisions occur in an automatized manner, in highly over-practiced situations. This does not diminish the larger role of consciousness in cognition, because, when necessary, decision makers retain the option of intervening consciously and deliberately to modify or fix their specific performances. Conscious supervision is thus the ultimate tribunal in cognition, a cutting-edge adaptation that is particularly important in the creative role of generating and changing the existing algorithms of culture that underlie most decisions.

Introduction

Decision making seems to be a very private thing: individualized, personal, and confined to the brain. Yet it has a cultural dimension. Culture defines much about the human brain, especially the so-called "higher-order" cognitive features that constrain and indeed, under some circumstances, mediate decisions. The human brain does not acquire language, symbolic skills, or any form of symbolic cognition without the pedagogical guidance of culture. Through its epigenetic impact, culture is a major determinant of how the brain self-organizes during development, both in its patterns of connectivity and in its large-scale functional architecture.

Individual decisions are made in the brain. Human brains, however, are closely interconnected with, and embedded in, the distributed networks of culture from infancy. These networks may not only define the decision-space, but also create, install, and constrain many of the cognitive processes that mediate decisions. Humans are collective thinkers, who rarely solve problems without input from the distributed cognitive systems of culture. For this reason, it is important to gain some perspective on the cultural and evolutionary context of decision making and its implications for building accurate models of neural and cognitive systems.

The Impact of Culture on Brain Development

The most obvious example of culture's impact on brain development is literacy skill. Literacy is a fairly recent historical change, with no precedent in archaic human cultures. The vast majority of the world's languages have never developed an indigenous writing system. Certain dominant modern cultures, by contrast, are not only literate, but heavily dependent on mass literacy for much of their cognitive work. Mass literacy is only spread by imposing modifications on the developing nervous systems of large numbers of individuals. These modifications are created by "educational" systems, which are basically systems of organized group pedagogy whose origins can be traced back to the beginnings of literate culture.

The cognitive subroutines that enable a person to become literate consist of chains of deeply automatized responses to visual symbols. These are hierarchically organized in functional brain architectures that support specific subcomponents of reading and writing skills, which are typically learned by prolonged immersion in educational systems that are highly idiosyncratic and culture-specific. The algorithms of educational systems are generated and transmitted collectively, and are formed by the governing ideas of the cultural environment. Literacy training is not easy; it takes a considerable amount of time and is not even close to becoming a species-universal skill for biologically modern humans.

Automatization of complex, fast response systems is the key to acquiring literacy skill. Non-automatized responses, such as those of someone who is learning a new language, do not allow the student to concentrate on the meaning of what is written. Automatization of all the stages of literacy training—including word recognition, grammar, vocabulary expansion, and expressive skill—can be achieved only after very extensive practice, to the point of overlearning, in successive stages of competency. During the acquisition phase of such skills, continuous conscious monitoring and corrective feedback is necessary. Once the basic skill has been learned to the point where the entire procedural system is automatic, conscious monitoring of the basic skill-set is no longer needed, and the response of the system becomes mandatory; that is, the reader cannot avoid responding to a visually presented word as a word. At that point, words and sentences can no longer be treated by the brain merely as a series of lines and contrasts; the meaning literally "pops out" of the marks on the page. Yet no one claims that these pop-out experiences are innate; they are culturally arbitrary and learned. They are also one of the most important interfaces with the distributed systems of culture, and they result in real physical changes to the brain, imposed by means of extensive cultural programming.

The physical reality of the culturally imposed automatic brain systems underlying literacy skill can be seen clearly in certain cases of acquired dyslexia and dysgraphia. In such cases, injury to the brain of a literate person selectively destroys a particular cognitive subcomponent of the literacy system, without damaging other closely related brain systems, such as speech and symbolic thought. Literacy-related brain systems thus appear quasi-modular in their organization: they can suffer partial breakdown of certain components, while leaving others intact. For example, one particular lesion might cause a patient to lose the ability to read while retaining the ability to write, and another patient might suffer the reverse. Specific lesions might even eliminate the ability to read irregularly spelled words, while the patient remains able to read words with regular spelling. These cases point to the existence of specificity of function in acquired brain architectures. This is incontrovertible evidence in support of the direct impact of culture on adult brain functional organization.

There are many other similar examples of cognitive skills that require extensive training, originate in culture, and depend upon acquired functional brain architectures (e.g., mathematical, musical, artistic and athletic skills). However, the neuropsychology of literacy skill stands as the strongest evidence that culture can impose radical cognitive reorganization on the brain.

This contrasts with a common alternative view of brain–culture interaction, which argues that the brain provides the basic mechanisms, whereas culture provides specific content. For example, in the theory of sexual behavior espoused by Behaviorism, innate brain mechanisms energize the human mating instinct, while culture shapes and defines the specific details of mating behavior in different times and places through conditioning. In the standard cognitive science approach to perception, the brain provides the innate neural machinery of perception, which defines the parameters of perceptual experience, and culture simply shapes the norms and expectations that influence specific perceptual experiences. Similarly, the neo-Chomskian view of language holds that language capacity is innate, universal, and brain-based, whereas culture provides the particular details of the native tongue.

These approaches share a common belief, which reduces the role of culture to that of content provider, and holds that cognitive capabilities are direct products of brain evolution. This is largely true of many aspects of common mammalian behavior and cognition. For example, the capacity to shift attention is innate and depends on specific brain systems; in a neurologically normal child, it will develop without cultural input. Culture may bias attention toward certain things and away from others, but the influence of culture is limited to specifying what to attend to, and it does not play a role in creating the capacity itself. The same applies to other basic functions, such as capacities for various kinds of perception and action.

This assumption, however, is not valid in the case of human higher cognition. For example, language does not emerge spontaneously in a socially isolated brain; unlike attention, it does not self-install. The raw capacity for language may indeed be there in the abstract sense that it is latent in every neurologically normal human, but it will remain unrealized unless culture has an opportunity to guide the brain through the very subtle and complex process of language acquisition. In this case, it is culture that enables the capacity itself. This is not a trivial distinction, because it reveals a unique evolutionary phenomenon: the development of cognitive capacities that are qualitatively more powerful than their predecessors, and originate not in a specific brain adaptation, but in a special coevolutionary event that involved a close feedback loop running from culture back to the brain, and vice versa.

It was no accident that, when asked to draw a diagram of the neural basis of language, Saussure drew two brains engaged in a circular interactive loop (Saussure 1908). Two brains constitute the minimal conditions for a culture, and their interaction adds up to more than the sum of the parts. Culture plays a crucial role in actually making language possible, because languages do not originate in individual brains; they emerge only in culture. They are negotiated, like treaties, and are assimilated by individuals. They never emerge in the isolated individual, and the process of language evolution, which started at least two million years ago, perhaps earlier, is literally inconceivable outside of the context of brain–culture coevolution. Thus, although the example of the culturally installed "literacy brain" demonstrates the vulnerability of the human neurocognitive system to cultural input in dramatic fashion, it is far from unique. The human brain has been wiring itself up through culture for a long time, and literacy skills are only the latest case in point.

Cultures as Distributed Cognitive Systems

What adaptive forces drove human cultures to invest so heavily in literacy education and, consequently, in the epigenetic reprogramming of millions of brains at great cost?

Human cultures are unique in their highly cognitive character: ideas and memories can be traded and shared among the members of a cultural group, and intellectual work can be shared. Groups can create cognitive outcomes, make decisions, influence perceptions, and generate worldviews. A useful perspective on this aspect of culture can be taken from computational modeling: culture can be compared in principle to distributed computational networks, in which many computers are interconnected in a network. The network can then acquire properties that were lacking in the individual computers making up the network, such as greater memory resources and a specialized division of cognitive labor. Membership in such a network can make each individual computer look "smarter" than it appeared before joining the network. By extension, this applies to human beings living in culture. Specialization and organization of work can be coordinated in a network, and the cognitive power of the coordinated group system can far exceed the reach of any individual. One could perhaps point to the Manhattan Project as the supreme example of what technologically enhanced cooperative cognitive work (including decision making) can achieve, when performed in distributed systems made up of specialized, symbolically coordinated components.

Distributed cognition is a useful paradigm in which to view the developing brain. From birth, the rapidly growing human brain is immersed in a massive distributed cognitive network: culture. The network "interface" of the brain to culture is usually a social one. It consists of interactions with the unwitting "carriers" of the particular culture in which the infant is raised: parents, relatives, and peers who convey crucial information about where to direct attention, what to notice, and what to remember. The human infant's brain is biased to seek such input from the start. One might say that it has evolved a specialized adaptation to seek out an early connection with cultural-cognitive networks (Tomasello 1999). Any serious failure to establish this social-cognitive connection can result in delayed development and in some cases, such as autism, in a permanent developmental disability. This early cultural bond is crucial; the human brain has evolved a dependency on culturally stored information for the realization of its design potential.

This dependency applies to the specific content of the knowledge stored in culture, but it applies especially to the process of gaining access to culture in the first place. The first priority of a developing human brain must be to acquire from culture the basic social and attentional tools that it needs to elaborate its cultural connection. Having done this in early infancy, it will then be in a position to acquire a massive amount of specific cultural content, some of which is procedural, in the form of skill, including language skill, and some of which is semantic. Even episodic and perceptual memories are affected greatly by culture, in the sense that they are heavily filtered and channeled; however, skills and many kinds of semantic representations literally cannot exist without culture, because they are generated there. Without completing the crucial early phases of connection and sharing of mind, much of the information in culture will remain unavailable to the brain throughout life. From the viewpoint of capacity development, social-cognitive skills are especially enabling and empowering in early life: they make possible and expand access to information stored in subtle and otherwise invisible cultural loci.

One of culture's most important by-products, technology, has further extended these prototypically human symbolic capacities by restructuring the distributed cognitive networks of culture, and opening up new possibilities for both representing knowledge and remembering it. A typical modern cognitive-cultural distributed network links together many human brains with communications technology, images, books, papers, and computers. These kinds of distributed networks perform much of the cognitive work of modern society, from landing aircraft, to predicting the weather, and planning educational curricula. Individuals must be attuned to these networks to function effectively in our society. Decision making occurs within tight network boundaries.

This raises a major scientific question: What are the specific domains in which the human brain attunes itself to culture? The major interface of the human brain and its cultures is undoubtedly a cognitive one. The uniquely cognitive nature of human cultures can only be explained in terms of a brain–culture symbiosis in the domain of cognition. Cognition can be appropriately singled out as the primary sphere in which culture and brain interact. Human cognition constitutes a complex core of subcapacities and operations, interconnected by means of an equally complex array of algorithms, shaped by cultural forces during development. This applies to both the individual brain and to the wider distributed systems of culture. The individual is transformed by immersion in a distributed system. In such systems, memory is distributed in many locations, and access paths proliferate.

One property of distributed systems is the division of labor across individuals. In a distributed system, an individual brain no longer has to contain within itself all of the skills and information needed for individual survival. Perceiving, remembering, recalling, searching, and attending are managed to a degree from the outside by means of various symbolic media, as are the specific learned algorithms of thought. As the division of cognitive labor in culture becomes more and more specialized, the adaptive task facing a young mind changes, and this has consequences for the deployment of the brain's resources. In particular, memory storage and retrieval is divided between brains and other media in the complex distributed systems of modern culture, as are many of the algorithms that drive thinking and problem solving. Since this modifies the habitual use patterns involved in cognition, and brain activity and growth directly reflect its habitual use patterns, it is reasonable to postulate that concomitant brain processes, such as synaptic growth and regional localization, are also immediately affected. Unfortunately, although brain plasticity has been well documented in humans, there is not yet very much direct empirical evidence from brain-imaging studies on precisely how habitual, culturally imposed use patterns affect growth and development throughout the life span. We have only begun to collect empirical data on the neuropsychological impact of our close interaction with the external symbolic environment. By collecting more evidence, perhaps we will come to know, more exactly, how early and deep immersion in the distributed cognitive networks of culture affects the development of the nervous system.

One way to refine the questions that need to be answered in this area further is to observe brain–culture interaction over long periods of time. The pattern of emergence of cognitive change and cultural differentiation in human ancestors might prove helpful in conceptualizing how internal cognitive activity, in the brain, is interwoven with cognitive cultural activity, in distributed networks. In turn, this might enable us to ask more telling questions of the brain.

A Model of Human Cognitive and Cultural Coevolution

The most unique innovation of human beings in prehistory was the evolution of distributed cognition to a new level, indeed, to several new levels that had no precedent in other species. The human brain is adapted to the existence of cognizing mind-sharing cultures that far exceed the individual in terms of their ability to store and transmit accumulated knowledge and skill. However, mind-sharing cultures could not have emerged by themselves de novo. They are the product of a spiraling interaction between brain evolution and cultural change. The following is a brief review of a specific model of brain–mind–culture coevolution in hominids (Donald 1991, 1993, 1995, 2001).

The methodology used to derive this model was inherently interdisciplinary, drawing from many fields that could provide relevant evidence. My basic technique was to test every hypothesis, whether it grew out of a single field of research, or several, against evidence from all other relevant fields of research, and to reject any hypothesis that was incompatible with any solid fact, whatever its origin. This tends to produce robust theories, since accidental convergences from quite disparate fields of inquiry are highly unlikely to occur, and multiple accidental convergences are even less likely (Donald 2004).

There was one additional core postulate driving this model: brain–culture coevolution, with cultural-cognitive evolution leading eventually to such innovations as language. If brain and culture coevolved, the result should have produced a universal architecture of cognition—both on the individual and the distributed levels—evident in all human cultures. Such a structure should endure, even in the modern context, because evolution is conservative and systems that are working well do not tend to be replaced. The larger architecture of distributed cognitive-cultural systems should be a relatively stable and universal structure. A large-scale cognitive-cultural hierarchy of mechanisms should form the basis for cognitive activity within the networks that support mind-sharing cultures.

In this model, there are three hypothesized "stages" of cultural-cognitive change in hominid evolution, during which the nature of hominid culture gradually shifted from the marginally symbolic to the proto-symbolic to the fully symbolic. This process was not conceived solely as a linear, gradualistic series of changes, but rather was characterized by several "punctuations" in an otherwise fairly stable hominid survival strategy. There was an archaic preadaptation about 2 million years ago when Homo first emerged, followed by a much more recent cognitive shift, within the past 400,000 years, that was radical and relatively rapid, and culminated in the fully symbolic cultures of biologically modern humans.

The physical evidence favoring this model came initially from two principal sources: fossils and material culture. An analysis of the fossil remains of human ancestors reveals two periods where there was a relatively rapid increase in hominid brain size and a change in body shape toward the modern pattern: the period from approximately –2 Mya to –1.5 Mya, when the species Homo first appeared, and a second period from –500 Kya to –150 Kya, when the species Homo sapiens first appeared.

Without necessarily conceding that increased brain size or body shape tells us anything in detail about the hominid mind, they do allow for some rough time markers and a partial reconstruction of their way of life. Such reconstructions suggest that these were periods of significant cognitive challenge, with a concomitant change in the survival strategies of hominids. The material cultural record left behind by hominids agrees with this picture. There were major changes in the cultural record during, and following, these two periods. The changes included changes in such things as toolmaking, firemaking and firetending, diet, hunting skill, migration patterns, and the location and construction of home bases and shelters. Cultural and anatomical changes have not always coincided, and there is much debate about such details as the number of hominid subspecies; however, the standard story of hominid emergence has not changed fundamentally during the last two decades.

There are compelling neural and cognitive considerations that greatly enrich this picture. Comparative anatomical evidence is an important clue here. Hominid evolution follows a trajectory from Miocene apes to modern humans. The starting and end points of brain anatomy are well known. Major differences between ape and human anatomy have been subjected to more detailed study, using advanced techniques, during the past decade, and the picture that emerges does not permit as much theoretical leeway as some might assume this field allows.

The cognitive networks that permeate all human cultures evolved in three stages, each of which added a new kind of representational "layer" to human culture and had its own evolutionary rationale. These networks dominate the brain and mind in epigenesis and impose a hierarchical structure on higher, or symbolic, cognition. Such networks might be labeled, for convenience, "cognitive-cultural networks" (CCNs). They influence significantly the developing brain of a child, through the mediation of parents and community. CCNs co-evolved with changes in various brain structures and cannot exist without the cerebral apparatus that allows the young brain to assimilate these representational systems. On the other hand, it appears that very little detail is specified in the genes at this level. Increasingly, as a result of human evolution, it is the interaction between a highly plastic genetic potential and cultural reality on the ground in any given generation that generates the actual cognitive organization of the individual brain.

Table 9.1 illustrates the key points of this evolutionary theory of human cognitive origins. It begins in Miocene primates who had cognitive capabilities that are assumed to be roughly similar to those of modern apes, and had capabilities that are labeled as episodic. The three successive stages of hominid cognitive evolution proposed in this scenario are labeled as mimetic, mythic, and theoretic. Note that hominid cognitive evolution has here been captured in three cultural stages, because the most radical innovation in the hominid line is distributed cognition, culminating in a system of language and symbolic communication that has cultural origins. The scenario is thus: first generate cognizing cultures of a proto-symbolic nature; then let these become more complex, until they "combust" spontaneously into systems of symbolic convention and, eventually, into full-fledged language.

This proposal may seem unfamiliar to many cognitive neuroscientists, but the "stages" of human cognitive-cultural evolution should not be too unfamiliar, because they were established on a rigorous cognitive criterion: each putative stage involved a novel form of memory representation, and a new style of cognitive governance at the top of the distributed cognitive system that was, quite literally, governing. Each new stage—mimetic, mythic, and theoretic—marked the genesis of a new medium, or domain, of memory representation in the distributed system, or CCN, and also in the individual brain. The latter effect was an epigenetic change due to "deep enculturation." Each CCN domain postulated in this model has a complex internal hierarchical structure dictated by the properties of the shared memory systems available to hominids at that stage. The superordinate descriptive labels (i.e., episodic, mimetic, mythic, and theoretic) express and capture the top, or governing, level of representation within each domain.

I would like to add that this is a "cascade" model inasmuch as it assumes (as Darwin did) a basically conservative process that retains previous gains. As hominids moved through this sequence of cognitive adaptations, they retained each previous adaptation, which continued to perform its cognitive work perfectly well. Mimetic cognition incorporates, and extends, prior gains at the episodic level; mythic, or narrative-based cognition, is built on top of a

Table 9.1 Key points of the evolutionary theory of human cognitive origins.

Stage	Species/ Period	Novel Forms of Representation	Manifest Change	Cognitive Governance
Episodic	Primate	Complex episodic event perceptions	Improved self-awareness and event sensitivity	Episodic and reactive; limited voluntary expressive morphology
Mimetic (1st transition)	Early hominids, peaking in *H. erectus* (4 M to 0.4 Mya)	Nonverbal action modeling	Revolution in skill, gesture (including vocal), nonverbal communication, shared attention	Mimetic: increased variability of custom, cultural "archetypes"
Mythic (2nd transition)	Sapient humans, peaking in *H. sapiens* (0.5 Mya to present)	Linguistic modeling	High-speed phonology, oral language, oral social record	Lexical invention, narrative thought, mythic framework of governance
Theoretic (3rd transition)	Recent sapient cultures	Extensive external symbolization, both verbal and nonverbal	Formalisms, large-scale theoretic artifacts and massive external memory storage	Institutionalized paradigmatic thought and invention

basically mimetic, or gestural, mode of thought and communication; and theoretic cognition evolved slowly out of the classic mythic-mimetic thought strategies of traditional human cultural networks, retaining the latter within it. The first two hominid transitions—from episodic to mimetic, and from mimetic to mythic—were mediated largely by neurobiological change, while the third transition to the theoretic mode was heavily dependent on changes in external, nonbiological, or artificial, memory technology. The fully modern mind retains all of these structures, both in the individual brain as well as in the distributed networks that govern cognitive activity in cultural networks.

Each of these stages was marked by complex modifications in hominid survival strategies that undoubtedly involved many different changes in skeletal anatomy, brain anatomy, emotional responsivity, intelligence, memory, social organization, reproductive strategies, and temperament, among many other factors. Cognitive evolution could not have taken place in a vacuum, and major changes in cognition undoubtedly had implications for many survival-related variables, including diet, intraspecific and interspecific aggression, heat dissipation, metabolic energy, disease resistance, physical size, sexual dimorphism, and so on. The cognitive stages listed above were derived in that very wide theoretical context. However, the prime driving force behind these changes was a cognitive one.

The reasons for labeling the primate cultures of the Miocene epoch as "episodic" have been spelled out in previous publications (Donald, 1991, 1993, 2001). The theory begins with the assumption that the early hominid brain, like its primate, and most probably australopithecine, predecessors, lacked language or any capacity for generating explicit symbolic representation in the wild. The archaic hominid brain, like most others in the primate line, shared the same basic design features that humans share with all primate brains. This means that the earliest predecessors of hominids would have been very clever social animals, with a remarkable ability to understand fairly complex social relationships, but limited expressive skill. In other words, they could understand social episodes and scenarios, but had no way of expressing this knowledge to one another.

The cognitive capacity that supports episodic intelligence is best described as "event representation." Events are the "atoms" of episodic cognition. Social life consists of events, clustered in episodes which define alliances, troupe membership, and power relationships. By this definition, primates have excellent event representations, or ERs. They can remember specific events in an episodic manner; that is, they remember vivid details that are specific to a particular episode (e.g., after a fight with a rival, they remember the principal agents, outcomes, and future social implications of the fight). That kind of vivid, detailed event memory in humans is usually called episodic memory, and it is anchored in concrete events. For this reason, the cognitive and cultural style of primates might be labeled "episodic."

The episodic mind-set of primates is non-symbolic or pre-symbolic in its expressive or representational style. There is no evidence that primates think or communicate in symbols in their natural state. The episodic mind is concrete, analogical, episode-bound, and anchored firmly in the perceived present. It acts largely within the span of working memory, using perceived similarities between situations (and also distinctions between them) as a means of choosing appropriate behavior.

Hominids, who shared an ancestor with chimpanzees about 6 million years ago, evolved beyond this mind-set at some point in their emergence. If we assume a Miocene starting point for hominids that was very close to the cognitive capacities of modern apes (A), and use biologically modern humans as the end point (B), the theoretical exercise becomes one of identifying the most probable sequence of events—neural, cognitive, and cultural—leading from A to B. The three transitions outlined in Table 9.1 constitute a coherent theory of the nature and approximate time course of the path from A to B. This provides a wide cognitive framework for reexamining the process of individual decision making in human beings.

Implications for Theories of Human Decision Making

The act of making a decision might be taken as one major paradigm with which to examine a very wide range of brain–culture interactions. Decisions are the final resolution events of a variety of cognitive scenarios that can engage, in theory, the entire voluntary action repertoire of human beings. Essentially, decisions occur at choice points in a cognitive sequence. Thus, one could, in theory, "decide" which memory to retrieve, which stimulus to attend to, which perceptual set to activate, which emotional attitude to assume toward a social scenario, as well as which pattern of action to pursue in a variety of contexts.

Decision making thus engages so many subroutines and subsidiary systems concerned with memory, symbolic representation, and thought as to constitute an abstract category that cuts across all of cognition. Decisions are sometimes imposed on innate brain systems (e.g., whether to smile in a particular social context) and are sometimes embedded in algorithms and mental habits with purely cultural origins (e.g., decisions involving numbers or other symbolic systems, or those that must obey complex symbol-based rules, such as buying stocks, filling out crossword puzzles, or choosing materials for a tool). Human decision making is most commonly a culturally determined process in which many basic cognitive operations play a part, and the mechanisms of such decisions must be regarded as hybrid systems in which both brain and culture play a role. When the individual "makes" a decision, that decision has usually been made within a wider framework of distributed cognition, and, in many instances, it is fair to ask whether the decision was really made by the distributed cognitive cultural system itself, with the individual reduced to a subsidiary role.

This is not a simple issue to resolve: the individual brain and mind contain within them a great deal of history and structure that can be brought to bear on how decisions are made in specific cases. The brain regions engaged in a specific kind of decision may be determined as much by this history as by innate brain growth patterns, both because of the epigenetic impact of culture on cognitive architecture and because the actual task imposed on the brain by a given decision can be changed by redistributive effects that occur within the networks of culture. Distributed systems are able to change where in the system each component that influences a certain decision is located. This applies to such things as the locus of memory storage for a specific item, of a specialized cognitive operation, and of the choice mechanism itself. When all of these components are located in a particular individual brain, decision making is one thing; when they are distributed across various people and information media, it is quite another, even if the final "decision" is made by one person. For this reason, and because decision making is so wide in its application, we should not predict the existence of a specialized brain region or subsystem that is devoted to resolving decisions in any general sense of the term. Rather, one might say that decisions can be made in many different ways that might involve different anatomical subsystems of the brain.

Better than Conscious?

The question of conscious versus unconscious processing in decision making can be better understood in the wider perspective of distributed CCNs and the brain's entrainment to them. The conscious mind is the mediator of novelty and learning. It has the capacity to guide mental development, but it is not the mediator of mundane routine, even in the highest aspects of symbolic thought. A professional mathematician does not think about his use of the elementary notations that mediate his creative thought process; if he did, he could not be creative at that level. Similarly, a writer who worried about forming individual letters, or composing correct grammatical sentences, could not focus on the level of narrative or characterization. Human cognitive prehistory is basically a scenario of downloading complex cognitive processes to the automatic mode. By creating a distributed system that carries the framework of collective cognition across generations, humans have reduced the load on consciousness. We have minimized the need for conscious monitoring of most thought and memory processes by forcing mastery in the individual to the point of automatization. This enables a person to move up to another level in the task hierarchy.

The decoupling of consciousness from attention is clear in cases of highly automatized skills, such as reading music. To master this task sufficiently to perform at a professional level, a complex chain of skills must be practiced for many years. This skill-set involves the entrainment of attention at an unconscious level, in the sense that a musician must not be self-conscious about elementary operations such as what a specific symbol on the page might mean. The performer must focus on interpretation, emotion, and coordination with accompanying musicians. The notes and phrasing must take care of themselves, meaning that they must not make demands on conscious capacity.

A musician has the option, however, of intervening consciously at those lower levels when necessary. Conscious attention has a "zoom" feature that allows intervention at many points in the task hierarchy. For instance, if a finger is locked, or the instrument is eccentric in some way, adjustment may have to be made at the level of fingering or some other technical skill. Those adjustments will be made with conscious guidance, because they are novel and unpredictable in outcome. The lesson is simple: the power of conscious intervention is available when needed. If the musician is well trained and in good health, all technical elements of the performance are well maintained, and the focus of conscious effort can be placed where it should be: at the top, where crucial decisions are being made online, as the performance unfolds.

A musician is often embedded in a larger distributed cognitive structure, such as an orchestra. That structure constrains the choices the musicians can make and dictates much about the performance. Individuals are still in control of their roles, but these roles are framed by a vast web of culturally enforced expectations and coordinated operations. The "zoom" function of consciousness is even more important in such situations, because monitoring must be simultaneously directed internally, at personal performance parameters, as well as externally, at coordination with the group.

The important conclusion is that the possibility of conscious intervention in every decision remains viable. Decisions may be made automatically, without conscious engagement, in highly overpracticed routine situations. Yet even in such situations, when necessary, the performer can intervene consciously at any level in the internal cognitive system. Certain kinds of decisions must be made consciously, especially those involving novelty or learning. However, for the larger distributed systems of culture to operate smoothly, the rule seems to be: the less conscious engagement, the better. Conscious intervention is needed for acquisition and feedback control, but most individual cognitive operations should be made as automatic as possible in such systems. This constitutes a kind of industrialized cultural-cognitive network coordination, with concomitant efficiencies and increased collective power.

At this Ernst Strüngmann Forum, much has been made of the superior powers of spontaneous "intuition" in decision making. Such intuitions are sometimes considered "unconscious"; however, this is a rigged argument. In most examples, cases of superior "intuitions" are clearly the outputs of deeply enculturated routines that have been acquired by means of conscious rehearsal and refinement. A highly automatized subroutine may indeed function better at times without conscious intervention: the musician example given above is a case in point. This applies, in principle, to many other examples: face recognition (an acquired, highly culture-specific skill), chess playing, various kinds of social judgment, business decisions, and the composition of poetry. In each case, the task hierarchy is typically acquired in the context of a distributed cognitive-cultural system, with extensive pedagogy and training, and highly conscious, or deliberate, practice and rehearsal (sometimes in the form of imaginative play), to the point of automatizing the response, which affords the temporary release of conscious monitoring. In short, one of the main objectives of human conscious supervision is to make itself less important in future performances of the same activity.

As in all things, however, there is an associated caveat: Although there are obvious advantages to abandoning personal conscious control in overlearned performances, under some circumstances (and especially in novel situations), there are equally obvious dangers. The conscious individual is still the ultimate arbiter of choice, and the CCNs that store algorithms in culture, and transmit them to new generations, cannot be constructed without a great deal of conscious deliberation. The short-term advantages of a loss of conscious control in many situations should not be allowed to overshadow the larger role of consciousness in assembling the elaborate, and uniquely human, distributed cognitive apparatus of culture, keeping it on course, and preventing it from becoming unstable.

References and Further Reading

Donald, M. 1991. Origins of the Modern Mind: Three Stages in the Evolution of Culture and Cognition. Cambridge, MA: Harvard Univ. Press.

Donald, M. 1993. Précis of Origins of the Modern Mind with multiple reviews and author's response. *Behav. Brain Sci.* **16**:737–791.

Donald, M. 1995. The neurobiology of human consciousness: An evolutionary approach. *Neuropsychologia* **33**:1087–1102.

Donald, M. 1998. Mimesis and the executive suite: Missing links in language evolution. In: Approaches to the Evolution of Language: Social and Cognitive Bases, ed. J. R. Hurford, M. Studdert-Kennedy, and C. Knight, pp. 44–67. Cambridge: Cambridge Univ. Press.

Donald, M. 1999. Preconditions for the evolution of protolanguages. In: The Descent of Mind, ed. M. C. Corballis and I. Lea, pp. 120–136. Oxford: Oxford Univ. Press.

Donald, M. 2001. A Mind So Rare: The Evolution of Human Consciousness. New York: W. W. Norton and Company.

Donald, M. 2004. The virtues of rigorous interdisciplinarity. In: The Development of the Mediated Mind: Sociocultural Context and Cognitive Development, ed. J. Lucariello, J. Hudson, R. Fivush, and P. Bauer, pp. 245–256. Cambridge: Cambridge Univ. Press.

Donald, M. 2005. Imitation and mimesis. In: Perspectives on Imitation: From Neuroscience to Social Science, ed. S. Hurley and N. Chater. Cambridge, MA: MIT Press.

Nelson, K. 1996. Language in Cognitive Development: Emergence of the Mediated Mind. New York: Cambridge Univ. Press.

Saussure, F. de. 1908/9. Introduction au deuxième cours de linguistique générale, ed. R. Godel. Geneva: Droz.

Shallice, T. 1988. From Neuropsychology to Mental Structure. New York: Cambridge Univ. Press.

Tomasello, M. 1999. The Cultural Origins of Human Cognition. Cambridge, MA: Harvard Univ. Press.

10

Marr, Memory, and Heuristics

Lael J. Schooler

Center for Adaptive Behavior and Cognition, Max Planck Institute
for Human Development, 14195 Berlin, Germany

Introduction

Michael Watkins has said that a cognitive theory "is a bit like someone else's toothbrush—it is fine for the individual's use, but for the rest of us…well, we would just rather not, thank you" (Watkins 1984, p. 86). To say whether people are behaving rationally requires a definition of what it means to behave rationally, and like a toothbrush everyone has their own. For the purposes of this chapter, I define rational behavior as follows:

> To behave rationally in some context is to display behavior that corresponds to a normative standard of behavior for that context.

The choice of the standard determines what constitutes rational behavior. For the economist, behaving rationally involves maximizing expected utility; for the logician, it is following the deductive rules of logic; and for the (Bayesian) statistician, it is acting according to Bayes's rule. One can even consider more ecologically minded views of rationality to be normative; that is, the rationality of a behavior is measured by how well it performs in a particular environment. One need not look far for demonstrations that people do not reason rationally with respect to a variety of normative standards. There are entire literatures on how and why people violate the rules of deductive logic and statistical inference. In the Wason (1968) card task, central to one such literature, people are given a rule of the form, "if p, then q," such as "if there is a vowel printed on one side of a card, then an even number is printed on the other." The participants are next presented with a set of cards (see Stevens, this volume, Figure 13.2), such as A, K, 2, 7. Their task is to choose only those cards that need to be flipped to check whether the rule holds. In this example, only the A-card (p) and the 7-card ($\sim q$) need to be checked. An odd number on the opposite side of the A-card would clearly violate the rule as would a vowel on the other side of the 7-card ($\sim q$). The rule says nothing about what is on the opposite side of a consonant, so flipping the K-card ($\sim p$) does not test the rule. Also, flipping the 2-card (q) cannot disconfirm the rule, because the rule does not restrict what is on the opposite side of an even numbered card. In general people perform terribly on this task, or at least their performance does not appear to be rational with respect to the rules of deduction. Oaksford and Chater (1996) surveyed 13 studies, covering a variety of Wason tasks. The proportions of people who flip the p(A), $\sim p$(K), q(2), $\sim q$(7) cards were 89%, 16%, 62%, and 25%, respectively. That is, people rarely flip the $\sim q$ card, which they should flip, and frequently flip the q card, which they need not do.

The generally low levels of performance in experiments using the Wason card task and in other reasoning tasks would seem to demonstrate that people are, in fact, irrational, when measured against accepted standard inferential rules. Anderson (1990) has proposed that apparent deviations from rationality may result from people employing optimal solutions to certain problems they face in their natural environments. However, behavior that is rational in natural environments may not necessarily be rational in the peculiar environments that experimental psychologists concoct. Next I discuss some of the roots of this idea.

David Marr's Levels of Explanation

Marr (1982) argues that fully understanding an information-processing system requires considering the system from multiple levels. Marr was interested in the visual system, which he argues evolved to "tell(s) us about shape and space and spatial arrangement" (Marr 1982, p. 36). The distinction that Marr makes among the levels of explanation can be more readily understood by referring to a far simpler information-processing system than vision: a clock. What does a clock do? It indexes time. How does it do it? It achieves this goal by measuring the passage of time by incrementing counters at fixed intervals. Marr says that descriptions like this are at the computational level.

The next level down, called the representation and algorithm level, describes how the goals should be achieved. In the case of a clock, it would map the cycles of an oscillator into seconds, minutes, and hours. Descriptions at this level of analysis require a specification of the representations and the algorithms that operate on them to achieve the goals specified at the computational level. Many combinations of representation and algorithms can achieve these goals; a 12- or 24-hour clock can index time. The choice of representation does constrain the choice of algorithm, such as how seconds are rolled over into minutes, and minutes into hours (e.g., what happens at 12:59). Further, not all representations and algorithms are equivalent; some computations may be simpler with one representation than another. Calculating the duration of a trip is simpler when the train leaves at 10:00 and arrives at 14:00 than when it leaves at 10:00 a.m. and arrives at 2:00 p.m.

The lowest level of description in Marr's hierarchy, the hardware implementation level, is concerned with describing the physical entities that carry out the computations of the representation and algorithm level. Here the current time could be represented by the configuration of hands on a clock face, the coordination of seconds and minutes handled by brass wheels, and the oscillator could be realized as a pendulum. Marr's point is that if you stumbled onto a morass of gears, you would be better able to make sense of these gears if you knew that they were part of a clock as opposed to a cash register, or a sewing machine. Similarly, one is going to be better able to understand people as information-processing systems, if one understands what those systems are trying to accomplish. As Marr puts it (Marr 1982, p. 27):

> Trying to understand perception by studying only neurons is like trying to understand bird flight by studying only feathers: It just cannot be done. In order to understand bird flight, we have to understand aerodynamics; only then do the structures of feathers and the different shapes of birds' wings make sense.

Marr (1982) demonstrated the utility of approaching the problem of vision from multiple levels, and particularly from the computational level. Anderson noted that most theorizing in cognitive psychology concerned representations and the processes that act on them, corresponding to Marr's representation and algorithm level. At that time relatively little theorizing in cognitive psychology was at Marr's computational level, though in the intervening years, models at this level have gained in popularity (e.g., Chater et al. 2006). Based on Marr's success with vision, Anderson (1990) suggested that the approach might work well for higher-level cognition, such as categorization and memory. Anderson relabeled Marr's computational level the rational level, because the computational level sounds like it should be describing the algorithm and representation level. His choice of the term *rational* also alludes to economic theorizing that often takes place at Marr's computational level. Economists focus more on the decisions agents make, rather than on the processes involved in coming to those decisions. In the economic realm, it is easy to appreciate that it is rational for firms to maximize profits or perhaps, as in the case of Ben and Jerry's (the famous American premium ice-cream maker), to maximize a combination of profits and social good. For the cognitive system, the currency is less clear. Thus, the critical step in what Anderson calls a rational analysis is to figure out what quantity the cognitive system might be optimizing, and to make predictions based on this about how people will behave in a particular situation, typically an experimental task.

A Computational (Rational) Level Analysis of the Wason Card Task

There would seem to be a weak case for the rationality of the cognitive system in light of people's irrational behavior on the Wason (1968) card task. However, Oaksford and Chater's (1996) rational analysis of the Wason card task shows that typical performance on the task, while violating traditional notions of rationality, is indeed quite rational when seen in the broader context of how people seek information in the world. Consider the following situations that parents may face. In one situation, hearing an utterance from the baby he was caring for, a young father might ask "was that just babbling," or if the baby says "baba," then the baby wants a bottle. If the mother comes home to find her husband giving the baby a bottle, and if she wanted to know whether "baba" was serving as the baby's signal it wanted a bottle, would it be rational for the mother to ask whether the baby had said "baba" before the feeding? Now imagine sixteen years have passed, and the mother is in the passenger seat teaching her son to drive. She wonders whether he knows that when the oil light is on, he should stop the car. Would it be rational for the mother to ask whether the oil light is on? It would seem quite natural for the young mother to ask about what the baby had said, and for the middle-aged mother to remain silent. Asking in the first case would be like flipping the 2-card, irrational with respect to deductive inference. Asking cannot disconfirm the hypothesis that the baby knows how to use the word, since logically many circumstances (e.g., fussing) can suggest an infant is hungry. In contrast, asking about the oil light would be like flipping the 7-card, rational with respect to the rules of logical inference. If the mother found that the oil light was on, this would be a violation of the rule. Our intuitions are at odds with logic.

Perhaps our intuitions are correct that the young mother is rational to ask about what the baby said, and the older mother is rational in remaining silent. The essential difference between the two situations is the amount of information the answer to the question is likely yield. Though asking whether the baby said "baba" could not provide a definitive answer, knowing what the baby said tells something about whether the baby knows the word. In contrast, asking about the oil light, though potentially highly informative in the unlikely event that the oil light is on, will tell nothing in the more likely event that the oil light is off.

Oaksford and Chater's (1996) analysis of the Wason task formalizes these intuitions. They assume that people apply experimental, information-seeking strategies to deductive tasks like the Wason. Though the details of their mathematical analysis are beyond the scope of this chapter, the flavor of it can be given here. As is true for nearly all rational analyses, they assume that people are behaving as if they are following Bayes's rule. They suggest that people are not treating the task as a test of logic, but rather are attempting to gauge the causal relation between two events. More specifically they assume what people are really trying to do in deductive tasks is to decide between two hypotheses: when *p* occurs (e.g., baby says "baba"), *q* must follow (e.g., baby wants a bottle), or the alternative hypothesis that event *p* is independent of event *q*. Sometimes the baby says "baba" and sometimes the baby is hungry, and it is only by chance that the baby says "baba" when it is hungry. In the case of the Wason task described earlier, the competing hypotheses are that an even number depends on a vowel or the alternative that evens and vowels are independent of each other. The question, then, is: Which card will provide the most evidence in terms of discriminating between these two rival hypotheses? Since people do not know in advance how useful an experiment (i.e., flipping a card) is going to prove to be in the end, they make their decisions based on how much information they expect to gain.

A critical difference between the parenting examples and the Wason (1968) task is that people have experience with how children learn words, but relatively little experience with numbered and lettered cards. Lacking any relevant experience about the cards, Oaksford and Chater (1996) assume that people treat them as if they are typical of causal relations they have seen in the past. When their model of information seeking is combined with the assumption that causally related events are relatively rare, it predicts the observed subject preferences for flipping cards, namely *p* (e.g., A-card) is chosen more than *q* (e.g., 2-card), *q* more than ~*p* (e.g., K-card), and ~*p* more than ~*q* (e.g., 7-card). The Wason (1968) task clearly demonstrates that people behave irrationally with respect to logic, whereas Oaksford and Chater's (1996) analysis shows that the behavior is rational with respect to how people seek information under " 'normal' life conditions" (Brunswik 1943, p. 259). In short, people can be seen to behave rationally with respect to the environment, but can appear to be operating irrationally with respect to a particular task, especially when the task that subjects are performing differs from the one intended by the experimenter.

The Representation and Algorithmic Level Places Bounds on Computational Level Analyses

The discussion of the Wason (1968) task was couched strictly at the rational (or computational) level. In practice, a rational analysis cannot focus strictly on the rational level, but must also consider the algorithm and representation level. The reason for this is that sometimes the rational solution requires calculations that would be physically impossible for any system to perform. In such circumstances a mapping needs to be made from the results of the rational level into algorithms and representations that approximate the computations called for by the rational analysis. In particular, assumptions have to be made about processing limitations. This relates with Simon's (1956) notion of bounded rationality; that is, people are rational within the constraints of their ability to process information. For example, Simon (1990) pointed out that ignoring processing limitations suggests that knowledge of the rules of chess should lead to perfect play. If a person or machine had an infinite amount of time to contemplate a chess move, and the potential countermoves of the opponent to that move, and the countermoves to all the opponent's potential countermoves, ad infinitum, then the person could select an initial move that would inevitably lead them to checkmate. The problem is that more board positions would have to be considered than there are molecules in the universe (Simon 1990).

There are some games, however, for which it is possible to know the game completely. For example, many adults know the moves and countermoves in tic-tac-toe to guarantee that they will at least not loose. Like tic-tac-toe, the Wason (1968) task is atypical. Thus the number of potential hypotheses and experiments raised by Oaksford and Chater's (1996) analysis of the task is relatively small compared to the number raised by problems people often face in their daily and work lives. For example, consider again the problem of interpreting what the baby means when he says "baba." The potential number of hypotheses for what "baba" means certainly exceeds the number of configurations of a chessboard. If Oaksford and Chater's information-seeking strategy were applied to the problem of vocabulary acquisition, where large numbers of hypotheses and experiments are potentially relevant, no system could cope with the computation.

Gigerenzer (2006) argues that these sorts of problems are not merely a nuisance for the rational analysis and other optimization approaches, but a fundamental flaw. Beyond their computational intractability, the optimization solutions require making simplifying assumptions about the problem for the sake of mathematical convenience. Brighton and Gigerenzer (2007) contend that these simplifications inevitably introduce error into the solution, which means that the optimization solution could be outperformed by simpler heuristics. In addition, even if the error introduced by simplification is not debilitating, the amount of data needed to estimate the parameters of the optimization solution may be so large as to be impractical. For example, DeMiguel, Garlappi, and Uppal (2007) compare a simple strategy of dividing investments equally among assets to optimize portfolio distribution. They report that with "parameters calibrated to U.S. stock-market data, we find that for a portfolio with only 25 assets, the estimation window needed is more than 3,000 months, and for a portfolio with 50 assets it is more than 6,000 months, while typically these parameters are estimated using 60–120 months of data" (DeMiguel et al., p. 25). In short, optimization can be problematic when (a) there are multiple criteria, (b) there is too little data to estimate parameters adequately, (c) the future does not look like the past, and (d) the assumptions underlying the optimization solution lead to significant errors. Under such circumstances, simpler strategies often fare better than more complex ones (Brighton, in preparation). To the extent that these conditions hold, the problem is not one of computational power; thus unconscious decision making, irrespective of its unbridled capacities, may still favor robust simple heuristics over more delicate complex ones. The critical point is that there is no decision strategy (or research methodology) that universally works better than another. The question is where and when are they appropriate.

It is important to understand when optimization solutions provide insight into cognition. As a start, we can flip critiques like Gigerenzer's; that is, consider situations in which (a) a single, or at least a dominant, criterion is shaping behavior, (b) there is extended experience with which to learn parameters, (c) the future looks like the past, and (d) the assumptions underlying the optimization solution adequately match the world. Alexander (1996) considers optimization examples from biology that provide insight into how organisms have evolved or learned to solve interesting problems. He discusses, for example, the optimal solutions to problems such as how thick bones should be, how fast a high jumper should run to maximize the height of their jump, and what size pores on an egg should be to permit adequate quantities of oxygen to enter while preventing the egg from drying out. Are there questions of decision making and information processing similar to the kinds of biological questions that Alexander considers?

Next, I consider an analysis of human memory, which, in my view, meets the constraints of a dominant criterion, extended experience, and a stable statistical structure of past and future events.

A Computational (Rational) Level Analysis of Human Memory Reveals the Benefits of Forgetting

Our astounding ability to retrieve information from memory must depend on "a powerful non-conscious mental apparatus" (Engel, this volume). Yet, we routinely run up against the limits of our memories. These limitations bar us from performing feats, such as reciting the *Iliad* from memory or, for many of us, remembering the three things we were to pick up at the store. Clearly, forgetfulness is among our most troublesome cognitive limitations over both the long ("What is his name?") and short term ("What temperature did the recipe say to set the oven?"). Next, I discuss how forgetting can be understood as the key property of a well-adapted memory system.

Anderson and colleagues (Anderson and Milson 1989; Anderson and Schooler 1991, 2000; Schooler and Anderson 1997) have argued that much of memory performance, including forgetting, might be understood as an adaptation to the structure of the environment. The key assumptions of this rational analysis are that the memory system (a) meets the informational demands stemming from environmental stimuli by retrieving memory traces associated with the stimuli and (b) acts on the expectation that environmental stimuli tend to reoccur in predictable ways. More generally, they argue that human memory essentially bets that as the recency and frequency with which a piece of information has been used decreases, the likelihood that it will be needed in the future also decreases in lawful ways. Because processing unneeded information is cognitively costly, the memory system is better off setting aside such little needed information by forgetting it. In this view, memory can be seen as making an endless series of decisions about what information to retrieve.

A simple time-saving feature that is common to many word processors can help illustrate how recency can be used to predict the need for information. When a user goes to open a document file, the program presents a "file buffer," a list of recently opened files from which the user can select. Whenever the desired file is included on the list, the user is spared the effort of searching through the file hierarchy. For this device to work efficiently, however, the word processor must provide users with the files they actually want. It does so by "forgetting" files that are considered unlikely to be needed on the basis of the assumption that the time since a file was last opened is negatively correlated with its likelihood of being needed now. The word processor uses the heuristic that the more recently a file has been opened, the more likely it is to be opened now. Though this simple rule does a remarkable job of putting the appropriate files on the list, it ignores other factors that likely predict whether a file will be needed, such as whether it has been opened frequently and the contexts in which it has been opened in the past.

This analysis implies that memory performance reflects the patterns with which stimuli appear and reappear in the environment. To test this implication, Anderson and Schooler (1991) examined various environments that place informational demands on the memory system and found a strong correspondence between the regularities in the occurrence of information (e.g., a word's frequency and recency of occurrence) in these environments (e.g., conversation) and the classic learning and forgetting curves (e.g., as described by Ebbinghaus, 1885/1964). In a conversational environment, for instance, Anderson and Schooler (1991) observed that the probability of hearing a particular word drops as the period of time since it was last used grows, much as recall of a given item decreases as the amount of time since it was last encountered increases. Other, more subtle effects have been observed as well (Schooler and Anderson 1997).

To appreciate the enormity of the optimization problem human memory is purported to solve, requires a few more details about rational analysis of memory. The basic setup is that information in long-term memory is stored in discrete records and that retrieval entails searching through these records to find a record that achieves some processing goal of the system. The explanatory power of the approach depends on the system estimating the probability that each record in long-term memory is the one sought, termed the need probability. The idea is that the memory system performs the equivalent of a Bayesian calculation of the posterior probability that any particular memory will be needed given how frequently and recently it had been needed in the past and the association of that memory to elements in the current context.

Records are considered in the order of their need probabilities, with the most promising records considered first. At some point, the memory system must terminate its search for further records. If p is the need probability, C is the cost of processing the record, and G is the gain associated with successfully finding the target, then the memory system should stop considering records when $pG < C$. In other words, the system stops searching through the memory records when the expected value (pG) of the next record is less than the cost of considering it. Even if memory contains only some 227 megabytes of information, as Landauer (1986) estimates, continuously attaching need probabilities to memory records and sorting through them seems implausible. The claim is not that these calculations are being carried out explicitly, but rather that the memory system functions this way.

A Memory-Based Heuristic at the
Representation and Algorithm Level

Motivated by concerns that optimization methods, such as those underlying the rational analysis of memory, are, for the most part, inappropriate for understanding cognition, the fast and frugal heuristics program examines simple strategies that exploit informational structures in the environment, enabling the mind to make surprisingly accurate decisions without much information or computation (Gigerenzer et al. 1999). The recognition heuristic illustrates the interplay between the structure of the environment and capacities of the human mind (Goldstein and Gigerenzer 2002). In short, the recognition heuristic uses the information about whether an object is recognized or not to make inferences about some criterion value of this object. More specifically, the recognition heuristic is designed for paired comparison between two objects: one recognized, the other not.

> Recognition heuristic: If one of two objects is recognized and the other is not, then infer that the recognized object has the higher value with respect to the criterion (Goldstein and Gigerenzer 2002, p. 76).

The recognition heuristic is simple because it can rely on recognition memory. Note that this does not mean that the process of recognition is simple per se, but rather the recognition heuristic is simple given the efficient recognition memory that humans possess.

The recognition heuristic will be successful in environments in which the probability of recognizing objects is correlated with the criterion to be inferred. This is, for example, the case in many geographical domains, such as city or mountain size (Goldstein and Gigerenzer 2002), and in many competitive domains, such as predicting the success of tennis players (Serwe and Frings 2006).

One reason why objects with larger criterion values are more often recognized is that they are more often mentioned in the environment.

To be successful the recognition heuristic requires that a person does not recognize too much or too little, since to be applied one of the alternatives needs to be recognized, but not the other. If a person recognizes too few or too many objects, then recognition will be uninformative because it will rarely discriminate between objects. In the classic example, U.S. residents recognize the names of nearly all U.S. cities, so they can rarely rely on recognition to infer which of two cities has the larger population. In contrast, for someone living in Germany, whether they recognize a city or not is a good predictor of population. Goldstein and Gigerenzer (2002) specified a less is more effect: conditions when people who recognize fewer objects and use recognition can out perform people who recognize more objects.

Schooler and Hertwig (2005) wanted to know whether forgetting could fuel the success of the recognition heuristic. The idea was that without forgetting, a person might, over time, recognize all objects of a certain kind (e.g., cities or companies). Then, recognition would no longer discriminate between objects. If, on the other hand, there was too much forgetting, the organism would not be able to recognize any of the objects, leaving it again unable to use recognition as a cue. The key to success lies in recognizing some, but not all of the objects, and forgetting helps to keep it that way, which will be demonstrated in more detail in the following. As it seems unlikely that forgetting was optimized to the problem of heuristic inference, this question is approached more appropriately from the representation and algorithm level, rather than the rational level.

To see why dropping down a level is appropriate, consider the analogy between how people search for information in memory and on the web. For many people, Google acts as an external memory; I cannot remember the last day at work in which I did not appeal to Google for some fact or another. It is no accident that the rational analysis of memory characterizes the problem facing human memory much like it is a search engine; the development of the rational analysis of memory depended heavily on work of library science and information retrieval (Burrel 1985). There are different ways in which you could use Google to decide which of two cities is largest. One approach would be to query Google directly with the name of a city, such as "Chicago" and population size, which returns: "nearly 2.9 million people," "there were 2,896,016 people." However, other approaches are also possible. For example, one could use the heuristic that larger cities tend to be mentioned on more web pages than smaller cities. This heuristic would give you the correct answer when comparing Chicago (web pages: 212,000,000; population: 2,833,321) to San Diego (web pages: 151,000,000, population: 1,256,951) or to San Antonio (web pages: 119,000,000 population 1,296,682), but would lead to the incorrect answer when comparing San Antonio to San Diego. Even if a search engine has been optimally tuned to retrieve relevant information, the search results can be used for entirely different purposes, such as answering forced choice questions about city populations. Similarly, even if human memory functions to retrieve relevant information optimally, it can also be exploited for other purposes. In the same way, it would be misguided to attempt to understand the performance of Google as the optimal solution to the problem of estimating city size. Similarly, it would be a mistake—assuming the rational analysis of memory has correctly characterized the primary function of memory—to try and understand the recognition-based heuristics from Marr's computational level. Instead, we need to drop down a level in Marr's hierarchy.

A Cognitive Architecture at the Representation and Algorithm Level

The ACT-R (Anderson and Lebiere 1998) is well suited to model cognition at Marr's representation and algorithm level. The ACT-R research program strives to develop an encompassing theory of cognition, specified to such a degree that phenomena from perceptual search to the learning of algebra might be modeled within the same framework. The core of ACT-R is constituted by the declarative memory system for facts (*knowing that*) and the procedural system for rules (*knowing how*). The declarative memory system consists of records that represent information (e.g., about the outside world, about oneself, about possible actions). These records take on activations that determine their accessibility; that is, whether and how quickly they can be retrieved. The activation of a record is higher, the more frequently and the more recently it has been used. Specifically, the activation equals the log odds (i.e., $\ln[p/(1 - p)]$) that the record will be needed to achieve a processing goal. Although these activations can be understood to reflect the need probability of the rational analysis of memory, they are calculated by an equation that strengthens and decays a record's activation according to the pattern with which it is used. One may ask a question, formulated hardware implementation, about how activation may be realized in the brain. Anderson (2007) has proposed that we can understand activation in terms of how long it takes a leaky-accumulator model to reach a threshold, an approach that has also been used to model neural firing data.

The procedural system consists of if-then rules that guide the course of actions an individual takes when performing a specific task. The if-side of a production rule specifies various conditions. These conditions can include, for example, the state of working memory and changes in perceptual information, such as detecting that a new object has appeared. If all the conditions of a production rule are met, then the rule fires, and the actions specified on the "then" side of the rule are implemented. These actions can include updating records, creating new records, setting goals, and initiating motor responses. This makes ACT-R a good framework within which to implement decision-making strategies in cognitively plausible ways.

L. J. Schooler

An Implementation of the Recognition Heuristic in ACT-R Reveals Additional Benefits of Forgetting

Bettman, Johnson, and Payne (1990) explored the relative cognitive complexity and effort that various decision strategies require by implementing them in production rules that describe simple cognitive steps, such as *read, add,* and *compare,* termed elementary information processes (EIPs). Building on this work, I will show how implementing the recognition heuristic, and potentially other decision making strategies, in ACT-R lets us explore how characteristics of the cognitive system, such as forgetting, affect decision making in specific environments.

According to Goldstein and Gigerenzer (2002), the recognition heuristic works because there is a chain of correlations linking the criterion (e.g., city population), via environmental frequencies (e.g., how often a city is mentioned), to recognition. The activation of ACT-R tracks such environmental regularities, so that activation differences reflect, in part, these frequency differences. Thus, it appears that inferences, such as deciding which of two cities is larger, could be based directly on the activation of associated chunks (e.g., city representations). This is prohibited, however, in the ACT-R modeling framework for reasons of psychological plausibility: subsymbolic quantities, such as activation, are held not to be directly accessible, just as people presumably cannot make decisions by directly observing differences in neural firing rates. Instead, though, the system could potentially capitalize on activation differences associated with various objects by gauging how it responds to them. The simplest measure of the system's response is whether a chunk associated to a specific object can be retrieved at all; this is what Schooler and Hertwig (2005) used to implement the recognition heuristic in ACT-R.

First, the model learned about German cities based on artificial environments that reflected how frequently the cities were mentioned in an American newspaper. Second, recognition rates for the model were calibrated against the empirical recognition rates that Goldstein and Gigerenzer (2002) observed. Recognizing a city was considered to be equivalent to retrieving the chunk associated with it. Third, the model was tested on pairs of German cities. To do this, the model's recognition rates determined the probability that it would successfully recognize a city. Finally, the production rules for the recognition heuristic dictated that whenever one city was recognized and the other was not, the recognized one was selected as being larger; in all other cases (both cities recognized or unrecognized), a guess was made. These decisions closely matched the observed human responses.

Using this model, Schooler and Hertwig (2005) asked whether forgetting can boost the accuracy of memory-based inferences, such as those made by the recognition heuristic? To find out, they varied forgetting rates, in terms of how quickly activation of a record decays in memory, and looked at how this affects the accuracy of the recognition heuristic's inferences. The results are plotted in Figure 10.1, which shows that the performance of the recognition heuristic peaks at intermediate decay rates. This happens because intermediate levels of forgetting maintain a distribution of recognition rates that are highly correlated with the criterion and, as stated earlier, it is just these correlations on which the recognition heuristic relies.

The recognition heuristic (and accordingly its ACT-R implementation) relies on a binary representation of recognition: an object is either simply recognized (and retrieved by ACT-R) or it is unrecognized (and not retrieved). This heuristic, however, essentially discards information when two objects are both recognized, but one is recognized more strongly than the other—a difference that could be used by some other mechanism to decide between the two objects, but which the recognition heuristic ignores. Considering this situation, Schooler and Hertwig (2005) noted that recognition could also be assessed within ACT-R in a continuous fashion in terms of how quickly an object's record can be retrieved. This information can then be used to make inferences with a related simple mechanism, the fluency heuristic. Such a heuristic for using the fluency of reprocessing as a cue in inferential judgment has been suggested earlier (e.g., Jacoby and Dallas 1981). Following this version of the fluency heuristic, if one of two objects is more fluently reprocessed, then this object is inferred to have the higher value with respect to the criterion.

The performance of the fluency heuristic turns out to be influenced by forgetting in much the same way as the recognition heuristic, as shown by the

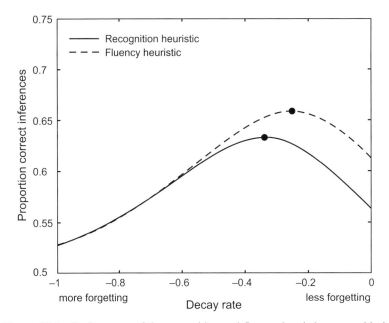

Figure 10.1 Performance of the recognition and fluency heuristics vary with decay rate (Schooler and Hertwig 2005).

upper line in Figure 10.1, which shows the additional gain in performance that fluency heuristic provides over and above the recognition heuristic. In the case of the fluency heuristic, intermediate amounts of forgetting increase the chances that differences in the retrieval times of two chunks will be detected. Part of the explanation for this is illustrated in Figure 10.2, which shows the exponential function that relates a chunk's activation to its retrieval time. Forgetting lowers the range of activations to levels that correspond to retrieval times that can be more easily discriminated; that is, a given difference in activation at a lower range results in a larger, more easily detected, difference in retrieval time than the same difference at a higher range.

Both the recognition and fluency heuristics can be understood as means to tap indirectly the environmental frequency information locked in the activations of chunks in ACT-R. These heuristics will be effective to the extent that the chain of correlations—linking the criterion values, environmental frequencies, activations and responses—is strong. By modifying the rate of memory decay within ACT-R, Schooler and Hertwig (2005) demonstrated the surprising finding that forgetting actually serves to improve the performance of these heuristics by strengthening the chain of correlations on which they rely. Implementing the recognition heuristic in ACT-R has shown concretely how conscious decision making can exploit the vast unconscious processing resources of human memory.

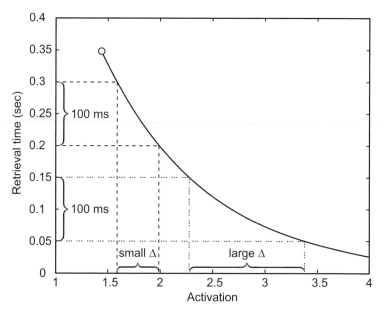

Figure 10.2   A chunk's activation determines its retrieval time (Schooler and Hertwig 2005).

Conclusion

I began by reviewing Marr's multilevel analysis of information-processing systems. His approach emphasizes understanding the function of the system, the algorithms and representations that can achieve that function, and how this might be realized in the brain. Next I reviewed Anderson's proposal that Bayesian optimization techniques are one way to specify the function of cognitive processes at Marr's computational level. I discussed some limitations and possible boundary conditions for optimization, which suggest when and why simple heuristics can out perform more complex decision strategies. I described the rational analysis of memory, one such optimization analysis, which views forgetting as an adaptation to the statistical structure of environmental events. Next, I reported an analysis at Marr's representation and algorithm level that shows how forgetting helps memory based heuristics work better. This analysis depended on implementations of the recognition and fluency heuristics in the ACT-R cognitive architecture, which includes an algorithmic description of memory retrieval that achieves the processing goals of the rational analysis of memory. These ACT-R models show how cognitive architectures, such as ACT-R, can be used as tools for understanding how heuristics and other decision-making strategies exploit and are shaped by basic cognitive capacities and the structure of the environment.

References

Alexander, R. M. 1996. Optima for Animal, 2nd ed. Princeton: Princeton Univ. Press.

Anderson, J. R. 1990. The Adaptive Character of Thought. Hillsdale, NJ: Lawrence Erlbaum.

Anderson, J. R. 2007. How Can the Human Mind Occur in the Physical Universe? New York: Oxford Univ. Press.

Anderson, J. R., and C. Lebiere. 1998. The Atomic Components of Thought. Mahwah, NJ: Lawrence Erlbaum.

Anderson, J. R., and R. Milson. 1989. Human memory: An adaptive perspective. *Psychol. Rev.* **96**:703–719.

Anderson, J. R., and L. J. Schooler. 1991. Reflections of the environment in memory. *Psychol. Sci.* **2**:396–408.

Anderson, J. R., and L. J. Schooler. 2000. The adaptive nature of memory. In: Handbook of Memory, ed. E. Tulving and F. I. M. Craik, pp. 557–570. New York: Oxford Univ. Press.

Bettman, J. R., E. J. Johnson, and J. W. Payne. 1990. A componential analysis of cognitive effort in choice. *Org. Behav. Hum. Dec. Proc.* **45**:111–139.

Brighton, H., and G. Gigerenzer. 2007. Bayesian brains and cognitive mechanisms: Harmony or dissonance? In: The Probabilistic Mind: Prospects for Rational Models of Cognition, ed. N. Chater and M. Oaksford. Oxford: Oxford Univ. Press, in press.

Brunswik, E. 1943. Organismic achievement and environmental probability. *Psychol. Rev.* **50**:255–272.

Burrell, Q. L. 1985. A note on aging on a library circulation model. *J. Documentation* **41**:100–115.

Chater, N., J. B. Tenenbaum, and A. Yuille. 2006. Probabilistic models of cognition: Conceptual foundations. *Trends Cogn. Sci.* **10(7)**:287–291.

DeMiguel, V., L. Garlappi, and R. Uppal. 2007. Optimal versus naive diversification: How inefficient is the 1/N portfolio strategy? *Rev. Financ. Stud.*, in press.

Ebbinghaus, H. 1885/1964. Memory: A Contribution to Experimental Psychology (trans. H.A. Ruger and C.E. Bussenius). New York: Dover.

Gigerenzer, G. 2006. Heuristics. In: Heuristics and the Law, ed. G. Gigerenzer and C. Engel, pp. 17–44. Cambridge, MA: MIT Press.

Gigerenzer, G., P. M. Todd, and the ABC Research Group. 1999. Simple Heuristics That Make Us Smart. Oxford: Oxford Univ. Press.

Goldstein, D. G., and G. Gigerenzer. 2002. Models of ecological rationality: The recognition heuristic. *Psychol. Rev.* **109**:75–90.

Jacoby, L. L., and M. Dallas. 1981. On the relationship between autobiographical and perceptual learning. *J. Exp. Psychol.: Gen.* **110**:306–340.

Landauer, T. K. 1986. How much do people remember? Some estimates of the quantity of learned information in long-term memory. *Cogn. Sci.* **10(4)**:477–493.

Marr, D. 1982. Vision. San Francisco: Freeman.

Oaksford, M., and N. Chater. 1996. Rational explanation of the selection task. *Psychol. Rev.* **103**:381–391.

Schooler, L. J., and J. R. Anderson. 1997. The role of process in the rational analysis of memory. *Cogn. Psychol.* **32(3)**:219–250.

Schooler, L. J., and R. Hertwig. 2005. How forgetting aids heuristic inference. *Psychol. Rev.* **112**:610–628.

Serwe, S., and C. Frings. 2006. Who will win Wimbledon? The recognition heuristic in predicting sports events. *J. Behav. Dec. Mak.* **19**:321–332.

Simon, H. A. 1956. Rational choice and the structure of the environment. *Psychol. Rev.* **63**: 129–138.

Simon, H. A. 1990. Invariants of human behavior. *Ann. Rev. Psychol.* **41**:1–20.

Wason, P. C. 1968. Reasoning about a rule. *Qtly. J. Exp. Psychol.* **20**:273–281.

Watkins, M. J. 1984. Models as toothbrushes. *Behav. Brain Sci.* **7**:86.

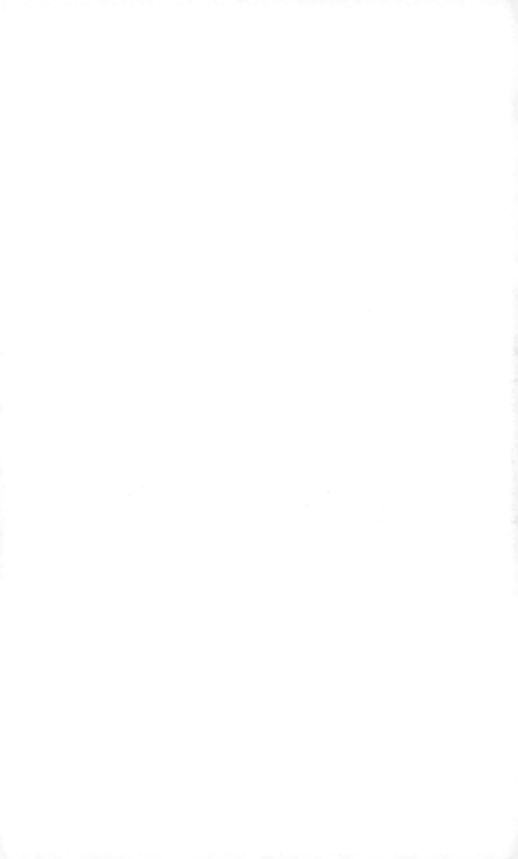

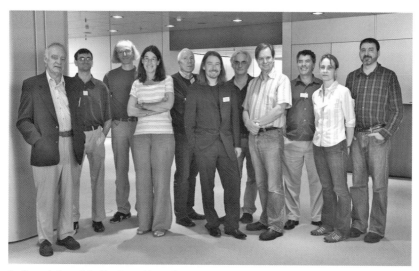

Left to right: Merlin Donald, Rob Kurzban, Michael Meyer-Hermann, Liz Spelke, Werner Güth, Christian Keysers, Jonathan Cohen, Eric Johnson, Jonathan Schooler, Julia Trommershäuser, Lael Schooler

11

Explicit and Implicit Strategies in Decision Making

Christian Keysers, Rapporteur

Robert Boyd, Jonathan Cohen, Merlin Donald,
Werner Güth, Eric Johnson, Robert Kurzban, Lael J. Schooler,
Jonathan Schooler, Elizabeth Spelke, and Julia Trommershäuser

Introduction

Human decision making may be best understood as a triad. At the level of a
single human individual, decision making depends on a variety of processes:
some are more explicit whereas others have a more implicit nature. These two
types of processes produce and are, in turn, influenced by, among other things,
human culture.

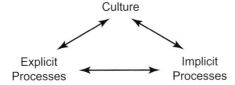

As the scope of our discussion group was to examine human decision making,
we begin with a discussion on the uniqueness of human cognition. Thereafter
we explore the nature of explicit and implicit processes, and how they interact,
and conclude by incorporating culture into decision making.

Uniquely Human

One way to hone in on an understanding of the relationship between implicit and explicit processes is to ask how animal cognition differs from human
thought. When we consider the sensory and motor systems of animals and the
brain systems that support them, humans look very similar to other animals

When we consider, however, the cognitive achievements of different species, we suddenly confront a chasm, for the products of human cognition far surpass those of any other animal. How should we intrepret this chasm? Does an appeal to the distinction between cognitive processes that are conscious versus unconscious, or implicit versus explicit, aid our understanding of the ever-increasing gap between humans and other species?

One attempt to address this question has focused on the capacities of human adults in relation to those of nonhuman animals. This research helps eliminate a number of intuitively plausible accounts of human uniqueness. For example, humans are not the only animals to use tools (as evidenced by the hooks of New Caledonian crows or termite fishing poles of chimpanzees; Hauser et al. 2002; Hunt et al. 2006) to communicate with symbols about aspects of the external world (e.g., the alarm calls of vervet monkeys; Cheney and Seyfarth 1990), or to reason about the epistemic states of others (as in gaze following and perhaps "theory of mind" reasoning in chimpanzees; Hare et al. 2001). Humans engage, however, in each of these activities far more extensively, systematically, and productively than any other animal. Along the timescale of evolution, the frequency and flexibility with which these capacities are used appear to show a sudden explosion in the transition from nonhuman primates to modern human beings (e.g., Mithen 1996), and this explosion needs to be explained. It is particularly visible in human infants and young children, who do not simply learn the specific tools, symbols, or patterns of behavior about which they get extensive information but who seek information from others actively so as to build encyclopedic knowledge about the world (e.g., a child who asks, "What is this for?" after every object in sight).

Accordingly, another set of attempts to address this question has focused on the capacities of human infants in relation to those of other animals. This research provides evidence that infants have systems from a very early age (in some cases at birth), for representing and reasoning about objects (Valenza et al. 2006), about other social agents (Farroni et al. 2002), and even about abstract entities in domains of geometry and number (Newcombe et al. 2000; Xu and Spelke 2000). For example, infants represent up to three inanimate objects exactly, they infer their motions and interactions in accord with basic physical constraints, and they maintain these representations when the objects move from view (e.g., Feigenson et al. 2004). As soon as children are able to locomote independently, they represent the distance and direction of their travel and make inferences about their changing position in accord with the rules of Euclidean geometry (e.g., Landau et al. 1981). In addition, infants represent the approximate cardinal value of large sets of elements, compare sets on the basis of cardinal value, and even perform operations on sets isomorphic to addition and subtraction (e.g., McCrink and Wynn 2004). In each of these cases, the cognitive systems found in infants continue to exist in older children and adults, and they support higher cognitive abilities such as physical, spatial, and numerical reasoning (e.g., Dehaene 1997; Scholl 2001). Nevertheless, nonhuman animals have been found to exhibit the same abilities, with the same signature patterns of performance (e.g., Hauser et al. 2003; for a review, see Spelke 2003a). These findings provide evidence that the cognitive systems underlying infants' achievements do not explain the species-specific cognitive capacities of humans.

Further attempts to illuminate human uniqueness focus on changes in cognitive capacities over human cognitive development. These studies provide evidence for both continuity and change in human cognition over development. On the one hand, the core cognitive systems found in human infants continue to exist and function throughout adulthood; they may also give rise to fundamental intuitions about the world as well as to rich systems of implicit knowledge. On the other hand, new systems emerge to bring about qualitative changes in human cognitive capacities that may underlie many of the hallmarks of mature, distinctively human cognition.

The development of number concepts serves as an example. As noted, infants have two systems for representing numbers: an exact system for distinguishing small numbers (1 vs. 2 vs. 3) and an approximate system for distinguishing large numbers with ratio precision (e.g., they discriminate 8 vs. 12 jellybeans as easily as 4 vs. 6). When children acquire the ability to count verbally, these two systems develop into one, which represents and operates over natural numbers. The stages of children's learning of counting are instructive (Wynn 1992): first they master the start of the list of number words (perhaps to "ten") and the meaning of "one." Then, in sequence, they learn the meanings of "two" and "three." Around four years of age, they induce that each word in the count list picks out a cardinal value that is one larger than the previous word. This induction appears to be beyond the grasp of the most highly trained animals (e.g., Matsuzawa 1985; Pepperberg 1987). In human children, this appears to result from systematically mapping the small exact number system, the large approximate number system, and the language of number words and verbal counting (Spelke 2003b).

In the case of numbers, therefore, uniquely human concepts and cognitive abilities result from the *productive combination* of concepts from preexisting "core" systems of representation that humans share with other animals. The same kind of developmental scenario appears to occur in other domains, including tool use (e.g., Bloom 2004), navigation (Spelke 2003b), and learning by observation. (Although nonhuman primates show rudiments of learning by observation and the mirror neurons that may be the prerequisite for imitation [Keysers and Perrett 2004; Keysers and Gazzola 2006], human adults can learn longer arbitrary sequences of actions far more rapidly and productively [e.g., Meltzoff and Prinz 2002].) Intuitively, it is appealing to suspect that this productive combinatorial capacity may relate to our capacity for explicit, conscious reasoning.

Language provides a particularly clear example of such productive, combinatorial explosion. Children first learn words, then very simple stereotyped

C. Keysers et al.

phrases, and then suddenly the combinatorial power explodes and adults can make phrases of almost unlimited length. Interestingly, such phrases are not simple strings of words; they obey syntactic rules. The difference between simple sequences and syntax has been formally investigated along the distinction between sequences generated by Markov decision processes and recursive, phrase-structure grammars. A Markov decision process is one in which each new element in the sequence is generated by drawing it from a fixed probability distribution over the list of possibilities, independent of prior elements in the list. In this respect, Markov decision processes have no "memory." In recursive, phrase-structure grammars, however, elements show that long-distance dependencies and structured sequences can be embedded within other structures of the same type. Phrase structure and recursion are central to language and other domains, including number and theory of mind. This provides critical, additional functionality, including recursion; that is, the ability to embed structured "subsequences" within a sequence. Accordingly, this distinction is critical for understanding sequential behavior such as, in particular, motor planning and language. Human behavior in these domains demonstrates clearly the capacity for recursion, as in the sentence: "The cat the dog chased meowed." This seemingly simple capability provides tremendous additional representational power and may be at least one factor at the core of the explosive combinatorial capacity so characteristic of human behavior.

A variety of neural network architectures have been proposed that can learn finite state grammars, such as simple recurrent networks (e.g., Elman 1990) and gated architectures (Hochreiter and Schmidhuber 1997). In some cases, these have been related directly to neural mechanisms (e.g., Botvinick and Plaut 2004; Braver and Cohen 2000; Frank et al. 2001). However, a comparison of these mechanisms across primate species remains an important challenge for understanding what changes may have occurred in these mechanisms in the human brain, or what additional mechanisms are needed to support the tremendous flexibility of human thought and behavior.

Current experiments on decision making in monkeys could lead to fundamental insights into some of the basic steps that may form prerequisites for this explosion. When a monkey learns to shift his eyes to the right when seeing a rightward movement, and to the left following a leftward movement, decision making is performed in a rather limited perception–action loop. Monkeys, though, can be trained to view the moving pattern, store the results of this analysis for a while, and then report their percept by seeking a green or a red target, which can appear in any location of the screen. In such a case, the standard perception–action loop is interrupted, and what is activated during the perceptual decision making is not a motor program but a rule: "saccade to the red dot" or "saccade to the green dot." When the targets finally appear, the decision making for the motor system is no longer based on a direct percept, but may rely on prefrontal storage of more abstract information. This detachment may represent the first step along a continuum that makes it possible for humans to make decisions based on explicit rules and representations.

The issue of syntax and flexibility may be linked also to another preadaptation present in nonhuman primates: their motor behavior already exhibits some of the embedded structure typical of human language and other domains of cognition. Let us consider the following sequence of actions: "grasp a fruit and bring it to the mouth." First, this sequence has a structure that clearly goes beyond that of a Markov process: the probability of "bringing to the mouth" depends on the previous action, being much higher after grasping food than after most other actions. Second, action sequences can be recursive: if the food that is grasped is a banana, then the action of peeling the banana is inserted into the sequence, thus becoming, "grasp the fruit, peel it, and bring the peeled fruit to the mouth." In addition, just as words in a phrase can be replaced while preserving the other elements, objects in actions can be replaced while preserving the rest of the action: "grasp the flea from another monkey's fur and bring it to the mouth." To make the structure of actions available to more general domains of human cognition such as language, the domain specificity of actions must be overcome. If the neural architecture enabling the flexibility of actions only receives input from regions representing concrete objects and would only have output onto motor structures, it would be unlikely for these areas to be of use for language and thought. This does not, however, appear to be the case: the premotor and supplementary motor areas of the brain have widespread connections, including prefrontal, temporal, and parietal areas, which are involved in many domains of decision making (Rizzolatti and Luppino 2001). The idea behind the importance of the motor system for other domains of cognition comes from the fact that the left ventral premotor region involved in hand and mouth actions in monkeys (area F5) is considered to be the homologue of the posterior aspects of Broca's area (Brodmann area 44 in humans), lesions of which cause language impairments, in particular, of language production and grammar but also inner speech (Aziz-Zadeh et al. 2005). In addition, human subjects appear to use ventral premotor regions for a number of perceptual judgment tasks that are not inherently motor (Fiebach and Schubotz 2006). One possible explanation for this may be that during evolution, the remarkable capacity of premotor structures to organize actions into sequences may have been employed for many domains of cognition, thus giving these domains the sense of effortful, serial control that is typical for actions.

If the combinatorial and recursive abilities of human cognition are so central for modern humans, it may prove fruitful to investigate specifically the neural substrate for this capacity by contrasting it against the seemingly less flexible behavior that other primates exhibit.

One open question concerns the causal relationship between language and other flexible mental capacities in humans. It remains uncertain whether flexible language is a prerequisite for flexibility in the other domains. For example, some languages lack words to express exact numerical values beyond "two" or "three," and native speakers of these languages do not spontaneously represent exact numbers beyond those limits (Pica et al. 2004; Gordon 2004). These speakers' abilities to represent approximate numerosity and to perform approximate addition and subtraction on these representations are, however, indistinguishable from that of adults and children whose language and culture includes a full verbal number system, and who have learned symbolic arithmetic. It is unclear whether these speakers fail to develop precise number concepts beyond the limits of language because they have no words for these numbers or because their culture fails to teach them the meaning of these numbers, with the absence of words reflecting the lack of cultural knowledge about these higher numbers. Another example involves subjects who do not possess language, either because they were born deaf and were not taught a sign language, or as a result of brain injury. Here, individuals develop many of the unique human capacities, such as complex imitation and tool use, which suggests that language is not a prerequisite for all uniquely human capacities.

Through the evolution of language, the human brain has created a medium that facilitates the communication of knowledge in dramatic ways. The capacity for imitation coupled with explicit pedagogy might be important antecedents of human cultural products that are far greater than that of any other animal. This has created a dense network of communication between individuals that renders society a distributed network in which the decisions of each individual are influenced heavily by the other individuals in a process that we term "cultural."

The combinatorial and recursive capacity of human cognition, of course, is not the only aspect that differentiates humans from nonhuman primates. The capacity to plan deliberately by thinking about events in the past and future is far more developed in humans than in other primates. During fruit foraging, primates often deplete a fruit tree and return to the tree after a time sufficient for the tree to replenish its fruit. Given the complexity of their habitat, it is unlikely that there are adaptations designed for each particular plant; this would suggest that nonhuman primates may have at least rudimentary capacities to plan across time. Humans, however, can reason about, and routinely plan into, the distant future. The Inter-Temporal Choice paradigm, in which subjects are asked to choose between a small amount today and a larger amount after a time delay ranging from seconds to years, demonstrates that the decisions of subjects change gradually as a function of the delay, with a discount function that is far flatter than that of even apes. This suggests that humans clearly have an extended capacity to plan into the future.

Based on cross-species comparisons, Donald (1991, 1993, 1995, 2001) has proposed that the complex of behaviors and phenomena commonly described as "conscious processing" evolved gradually through a series of adaptations in various vertebrate species, each of which served to increase the degree of autonomous control over its own cognitive activities. Various aspects of conscious processing, such as alertness, selectivity, self-monitoring, and metacognitive oversight, may have evolved at different stages of evolution, for different adaptive reasons, and with different neural underpinnings. As a result, human conscious processing is enabled by a complex of neural structures, each of which has a unique function and evolutionary history. Human beings have a special kind of conscious control, distinguished by oversight, as shown in their exceptional human ability to self-rehearse skill and, especially, to automatize very complex skills that involve automatic serial attentional control. The primary adaptive purpose of conscious supervision of skills is not only to acquire skills, but to automatize them in a deliberate and consciously supervised manner. This capability emerged early in human evolution and was a precondition for the later evolution of language, and even of protolanguage (Donald 1998, 1999, 2005). It was also a precondition for the emergence of other kinds of advanced symbolic thought-skills, such as mathematics. Although this was not the only unique feature of conscious control in humans, it is perhaps the most characteristic one.

Overall, humans differ from nonhuman primates in a number of ways pertinent to decision making. They have a combinatorial capacity that is reflected in language, mathematics, and other domains. Their language and imitation capacities enable them to communicate more effectively than any other animal, and their tendency to teach each other deliberately may have enabled the development of a rich culture. These processes may have equipped humans with explicit mechanisms for coping with more complex cognitive demands than those of other animals, and these capacities have important implications for their decision-making processes.

Explicit—Implicit

Intuitively, human individuals believe that two types of processes occur in the mind. An example of the first process would be the act of tying shoe laces. Conscious control does not seem to be required, as one can, for example, talk about an unrelated topic while performing the task. In addition, it is difficult to verbalize the procedure. An example of the second process would be arithmetic calculation: $3 + 7 + 12 + 23$. Here, conscious control is required, as evidenced by the degree to which performing another conscious operation (e.g., reciting the alphabet) interferes. Subjects can verbally describe parts of this process easily as well as carry out a continuous description of the operations; they also perceive that they are consciously aware of "what goes on in their heads" while performing the task. Nevertheless, research provides evidence that even the most explicit mathematical calculations are made possible, in part, through a host of automatic processes that are inaccessible to consciousness, including the automatic activation of core processes and approximate representations of numerical magnitude (e.g., Stanescu et al. 2000; for a review, see Dehaene 1997). When the core processes are impaired, mental arithmetic suffers greatly (e.g., Lemer et al. 2003). This illustrates that explicit cognitive processes cannot operate in isolation from implicit ones.

The *implicit association task* (Greenwald et al. 1998) is potentially interesting because it purports to assess the first type of process; namely, the association between, for example, a category and attitudes. In the canonical version, a subject is given a list of, say, African-American and European-American names as well as words with either good (happy) or bad (death) connotations. The task involves placing a word into a category depending on its content. In one condition, if the word is either the name of an African-American or something negative, one choice is indicated; if the word is either the name of a typical European-American or something positive, the other choice is selected. In another condition, if the word is the name of an African-American or positive, it is placed into one category, whereas if the word is either European-American or negative, it is placed into the other. Reaction times are measured and the difference in speed between the two tasks is taken to be a measure of the (implicit) association between the social category and negative (or positive) views. Reaction times are longer when African-American names are paired with positive words or European-American names are associated with negative words.

Subjects who show this implicit association will claim, however, to be unprejudiced, as measured by self-report scales (Greenwald et al. 1998). This is taken to be evidence that on one level—the implicit level—there is an association that is denied at another level—the explicit level—by the subjects. The implicit association task illustrates how psychologists have viewed and addressed empirically the implicit/explicit distinction.

It also reveals how a multisystem structure, with subsystems representing similar information in different forms (in this case, racial stereotypes), can be present in the brain as a whole, even though the subsystems conflict with one another (Kurzban and Aktipis 2007). To the extent that the computational mechanisms responsible for verbal report about the relevant questions do not have access to the information contained in the implicit associations that produce the experimental result, these associations do not influence verbal reports.

A number of different terminologies have been proposed for distinguishing these two types of processes (Table 11.1). Originating from different scientific traditions, these distinctions do not map perfectly onto each other. Defining subcategories of mental processes by several of these distinctions would suggest, for our purposes, a distinction that is too fine.

At this stage of research, it would be a vain enterprise to attempt to define unambiguously a set of features common to all processes placed either in the right- or left-hand columns of this table. Thus, to avoid bias in our discussions as well as in earlier versions of this report, we referred to processes as being those that fall within the left- or right-hand columns. This terminology, however, was felt to be cumbersome for the publication, and thus we refer to the processes as being reflexive or reflective.

Table 11.1   Separation of mental processes, originating from numerous scientific traditions, into two types of processes.

System 1 / Reflexive Processes	System 2 / Reflective Processes
Implicit	Explicit
Nonconscious	Conscious
Compiled	Interpreted
Procedural	Declarative
Automatic	Controlled
Habitual	Deliberate
Involuntary	Voluntary
Pre-preceptual	Perceptual
Pre-attentive	Attentive
Not registered	Remembered
Encapsulated	Accessible
Domain-specific	Domain-general

It is often felt that reflective processes are represented in a propositional format that can be transformed easily or explained in natural language, whereas reflexive processes are not. It is easy to explain how $(1 + 2) - (2 - 3)$ is equal to $1 + 2 - 2 + 3$, but it would be difficult for most of us to explain the motor process that allows us to run.

Behavioral performance in tasks that require reflective processes generally suffer if subjects are asked to perform attention and working memory-dependent tasks simultaneously, such as mental arithmetic (e.g., counting backwards in steps of 7 from 322), while reflexive processes are relatively less affected by such manipulations. Most activities require both and therefore suffer to some extent from interference from attention and working memory-dependent tasks. Consider the act of riding a bicycle: most people are able to ride while counting backward by threes, which shows that core skills involved in this activity might fall under reflexive processes. The speed at which you might ride, however, may be reduced by the dual task, and the risk of having an accident may increase, suggesting that skill can benefit from engaging reflective processes to complement reflexive processes.

Most people are generally aware of the source of information that governs reflective processes; however, they are often unaware of the sources of information governing reflexive processes. For instance, consider the following moral quandary:

Christel and her brother John go to Europe. In the romantic atmosphere of Europe, they have protected sex. Do you think this is morally wrong?

Subjects generally answer yes, but when asked to verbalize the basis for their decision, most give reasons that are unlikely to be the true grounds for their decision (e.g., "because if they had a child, the child would be at risk of showing genetic deficiencies"). They might be unaware of key elements that drove their decision, which would point toward the existence of reflexive processes within their decisions (Haidt 2001). Alternatively, they might be truly aware of the motives behind their decision but fail to report these because they assume that a different rationale would be more desirable.

Our ultimate goal is to understand the neural mechanisms that underlie these two types of processes and the differences between them. Dimensions such as neural activity versus synaptic connections as well as local versus distributed representations are thought to be important (e.g., Cohen et al. 1996). For example, the flexibility of reflective processes, and their accessibility to report, may reflect their reliance on discrete patterns of neural activity used to represent critical components of the process (e.g., the intermediate products of a mental calculation or the subgoals of a sequence of actions). One feature of such representations may be the ability to activate them relatively independently of one another, and in arbitrary combination with others. This can be achieved in neural networks by local or functionally independent representations. This contrasts with distributed representations, which share overlapping feature sets. Distributed representations afford efficiency of coding (similar concepts share overlapping representations) and the ability for inference (activating a concept primes related ones). However, for the same reasons, they are less flexible. This distinction between local or functionally independent versus distributed representation may be an important factor underlying differences between both types of processes.

Another dimension may be the state versus weight distinction; that is, the difference between storing information in patterns of neural activity (states) versus changes in synaptic connection strengths (weights). Storing information as a pattern of activity in working memory (again, whether it be an item or a goal) is tremendously flexible (e.g., it can be modified quickly), but not very durable. Of course, information can also be stored in the nervous system through synaptic modification. Although in some cases this can happen quickly (e.g., in the hippocampus and amygdala), learning is thought to be more durable, but more gradual in the neocortex (e.g., McClelland et al. 1995). Such learning could support efficient processes (e.g., the execution of a routine sequence of actions), but would take time to learn and be less flexible. For example, when first learning to play the piano, a sequence of notes might be represented separately as distinct patterns of neural activity that activate other patterns of neural activity corresponding to the action needed to play that note. As a musical piece is learned, the entire sequence may come to be represented as a single pattern of neural activity as well as synaptic connections that allow the pattern of activity associated with each action to trigger the next action, thus bypassing representations of the notes themselves. The player, therefore, would have learned to replace an "explicit" or "declarative" representation of the notes (that may be consciously accessible) with a more "implicit" or "procedural" representation of the entire sequence. This would allow the actions to proceed quickly and efficiently from one to the next, presumably without direct involvement of the representation of each note by itself (and therefore perhaps less conscious awareness of, or access to, this information). This scenario corresponds closely to the perspective offered by some of the formal models described below.

Domain specificity may also be important for the distinctions. While reflexive processes are often specific for a particular cognitive domain, reflective processes might transcend the border of domains. Using the example above, representing the sequence as patterns of activity associated with each note, the person could play that sequence on any instrument for which they know the relevant actions. However, once this has been learned as a sequence of particular actions, it is specific to the instrument for which those actions are appropriate. This is similar to compiling a program for a particular machine. Written in a suitable language, the program can run on any machine that has a compiler for that language. However, once it has been compiled, it can only run on the type of machine for which it has been compiled.

The distinction between domain generality and domain specificity may also explain other phenomena. For example, because of their domain generality, reflective processes may have the peculiar characteristic of "disliking" contradictions. Thus, a series of propositions based on reflective processes (e.g., "I don't like my new neighbor," "My new neighbor is from the Congo," "Racism is bad") potentially creates cognitive dissonance that will lead to changes in some of these propositions in order to reach internal consistency. In contrast, because of their domain specificity, this is seen less often in reflexive processes: while observing the waterfall illusion, subjects report seeing movement but also report that individual features stay in the same location. Realizing this discrepancy creates a conscious sense of "oddness," which may be a reflective process, but does not lead to a change in the perception itself (reflexive processes), which appears to be immune to this dissonance. At the same time, when conflicting information occurs within the domain of reflexive processes, inconsistencies and instabilities can arise. Binocular rivalry and the Necker cube are good examples of this: incompatible sources of information produce unstable perceptual representations.

Reflective processes may also have the peculiarity of being deliberately triggered. For example, if someone nudges your back while you are standing, you will step forward to maintain your balance without feeling that you did so deliberately. If I ask you, "please step forward," you will take a similar action, but this time you will have the feeling that although I encouraged you to do so, you triggered the movement deliberately. The same action—stepping forward—can be accompanied by a feeling of automaticity or deliberate, self-triggering. This difference has some correspondence with neurology: patients with Parkinson's disease, for example, will step forward to maintain their balance, but they find it very difficult to step forward in a deliberate, self-triggered manner. A similar distinction can be applied to other modalities. Memories can be triggered externally (e.g., the smell of a Madeleine dipped in tea can trigger memories of the past) or self-triggered (the act of reviewing previous actions to recall where you left your keys). The latter process happens frequently in humans, but animals are also capable of deliberately conjuring visual memories (Naya et al. 1996).

Some of these distinctions depend on whether the process is accompanied by a feeling of "awareness"—a criterion that is both important and difficult. We feel intuitively that awareness is an important dimension of our psychological life, and referring to consciousness links research to the interest of the general public. Consciousness carries important implications for our legal system. A crime committed without realizing what one is doing is treated very differently to a similar crime committed without conscious understanding of one's act, for instance, under the influence of a drug (see Glimcher, this volume). Consciousness is, however, challenging to measure, as ultimately all appraisals must rely directly or indirectly on self-reports. The challenges of appraising consciousness can be readily seen by considering the different ways in which a person might be conscious of a cognitive event. An individual may be able to report that they experienced an event (e.g., the appearance of a recently presented face) without being able to describe the quality of that experience. Moreover, even the sheer judgment of whether or not the event was experienced may be subject to criterion factors (e.g., how conscious a signal must be for a person to characterize that experience as "conscious" depends on perceptions of the relative costs and benefits of a hit vs. a false alarm). Even if an individual is unambiguously experiencing a cognitive event (e.g., mind wandering while reading), it may take some time before that person notices explicitly that such events have taken place. Such subtleties in the measurement of consciousness raise important questions regarding the value of using consciousness per se as a heuristic for classifying processes, and thus is an area in which reasonable people can disagree. In our discussions, there was significant dissension regarding how pivotal the consciousness criterion should be in classifying cognitive operations. Some felt that consciousness itself is a red herring, and that the classification of cognitive states and processes should be based on more scientifically tractable constructs such as underlying neural substrates or computational processes. Others felt that despite its challenges, exploring the mapping between cognitive processes and consciousness is a worthwhile undertaking that can be enhanced through the careful recognition of the different types of conscious classification (e.g., detection vs. description, simply experienced vs. metacognitively appraised).

Although we disagreed on the degree to which consciousness should be viewed as pivotal in the classification of cognitive processes in Table 11.1, we agreed that two approaches seemed promising. First, systematically examining in which respects the different distinctions proposed in Table 11.1 overlap may help us explore the core properties of what we believe to be the two main clusters of processes. Second, the identification of particular examples of processes that systematically fall within the right- or the left-hand column of Table 11.1, independent of terminology, could provide prototypical examples of these processes. These examples could then be studied using evolutionary, neuroscientific, and computational approaches to provide snapshots of how our brain implements these different processes and why, in evolutionary terms, we have such mechanisms. The resultant understanding could be used to form the basis of a better understanding of the clusters they represent.

An additional approach is to map this distinction—whether categorical or representational of an underlying continuum—onto underlying neural mechanisms. In doing so, however, we need to exercise caution. Although the distinctions in Table 11.1 have received considerable support in the behavioral sciences, they may not map neatly onto neural mechanisms or architectures. In particular, it seems likely that performance of any *task* will involve a mix of *processes* from each column. It may therefore be useful to distinguish between tasks and processes. For example, even the most commonly used examples of automatic *tasks* (e.g., driving a car), which involve mostly unconscious or procedural *processes*, typically require an explicit and conscious intent to initiate the task. Conversely, tasks commonly used to highlight reflective processes (e.g., novice performance on a musical instrument) involve many automatic, unconscious, and procedural processes (e.g., the actions associated with playing each note, each of which is itself composed of a complex sequence of precise motor commands). Even the earliest efforts to identify the neural mechanisms underlying both types of processes have revealed a high degree of overlap, such as the role of dopamine in simple conditioning (Montague et al. 1996) and its role in gating of representations into working memory (Braver and Cohen 2000; Frank et al. 2001).

Even if the relationships in Table 11.1 and the underlying neural mechanisms are complex, this does not mean that the distinctions in Table 11.1 are useless. For some purposes, at other levels of analysis, these distinctions may reflect useful functional abstractions that serve as valuable heuristics for understanding higher-level phenomena (e.g., social interactions). Accordingly, the approaches we have described are not limited to decision making: in the understanding of social cognition, progress has been made even without clear definitions of the object of study. The need for terms such as explicit and implicit may actually disappear as a better understanding of the processes emerges.

Transfer between Processes

Interestingly, during behavior, human beings routinely change how strongly they rely on reflexive and reflective processes. One example in representational format is the learning of a motor skill. As described above, at first, representations about playing a piano might be in propositional form: "play middle C with the index finger of your right hand." The novice might experience playing the piano in the early stages as the feeling of executing these sorts of propositions and may indeed interpret notes in this way, as propositions directing their actions. Later, with practice and repetition, an expert piano player's movements will be caused by procedural representations, not in propositional form, but rather in the format of procedural memory. A reasonable characterization of the causal etiology of a novice playing the piano is a set of propositional representations, whereas the causal etiology of the muscle movements in the expert is a set of representations in procedural formats (Squire 1987).

In sum, it is fruitless to ask whether reflexive and reflective processes generally lead to better performance. It would be better to ask what mix of processes is involved in different circumstances. A number of approaches have allowed us to examine the contribution of the two types of processes in different situations.

Neuroscience

Functional neuroimaging allows us to examine the brain circuits involved in a number of tasks which, in turn, can be helpful in identifying the processes involved. Consider the footbridge scenario (Cohen 2005):

> As a bystander on a footbridge that crosses over a track, you see an oncoming trolley that will most certainly kill five individuals working down the track. You must decide whether to push a large worker, who is standing on the bridge close to its edge, off the bridge to block the oncoming trolley. You realize that this will certainly kill the large worker but that the action will spare the five workers further down the track.

At least two streams of information processes would be activated in this process: one is similar to that observed when certain emotional processes are engaged; the other is commonly associated with more deliberative forms of processing (Greene and Haidt 2002; Cohen 2005). Similar dissociations can be found when subjects have to decide whether they prefer to receive $10 today or $12 in a week's time (inter-temporal choice). Generally, these findings have been taken as evidence that many decision problems are influenced by both controlled, deliberative, reflective processes and emotional, less-controlled mechanisms that might better be classified as reflexive processes.

What can we deduce from fMRI experiments? By measuring the disruptive effect of deoxyhaemoglobin on the spin of protons in the brain, fMRI can indirectly localize changes of metabolic demands in the brain. The spatial resolution of the method is higher than that of many other neuroimaging techniques (e.g., EEG, MEG and TMS) but remains coarse compared to the size of the neurons and synapses that actually process information in the brain: fMRI typically measures activity in spatial units of 3 mm × 3 mm × 3 mm = 27 mm³. Within this volume, the method averages the metabolic demands of about 2500 million synapses and 25 million neurons organized in approximately 10 distinct functional columns. This spatial limitation constrains the interpretation of fMRI findings substantially. If one finds, for instance, that lowering the amount offered in an ultimatum game results in the recruitment of additional brain areas (Sanfey et al. 2003), it is reasonable to conclude that additional *processes* have been recruited by the new task parameters. What is difficult to do with fMRI, on the other hand, is to gain information about the *nature* of the additional processes that have been recruited: looking *where* in the brain the task causes activity cannot tell us directly *what* happens in that location of the brain. Many researchers interpret activation of a particular brain region "A" (e.g., the anterior insula) by referring to evidence that the same brain region was recruited in a number of other tasks, all of which are thought to share a certain process X (e.g., processing aversive emotional material; Wicker et al. 2003). This evidence is then used to suggest, for example, that brain activity in the insula during the ultimatum game indicates that the task involves the processing of one's negative emotional responses during unfair offers. This line of thought is tempting, because rejecting unfair offers often goes hand in hand with a negative emotional feeling, and the anterior insula is indeed active while rejecting ultimatum offers (Sanfey et al. 2003) and while subjects smell disgusting odors (Wicker et al. 2003). This can be taken to suggest that processing one's own feeling of disgust *might* be an element in rejecting unfair offers. It is, however, important to realize that areas such as the anterior insula contain hundreds of millions of neurons, and finding that such an area is recruited during the experience of disgust is not evidence that all of these neurons participate exclusively in the experience of disgust. Indeed, the anterior insula is involved in processing a range of emotions, including pain and positive emotions (Jabbi et al. 2007) as well as disgust and a variety of more cognitive tasks involving language. With that caveat in mind, finding that a task activates the anterior insula, which has often been found to be involved in emotional processes, *suggests* that the task requires emotional processing, but it does not *prove* that it involves such a process. At present, for many brain areas, our understanding of their function remains too scant to allow us to conclude *what* processes are involved in a task based on the location of activation. This interpretative limitation is common to all neuroimaging studies, and there is an awareness of this throughout the neuroscientific community. At the border between disciplines, however, neuroimaging studies are increasingly referred to by scholars outside the field of neuroscience. It is thus important for these scholars to be aware of the tentative nature of the interpretation of neuroimaging data.

Modeling

The development of formal models of decision making and their implementation in artificial systems has provided a fruitful testing ground for our understanding of decision making. In particular, it has helped identify the advantages and disadvantages of the processes shown in Table 11.1.

One fundamental trade-off between processes is the efficiency but rigidity of reflexive processes versus the flexibility but inefficiency of reflective processes. This distinction has been captured by several formalisms: model-free versus model-based learning mechanisms (Daw et al. 2007). Standard reinforcement learning algorithms provide an example of a model-free mechanism (sometimes referred to as "habit learning"). These models learn to represent the future value of each state in an environment. With sufficient time and stability of the environment, reinforcement learning algorithms can be shown to converge on an accurate representation of the expected future value of every state based on the future rewards with which each is associated and their probability of occurrence. However, learning the state-value associations is slow (requiring an exploration of all states in the environment), and if the environment changes (e.g., the probabilities of states changes), then the value representations can quickly become obsolete. In this sense, the system is inflexible—it has a hard time adapting to new environments. This contrasts with a mechanism that has a reflective-type representation (i.e., a model) of all perceived states in the world (and their associated rewards) and can simulate the various sequences of actions that can be taken from a given state to determine its future value. This system is flexible, inasmuch as it can compute the value of any state "on the fly." It is thus robust to changes in the environment, since the model can be quickly updated when the world changes. However, its ability to carry out simulations is limited both by its memory capacity (i.e., the length of sequences that it can simulate) and the time it takes to carry out such simulations, and thus it is less efficient than a model-free system. This trade-off between efficiency and flexibility seems to capture an important distinction between both types of processes.

ACT-R theory provides another formalism within which to describe this trade-off between efficiency and flexibility in reflexive versus reflective processes. In ACT-R this can be explained by the relative degree to which a process relies on each of two fundamental memory mechanisms: declarative and procedural memory. The core of ACT-R is constituted by the declarative memory system for facts (knowing what) and the procedural system for rules (knowing how). The declarative memory system consists of records that represent information, for example, about the outside world, about oneself, or about possible actions. The procedural system consists of if-then rules that guide the course of actions an individual takes when performing a specific task. The "if" side of a production rule specifies various conditions: the state of working memory, changes in perceptual information (e.g., detecting that a new object has appeared). If all conditions of a production rule are met, then the rule fires and the actions specified (the "then" side of the rule) are executed. These actions can include updating records, creating new records, setting goals, and initiating motor responses.

To see how processing in ACT-R relates to the distinction between model-free and model-based learning mechanisms, consider the situation of trying to guess your friend's two-letter pin code to access his bank account. Initially, you would explore the environment, trying out different pin codes. This could be accomplished by trying out various sequences: if want-pin then try "3" as first number; if want-pin then try "8" as second number, etc. This yields a highly flexible system that would eventually find the pin, say, "13" and produce a production of the form: if want-pin, then try "13." Over time, as you consistently gain access to your friend's account with this sequence, guided by a process of reinforcement learning, the "13" production would be strengthened, increasing the likelihood of firing and the speed with which it fires. Thus, it would win out over the simpler but more flexible productions that lead to exploration. However, this would lead to a problem if your friend changes his pin code. Here, the system would do well to return to the more flexible, but slower model-based production that can explore the environment. Notice, however, that in the ACT-R implementation, there would not be two independent systems. Instead, in reflective processes, processing relies more heavily on the declarative system (corresponding to the representation of the model in model-based learning), whereas in reflexive processes there is greater reliance on the procedural system. The general point is that there are trade-offs between more automatic, ballistic (i.e., procedural, in ACT-R) processes and more controlled, flexible ones that rely more on declarative memory. Which works best depends on the structure, stability, and experience with the environment.

If we include the reasonable assumption that we are consciously aware of changes to the goal representation that guides our behavior, we would end up with a situation where we are conscious of fishing around for the pin code by using explorative production, but unconscious of typing the pin when using the chunked "13" production. Consciousness—a distinction that has been used to distinguish system 1 and system 2—in the ACT-R implementation falls out of a single set of mechanisms, but understanding how this translates to the human brain remains uncertain.

Behavior

As discussed above, infants have approximate concepts of number that continue in adulthood. In addition, however, adults have precise number concepts. Adult number processes suffer from attentional load and would thus be classified as reflective processes, whereas the former do not. Both number processes could be used to investigate the dual nature and interaction of decision making. For instance, many models of decision making suggest that quantities are integrated *as if* they were processed using an explicit arithmetic strategy. Outcomes, for example, are weighted by their probabilities, or amounts are discounted by delay time. There are many reasons to suggest that various decisions are not made using an explicit arithmetic strategy: Protocol analysis shows that such explicit multiplication is rare, and analysis of reaction times does not seem consistent with explicit multiplication. In addition, analyses of information acquisition show that people seem to look at probabilities and payoffs contiguously, which seems inconsistent with the use of explicit arithmetic strategies. This suggests that behavioral experiments can be used to examine the degree to which decisions follow the psychometric laws of reflective processes, explicit arithmetic of reflexive processes, and approximate numerosity. An example might be to measure the subject's psychometric sensitivities along their intuitive sense of numerosity and to examine whether their choice behavior in economic decisions is better predicted by the characteristics of their approximate or explicit mathematical capacities, or a weighted combination of both. Placing subjects under constraints of high attentional load or allowing them only a brief instant to make decisions may be another way to probe the role of approximate numerosities in decision making.

The Impact of Making Implicit Knowledge Explicit

One strategy to study the relationship between implicit and explicit knowledge is to ask: What is the impact of making implicit knowledge explicit? The core intuition that can be affected by the use of implicit knowledge to make it explicit is illustrated using the example of motor processes. Everyone has had experience with trying to decompose a well-learned motor skill (e.g., explaining how to perform a tennis serve) only to find that in the attempt to characterize the process, it loses its automatic fluency. The basic claim that implicit processes can be affected (often negatively) by explication has been empirically illustrated in a variety of different domains, including memory, problem solving, and decision making.

Memory

Numerous studies have shown that attempting to describe a nonverbal stimulus can impair subsequent recognition performance. For example, Schooler and Engstler-Schooler (1990) showed participants in a study a video of a bank robbery. Some participants were subsequently asked to describe the appearance of the face of the robber in detail, while others were given an unrelated filler activity. Finally, all participants were given a forced choice recognition test, including a photo of the previously seen robber and seven similar distractor faces. The results revealed that describing the face led to a markedly impaired recognition performance relative to those who did not describe the face. Since the original demonstration of this negative consequence of explicit verbalization (termed verbal overshadowing), the approach can be generalized to other types of nonverbal stimuli, including memory for colors (Schooler and Engstler-Schooler 1990), music (Houser, Fiore, and Schooler, unpublished), voices (Perfect et al. 2002), abstract figures (Brandimonte et al. 1997), wines (Melcher and Schooler 1996), and mushrooms (Melcher and Schooler 2004).

One critical issue in understanding the impact of experiences that are not able to be explained involves the question of how expertise mediates this effect. A reasonable hypothesis is that when individuals are first acquiring a skill, explicit verbal description should be at a minimum benign and quite possibly helpful. However, as the skill becomes proceduralized, it may become more vulnerable to verbal explication. At the same time, if in the process of gaining expertise individuals also gain skill in verbally describing their knowledge, verbalization might not be disruptive. A study on the effects of verbalization on memory for the tastes of wine illustrates these points. Melcher and Schooler (1996) asked participants to taste a wine and either verbalize it or perform a control task prior to identifying the tasted wine among distracters. Participants were non-wine drinkers, untrained wine drinkers, or trained wine experts (i.e., professionals or those who had taken wine seminars). This study showed that verbalization only impaired untrained wine drinkers. Trained wine drinkers have the verbal ability to describe the various aspects of wine detected by their palates and do not experience verbal overshadowing, ostensibly because their experiences and verbalizations correspond. Similarly, non-wine drinkers have neither the expertise to perceive wines in depth nor the verbal tools to describe them, and thus their experiences and verbalizations do not interfere with each other. Untrained wine drinkers' perceptual expertise in wine tasting exceeds their verbal expertise in describing wine, and thus they do not have the verbal tools to describe all of the nuances that their palates detected.

Problem Solving

Over the years, various researchers have speculated that the processes leading to solutions on insight problems, in which the solution seems to pop out of the blue, are markedly less explicitly reportable relative to more logical or analytical problem-solving tasks. Accordingly, if verbal explication of implicit processes can interfere with those processes, then verbal description of insight problem solving might be disruptive. Consistent with this prediction, Schooler et al. (1993) found that participants who were asked to think aloud while trying to solve insight problems were significantly less successful than participants who worked on the problems silently. In contrast, thinking aloud had no effect on participants' ability to solve logical problems. Furthermore, in a protocol analysis, Melcher and Schooler (1996) found that the contents of participants' verbal transcripts were predictive of their success at solving logical problems, but not insight problems. This suggests that the source of the disruptive effects of explicating insight problem solving stems from the fact that the processes contributing to successful solutions are not available for verbal report.

Decision Making

A number of studies have demonstrated that verbal reflection can disrupt the quality of affective decisions. In one study, participants were given the opportunity to taste various strawberry jams (Wilson and Schooler 1991). In one condition, participants analyzed why they felt the way they did about the jams, whereas in another they did not. Thereafter, all participants rated the jams. When compared with the ratings of jam experts (who were from the Consumers Union), participants who went simply with their intuitions were in marked agreement with the experts. However, participants who analyzed their reasons generated evaluations that did not correspond with expert opinion. A follow-up study examined the impact of analyzing reasons on post-choice satisfaction. Participants were shown various art posters and were allowed to select one to take home. Prior to their decision, half of the participants analyzed why they felt the way they did about the posters. When contacted two weeks later, these individuals were less satisfied with their choices and less likely to have the posters hung on their walls. Such findings suggest that, as in the case of memory and problem solving, explicit reflection about decisions that typically draw on nonreportable processes can disrupt the quality of those decisions.

Summary

In considering the evidence for disruptive effects of explicit reflection on tasks that draw on implicit knowledge, several critical issues arise. First, what are the underlying mechanisms driving these effects? Two general classes of mechanisms have been proposed. According to a specific *content account*, verbal reflection is disruptive because in the course of describing an experience, individuals generate explicit verbal content that leads them astray. For example, individuals might erroneously describe the appearance of a face and then choose one that best fits their flawed description. According to a general *processing account*, verbal reflection leads to a generalized shift in the basic cognitive operations in which participants engage. For example, verbalization could cause participants to shift from an automatic holistic face recognition strategy (e.g., choosing the face that "pops out") to a more strategic analytic strategy (e.g., systematically comparing the faces feature by feature). At present, there is debate regarding which of these accounts best characterizes the findings, although it is notable that there are some results that are very difficult to accommodate with a processing account. For example, if, following verbal reflection, individuals rely on the specific content of what they said, then it is not self-evident why describing one face would interfere with the recognition of a different face that had not been described.

Importantly, the existence of suggestive (if not conclusive) evidence supporting a processing account of the disruptive effects of verbalization in the case of face recognition does not rule out the possibility that verbal overshadowing effects in other domains might not be more driven by the specific content of the verbalizations. This observation highlights a more general point, which is that there are a variety of notable differences among the domains in which the negative effects of explicit reflection have been observed. In the area of memory, the qualities that make stimuli difficult to describe most likely stem from their perceptual nature. It is not that the experience of a face or a taste is unconscious, it is simply that such experiences do not readily lend themselves to translation into words. In contrast, in the domain of insight problem solving, the nonreportable processes that lead to a solution may genuinely be unconscious in nature. Finally, in the case of decision making, the source of the disruption of verbal reflection may stem not from the perceptual nature of the stimuli but rather from the fact that the decisions are being based on an affective intuitive reaction to the stimuli that may simply not lend itself to reflective penetration. The reasons behind the lack of capacity for explicit reporting may vary markedly, highlighting the main point; namely, that implicit knowledge does not necessarily originate from the same underlying cognitive mechanisms.

Although caution is advised in considering the shared mechanism and underlying representations leading to verbal overshadowing effects across domains, there are some commonalities. In the memory domain, verbal overshadowing effects are attenuated if, following verbal description, participants are forced to make their recognition decisions quickly. Similarly, in the domain of affective decision making, if individuals are forced to make snap decisions, the negative consequences of previously having reflected verbally on the basis of their preferences can be attenuated. This suggests that despite the disparities between the domains, forcing individuals to reapply implicit processes negates the negative consequences of making implicit explicit.

Too Bad—Two is Bad: Problems with a Dual Process Perspective

Many lines of thought converge to the idea that humans have two distinguishable *types* of processes that occur in the brain and that these two types are not mutually exclusive. The process of decision making, however, can also be examined at an even more global or local perspective.

Two Is Too Many: Two Horses but a Single Cart

When adopting the perspective of the organism as a whole, it becomes obvious that the organism has to settle ultimately for a single decision at a given moment in time. In a moral dilemma, as in the footbridge scenario, one has to decide whether to push the large person from the bridge in order to save five individuals, or to refrain and let the five individuals die. If one assumes that a more emotional process would tend toward not pushing the person over the bridge, while a more deliberate calculating process would favor this act, the question remains as to how these two processes are integrated to reach a final decision. A similar line of reasoning may apply to the decision of whether to accept $10 today or to wait and receive $12 in a week's time.

The two proposed processes may perform entirely distinct computations and compete in an unsupervised fashion against each other. This may be the case if both processes feed onto the same output node, with one sending more excitatory inputs toward nodes that would push the large individual, while the other sends more inhibitory inputs toward these nodes. The two processes may also have direct inhibitory connections between each other. In such a case, it could be argued that the system will ultimately reach a single conclusion and that relatively little integration occurs between the processes.

Viewed differently, the two sets of processes calculate their own decisions but, in addition, another process is added before access is granted to motor output. This additional decision process could decide, based on the particular situation, how to weigh the decision of the two processes. For instance, a trained magistrate may have learned not to trust his emotions when making moral decisions and may thus base his decision entirely on the outcome of the deliberate calculating process ("one death is better than five"). Alternatively, after reading scientific publications, the same magistrate may decide to trust his gut feeling when deciding what painting to buy for his living room. Under such a perspective, the system may be seen as less competitive and more as an integrated whole that draws on multiple subsystems. A clear challenge for such an architecture is that the superordinate decision process would need to optimize some form of general utility function. Some have interpreted existing data as suggesting that humans do not maximize a single, simple utility function, which in turn would imply that it is unlikely that the brain routinely implements fully rational superordinate decisions (see, e.g., Camerer 2003). Perhaps individual computational processes generate outputs—such as a decision—as well as a probability that the decision is the correct one (on some standard).

Overall, it should be noted that the idea of integrated decision making does not mean that the brain implements a single uniform decision process per se. The brain is a mosaic of regions with different patterns of input and output and distinct cytoarchitectonics. Brain regions, therefore, differ in the types of computations they can perform. These unique processes are then integrated through an intricate network of synaptic connections between brain areas.

A potential mechanism through which different processing streams of decision making in the brain could integrate with each other is linked to the fact that most brain areas have reciprocal connections with each other. If area A and area B both provide independent decisions and feed these decisions to a subsequent area C, then the influence of area A on the decision in C will be sent back not only to area A but also area B; the same applies to the influence of area B on the decision in C. A single stable decision state in the system can then be achieved through the forward and backward propagation of evidence for a particular decision, providing more integration than would be assumed without backwards connections.

Two Is Too Few!

Table 11.1 conveys a set of distinctions that are common and long-standing in the behavioral science literature. Although these broad distinctions may be useful, it is worth questioning just how similar the mechanisms are that underlie the processes of each type. With regard to reflexive processes, there is general consensus that different processes must engage distinct mechanisms. That is, specific instances of automatic or implicit processes (e.g., driving a car, playing a musical instrument, or responding emotionally to a movie scene) certainly involve very different mechanisms, even if they share commonalities at some level. This is consistent with the high degree of domain specificity of such processes, as discussed earlier. Detailed mathematical and computational models are beginning to emerge that characterize formally the mechanisms involved in such processes (e.g., retrieval from episodic memory, semantic priming, sequential action). This should help illuminate both the differences and commonalities among such processes (e.g., Botvinick and Plaut 2004; McClelland, McNaughton and O'Reilly 1995; Ratcliff and McKoon 1988, 1996, 1997).

There is less consensus about reflective processes. Traditional cognitive psychological theory postulated that these share a central attentional resource (e.g., Posner and Snyder 1975; Shiffrin and Schneider 1977; Baddeley 1981), as evidenced by their ability to interfere with each other (for dissenting arguments, see Allport 1982; Navon and Gopher 1979). This would suggest that reflective processes rely on a common set of mechanisms, such as a single attentional and working memory mechanism with limited resources. However, more recent work suggests that there may be greater diversity than had previously been thought, including evidence for domain specificity in working memory processes (e.g., Shah and Miyake 1996) and the operation of different types of control mechanisms (e.g., Cohen and O'Reilly 1996; Braver et al. 2003). Thus, it seems likely that both types of processes have diverse mechanisms that share a common but not identical set of properties. Again, the specification of formal models in conjunction with a search for neural mechanisms will help refine our understanding of the relationship between and within these categories.

Summary

Although it may be helpful for current research to use the heuristic that there might be two *types* of processes contributing to decision making, we feel that it is imperative to collect further empirical evidence through a multidisciplinary approach. Such investigations will need to integrate the neurosciences, the study of behavior, and computational modeling. The resulting empirical evidence will focus our thinking and hopefully permit an understanding of the formal structure of decision making to emerge.

Culture

Individual decision making appears to be composed of multiple processes, yet the complexity of human decision making does not stop with the individual. The human brain and the decisions that humans have made have shaped our environment and our culture dramatically. The unique properties of human cognition outlined above enable us to talk to each other in high-rise buildings and to generate reports. No other animal has produced a culture of that sophistication or shaped its environment as much as we have.

One way to examine the effect of our own decisions on culture is to view culture as a result of individuals linked together through language, imitation, and learning by observation. This link transforms us as individuals into a network of brains that is more complex than the simple sum of its parts (Donald, this volume) and represents one of the major evolutionary cognitive innovations of hominids. Human beings perceive, remember, and make decisions in groups. They also trade memories and ideas, and build systems and technologies that regulate, and sometimes radically modify, the nature and patterning of cognitive activity in groups. Human culture has thus evolved into a storehouse of knowledge and procedures that are collectively available.

Human adult brains are the result of an intimate interaction between brains and culture, and the human brain is specifically adapted for connecting to cognitive–cultural networks (CCNs). Many of the capabilities that comprise "higher cognition," including language, do not appear in development without an efficient connection to CCNs. Some of the skills needed for building an effective connection with culture (e.g., joint attention, theory of mind, and perspective taking) are themselves dependent on cultural input. In that sense, the human brain cannot realize its design potential without extensive cultural input.

Culture Influences Decision Making

The relationship between brain and culture is bidirectional. Obviously, the brain influences culture. Canine brains produce canine cultures, primate brains primate cultures, and human brains human cultures. For humans, however, the reverse influence is much greater than in other species: the human brain receives from culture a great deal of specific formatting that enables it to use symbols. Moreover, the symbols themselves are conventions generated in cultural networks.

The clearest and best-documented case of culture influencing the brain is literacy. Writing is relatively new in human history and still far from universal in human society. Since the vast majority of human languages have no indigenous writing system, a specific brain adaptation for literacy could not have evolved. Literacy skill is a cultural innovation, imposed by culture through prolonged education, and yet it results in a quasi-modular brain architecture (Donald 1991). The neuropsychology of literacy has been well documented in cases of acquired dyslexia, and the brain systems that support literacy skill can break down in a double-dissociated manner, with patients selectively losing only part of the system. Thus, one can lose the ability to read irregular words independently of the ability to read regular words, and vice versa (Shallice 1988). Brain imaging studies further demonstrate the impact of literacy on brain organization (Petersson et al. 2000; Li et al. 2006; Stewart et al. 2003), in particular by showing that a visual area in the left occipito-temporal sulcus becomes partially specialized for visual word recognition in a given script during reading acquisition (Baker et al. 2007; McCandliss et al. 2003; Vinckier et al. 2007).

From this example alone, one can conclude that culture is able to affect significantly the functional architecture of the nervous system. Note, however, that this influence stays within bounds. Comparative fMRI studies indicate that a universal brain network is activated in readers of writing systems as different as English, French, Hebrew, or Chinese, with minor differences as a function of script (Bolger et al. 2005; Nakamura et al. 2005; Paulesu et al. 2001). Dehaene (2007) argues that the invention of writing systems was tightly constrained by the prior functional architecture of the brain and thus the interaction between brain structures and cultural inventions is bidirectional: cerebral networks can be partially "recycled" to a novel cultural use, but they also impose important constraints on which cultural inventions are successful (Dehaene 2007; for a similar argument concerning mathematical invention, see Dehaene 1997).

Developmental theorists have proposed that culture provides essential input in the development of such fundamental cognitive capacities as joint attention, word-finding, and social cognition (Nelson 1996; Tomasello 1990). These capacities are highly evolved in humans, but can only develop normally with extensive cultural guidance. Because culture influences the functional organization of the cognitive system so deeply in ontogenesis, *ipso facto* it affects the apparatus of decision making.

Inherent in the idea that human cognition is closely interdependent on CCNs is the realization that our brains and decisions are also heavily influenced by our culture in very specific contexts. Over the last years, this effect has been extensively investigated.

One example of how explicit cultural concepts can influence individual decision making is illustrated by examining the relationship between beliefs about free will and moral action. In a recent study (Vohs and Schooler 2007), participants were given an excerpt drawn from Francis Crick's, "*The Astonishing Hypothesis,*" in which he argues that humans are simply machines and lack any real sense of free will. Other participants were given a comparably long section of text that made no reference to the issue of free will. All participants were then given a mental arithmetic task for which there was an opportunity to cheat. Vohs and Schooler found that participants who read the article were significantly more likely to cheat, and that this increased cheating behavior was mediated by a reduced belief in free will. In another study, participants who were given deterministic statements were more likely to overpay themselves for their performance on a problem-solving task. Together, these studies illustrate how establishing certain assumptions explicitly about human nature can impact powerfully, and in some cases perhaps detrimentally, people's moral decisions.

One can also compare decision-making behavior in different cultures. Recently, a team of anthropologists and economists performed two rounds of experimental games in a wide range of small-scale societies, including foragers, small-scale horticulturalists, pastoralists, and sedentary farmers (Henrich 2000; Henrich et al. 2004, 2005). One of the tasks was the ultimatum game, which allows two parties (the proposer and the responder) to share a gross positive amount of money. The proposer suggests a distribution of this amount among the two, which the responder can either accept or reject. Acceptance results in the proposed distribution, whereas rejection leaves both parties empty-handed. Another task was the dictator game, where there is no veto power (i.e., whatever the proposer suggests is automatically implemented). The third type of game was the so-called public goods game. Here each of several players can either invest a part of their capital into the "public good" or keep all of their money. At the end of each round, a player earned what he kept plus what he got from the sum of all contributions after the contributions had been multiplied by a certain factor determining the amount of the public good. Parameters are such that individually it pays to keep everything (i.e., contribute nothing), although the group of all players would gain by contributing. Under certain conditions, third-party punishment was implemented by letting a third party watch how the money amount is allocated in the dictator game. Being aware of the distribution, the third party had the choice of subtracting a gross positive punishment from what the "dictator" took. In case of punishing, this subtracted amount was lost (i.e., it was neither given to the recipient nor collected by the third party).

In the first round, the ultimatum game was performed in all societies, whereas the public goods game and the dictator game were performed only in a subset of societies. In the second round, ultimatum, dictator, and third-party punishment games were performed in all societies. These experiments reveal a number of interesting results:

1. *Behavior in the ultimatum game varies widely.* Modal offers (i.e., how much proposers assign to responders) vary from above 50% to as low as 15%, and in some societies such low offers were usually accepted. This behavior is closer to predictions based on opportunism in the sense of own money maximization than the behavior of Western university subjects.

2. *Behavioral differences are correlated with group characteristics but not individual characteristics.* Individual ultimatum game offers were not significantly correlated with individual characteristics (e.g., income, wealth, education, market contact, age or sex). However, multiple linear regressions showed that more average aggregate market contact and cooperation in subsistence increases significantly average ultimatum game offers, and together the two variables accounted for more than half of the variance in average offers among groups.

3. *Variation in punishment predicts variation in altruism across societies.* In the third-party punishment game, the average acceptance threshold (the minimum offer not punished by the third party) provides a measure of the level of punishment in that society. This measure of punishment also predicts the level of altruism as measured by dictator generosity (the size of offers in the ordinary dictator game) across societies.

Taken together, these experiments indicate how institutions (e.g., punishment) and culture can strongly affect individual decision making.

Research on concepts of number and geometry show an interesting pattern of cultural variability and invariance in human concepts. Studies of several remote human groups provide evidence that verbal counting systems are not universal: there are languages that lack words for any exact numerical values beyond "two" or "three," and native speakers of those languages do not spontaneously represent exact numbers beyond that limit (Pica et al. 2004; Gordon 2004). Nevertheless, these speakers' abilities to represent approximate numerosities, and to perform approximate addition and subtraction on these representations, are indistinguishable from those of adults and children whose language and culture includes a full verbal number system and who have learned symbolic arithmetic. This suggests that the core representations of number that emerge in infants are universal across human cultures and provides a common foundation for culturally variable, higher level skills. A similar set of findings has been obtained with regard to geometric representations (Dehaene et al. 2006). If explicit calculations play a fundamental role in decision making, then the effect of culture on numerical concepts may be expected to have a fundamental impact on decision making. If decision making depends, however, on implicit calculations through the culturally invariant systems of number representation, as some evidence suggests (e.g., Chen et al. 2006), then patterns of decision making should show cultural invariance as well.

Intercultural comparisons that attempt to correlate differences in numerical concepts with decisions in games may be a fruitful way to test these ideas. More generally, experimental integration of cross-cultural, developmental, and cross-species comparisons may be extremely fruitful in specifying the elements of decision making.

Rate of Change

An important challenge to human decision making that directly relates to culture is the timescale over which biological and cultural evolution proceeds. Biological evolution gave rise to the neural mechanisms underlying the power of human cognition. The development of these mechanisms seems to have occurred relatively rapidly during biological evolution. However, the technological and social innovations to which these structures have given rise (i.e., the process of cultural evolution) have developed even faster and may outpace the process of biological evolution (Cohen 2005). Changes in the physical and social environment produced by cultural evolution may now be creating circumstances for which the older mechanisms in our brains are not fully adapted. This, in turn, may account for many of the idiosyncrasies and/or inconsistencies we observe in human behavior. Many modern circumstances may confront the human brain with decisions that can be made both by older mechanisms that were not adapted to the present circumstance as well as the more recently evolved mechanisms that support higher cognitive faculties which, in turn, could lead to conflict and inconsistency in behavior: competing responses to the unlimited availability of high caloric foods from our appetitive systems and from those that can take account of longer-term goals and consequences (Burnham and Phelan 2000).

In view of these rapid changes, there is a positive message in that humans have specifically evolved to respond to fast changes. It is likely that human populations have been subjected to rapid, high amplitude environmental changes for at least the last 800,000 years. Data from the Greenland ice caps provides a record of world temperatures over the last 120,000 years at a minimum resolution of ten years. Unlike the current interglacial climate period, these records indicate that glacial periods were characterized by fluctuations of world temperature from glacial cold to almost interglacial warmth, often over a period of a few hundred years. Lower resolution records from deep-sea cores suggest that human populations have been subjected to this varying climate regime for at least the last 800,000 years. It is plausible that the evolution of the capacity for social learning is an adaptation to such climate fluctuations, though of course climatic variation is but one element of the environment shaping cognitive adaptations. Unlike any other mammal, humans have the capacity to learn complicated skills easily by observing others. This is likely to be a refinement of the ability of primates to learn by observations, the neural basis of which may rely on mirror neurons that are found both in humans and monkeys. The much more efficient capacity of humans to learn skills through observation, however, allows for the rapid, cumulative evolution of locally adaptive skills—a trick that allowed human foragers to occupy almost every terrestrial habitat. Human intelligence alone has not equipped us to learn to live in such a diverse range of habitats, rather social learning has allowed human populations to accumulate gradually, but rapidly (by the standards of genetic evolution), highly habitat-specific technologies and knowledge. It is impossible, for example, for a single individual to find out how to make a kayak in the Arctic or a blow gun in the African desert without the benefit of the long line of cultural exchange between teachers and students. It has been argued that this specific adaptation may be both the source of our fast cultural evolution and the preparation to address the resulting challenges (see Boyd and Richerson, this volume).

Conclusions

Our uniquely human capacities have created a dense web of social interactions and a complex, rapidly changing cultural environment. Human culture differs in space and time, as do differences in explicit mathematical skills and institutions (e.g., morals, punishment and mandatory social securities). These differences have been shown to have dramatic effects on decision making. Examining the pathways in which culture interacts with reflective or reflexive processes within individuals and developing a better understanding for the dynamics of the complex interactions occurring in social networks remain important topics for further investigation. A better understanding of decision making at all levels will have important implications for our legal system, as it will inform our understanding of concepts such as responsibility and negligence.

Acknowledgments

We wish to thank Stan Dehaene for his precious input and Julia Lupp for her invaluable help in generating this report. Christian Keysers was supported by a Marie Curie Excellence Grant of the European Commission and a VIDI grant of the dutch N.W.O.

References

Allport, D. A. 1982. Attention and performance. In: New Directions in Cognitive Psychology, ed. G. I. Claxton. London: Routledge and Keagan-Paul.

Aziz-Zadeh, L., L. Cattaneo, M. Rochat, and G. Rizzolatti. 2005. Covert speech arrest induced by rTMS over both motor and nonmotor left hemisphere frontal sites. *J. Cogn. Neurosci.* **17**:928–938.

Baddeley, A. 1981. The concept of working memory: A view of its current state and probable future development. *Cognition* **10(1-3)**:17–23.

Baker, C. I., J. Liu, L. L. Wald, K. K. Kwong, T. Benner et al. 2007. Visual word processing and experiential origins of functional selectivity in human extrastriate cortex. *Proc. Natl. Acad. Sci.* **104(21)**:9087–9092.

Bloom, P. 2004. Descartes' Baby: How the Science of Child Development Explains What Makes Us Human. New York: Basic Books.

Bolger, D. J., C. A. Perfetti, and W. Schneider. 2005. Cross-cultural effect on the brain revisited: Universal structures plus writing system variation. *Hum. Brain Map.* **25(1)**:92–104.

Botvinick, M., and D. C. Plaut. 2004. Doing without schema hierarchies: A recurrent connectionist approach to normal and impaired routine sequential action. *Psychol Rev.* **111(2)**:395–429.

Brandimonte, M. A., J. W. Schooler, and P. Gabbino. 1997. Attenuating verbal overshadowing through visual retrieval cues. *J. Exp. Psychol.: Learn. Mem. Cogn.* **23**:915–931.

Braver, T. S., and J. D. Cohen. 2000. On the control of control: The role of dopamine in regulating prefrontal function and working memory. In: Control of Cognitive Processes, ed. S. Monsell and J. Driver, pp. 713–737. A Bradford Book. Cambridge MA: MIT Press.

Braver, T. S., J. R. Reynolds, and D. I. Donaldson. 2003. Neural mechanisms of transient and sustained cognitive control during task switching. *Neuron* **39(4)**:713–726.

Burnham, T., and J. Phelan. 2000. Mean Genes: From Sex to Money to Food, Taming Our Primal Instincts. Cambridge, MA: Perseus Publ.

Camerer, C. F. 2003. Behavioral Game Theory: Experiments on Strategic Interaction: Princeton, NJ: Princeton Univ. Press.

Chen, M. K., V. Lakshminaryanan, and L. R. Santos. 2006. The evolution of our preferences: Evidence from capuchin monkey trading behavior. *J. Pol. Econ.* **114(3)**:517–537.

Cheney, D. L., and R. M. Seyfarth. 1990. How Monkeys See the World. Chicago: Univ. of Chicago Press.

Cohen, J. D. 2005. The vulcanization of the human brain: A neural perspective on interactions between cognition and emotion. *J. Econ. Persp.* **19(4)**:3–24.

Cohen, J. D., T. S. Braver, and R. C. O'Reilly. 1996. A computational approach to prefrontal cortex, cognitive control, and schizophrenia: Recent developments and current challenges. *Phil. Trans. Roy. Soc. Lond. B* **351(1346)**:515–1527.

Cohen, J. D., and R. C. O'Reilly. 1996. A preliminary theory of the interactions between prefrontal cortex and hippocampus that contribute to planning and prospective memory. In: Prospective Memory: Theory and Applications, ed. M. Brandimonte, G. O. Einstein, and M. A. McDaniel, pp. 267–295. Hillsdale, NJ: Erlbaum.

Daw, M. I., M. C. Ashby, and J. T. R. Isaac. 2007. Coordinated developmental recruitment of latent fast spiking interneurons in layer IV barrel cortex. *Nature Neurosci.* **10(4)**:453–461.

Dehaene, S. 1997. The Number Sense. New York: Oxford Univ. Press.

Dehaene, S. 2007. Reading in the Brain. New York: Penguin, in press.

Dehaene, S., V. Izard, P. Pica, and E. S. Spelke. 2006. Core knowledge of geometry in an Amazonian indigene group. *Science* **311**:381–384.

Donald, M. 1991. Origins of the Modern Mind: Three Stages in the Evolution of Culture and Cognition. Cambridge, MA: Harvard Univ. Press.

Donald, M. 1993. Précis of "Origins of the Modern Mind" with multiple reviews and author's response. *Behav. Brain Sci.* **16**:737–791.

Donald, M. 1995. The neurobiology of human consciousness: An evolutionary approach. *Neuropsychologia* **33**:1087–1102.

Donald, M. 1998. Mimesis and the executive suite: Missing links in language evolution. In: Approaches to the Evolution of Language: Social and Cognitive Bases, ed. J. R. Hurford, M. Studdert-Kennedy, and C. Knight, pp. 44–67. Cambridge: Cambridge Univ. Press.

Donald, M. 1999. Preconditions for the evolution of protolanguages. In: The Descent of Mind, ed. M. C. Corballis and I. Lea, pp. 120–136. Oxford: Oxford Univ. Press.

Donald, M. 2001. A Mind So Rare: The Evolution of Human Consciousness. New York: W. W. Norton.

Donald, M. 2005. Imitation and mimesis. In: Perspectives on Imitation: From Neuroscience to Social Science, ed. S. Hurley and N. Chater. Cambridge, MA: MIT Press.

Elman, J. L. 1990. Finding structure in time. *Cogn. Sci.* **14**:179–211.

Farroni, T., G. Csibra, F. Simion, and M. H. Johnson. 2002. Eye contact detection in humans from birth. *Proc. Natl. Acad. Sci.* **99(14)**:9602–9605.

Feigenson, L., S. Dehaene, and E. S. Spelke. 2004. Core systems of number. *Trends Cogn. Sci.* **8**:307–314.

Fiebach, C. J., and R. I. Schubotz. 2006. Dynamic anticipatory processing of hierarchical sequential events: A common role for Broca's area and ventral premotor cortex across domains? *Cortex* **42**:499–502.

Frank, M. J., B. Loughry, and R. C. O'Reilly. 2001. Interactions between frontal cortex and basal ganglia in working memory: A computational model. *Cogn. Aff. Behav. Neurosci.* **1(2)**:137–160.

Gordon, P. 2004. Numerical cognition without words: Evidence from Amazonia. *Science* **306**:496–499.

Greene, J., and J. Haidt. 2002. How (and where) does moral judgment work? *Trends Cogn. Sci.* **6(12)**:517–523.

Greenwald, A. G., D. E. McGhee, and J. L. K. Schwartz. 1998. Measuring individual differences in implicit cognition: The implicit association test. *J. Pers. Soc. Psychol.* **74**:1464–1480.

Haidt, J. 2001. The emotional dog and its rational tail: A social intuitionist approach to moral judgment. *Psychol. Rev.* **108***:*814–834.

Hare, B., J. Call, and M. Tomasello. 2001. Do chimpanzees know what conspecifics know? *Anim. Behav.* **61**:139–151.

Hauser, M. D., H. Pearson, and D. Seelig. 2002. Ontogeny of tool use in cotton-top tamarins (*Saguinus oedipus*): Innate recognition of functionally relevant features. *Anim. Behav.* **64**:299–311.

Hauser, M. D., F. Tsao, P. Garcia, and E. S. Spelke. 2003. Evolutionary foundations of number: Spontaneous representation of numerical magnitudes by cotton-top tamarins. *Proc. Roy. Soc. Lond. B* **270**:1441–1446.

Henrich, J. 2000. Does culture matter in economic behavior? Ultimatum game bargaining among the Machiguenga. *Am. Econ. Rev.* **90(4)**:973–979.

Henrich, J., S. Bowles, C. Camerer, E. Fehr, and H. Gintis. 2004. The Foundations of Human Sociality: Economic Experiments and Ethnographic Evidence from Fifteen Small-scale Societies. New York: Oxford Univ. Press.

Henrich, J., R. Boyd, S. Bowles, H. Gintis, E. Fehr et al. 2005. "Economic man" in cross-cultural perspective: Behavioral experiments in 15 small-scale societies. *Behav. Brain Sci* **28**:795–855.

Henrich, J., R. McElreath, A. Barr, A. Ensimger, J. Barrett et al. 2006. Costly punishment across human societies. *Science* **312**:1767−1770.

Hochreiter, S., and J. Schmidhuber. 1997. Long short-term memory. *Neural Comp.* **9(8)**:1735–1780.

Hunt, G. R., M. C. Corballis, and R. D. Gray. 2006. Design complexity and strength of laterality are correlated in New Caledonian crows' pandanus tool manufacture. *Proc. Roy. Soc. Lond. B* **273**:1127–1133.

Jabbi, M., M. Swart, and C. Keysers. 2007. Empathy for positive and negative emotions in the gustatory cortex. *Neuroimage* **34**:1744–1753.

Keysers, C., and V. Gazzola. 2006. Towards a unifying neural theory of social cognition. *Prog Brain Res.* **156**:379–401.

Keysers, C., and D. I. Perrett. 2004. Demystifying social cognition: A Hebbian perspective. *Trends Cogn Sci.* **8**:501–507.

Kurzban, R., and C. A. Aktipis. 2007. Modularity and the social mind: Why social psychologists should be less self-ish. *Pers. Soc. Psychol. Rev.* **11**:131–149.

Landau, B., H. Gleitman, and E. S. Spelke. 1981. Spatial knowledge and geometrical representation in a child blind from birth. *Science* **213**:1275–1278.

Lemer, C., S. Dehaene, E. S. Spelke, and L. Cohen. 2003. Approximate quantities and exact number words: Dissociable systems. *Neuropsychologia* **41**:1942–1958.

Li, G., R. T. F. Cheung, J. H. Gao, T. M. Lee, L. Tan et al. 2006. Cognitive processing in Chinese literate and illiterate subjects: An fMRI study. *Hum. Brain Map.* **27**:144–152.

Matsuzawa, T. 1985. Use of numbers by a chimpanzee. *Nature* **315**:57–59.

McCandliss, B. D., L. Cohen, and S. Dehaene. 2003. The visual word form area: Expertise for reading in the fusiform gyrus. *Trends Cogn. Sci.* **7**:293–299.

McClelland, J. L., B. L. McNaughton, and R. C. O'Reilly. 1995. Why there are complementary learnings systems in the hippocampus and neocortex: Insights from the successes and failures of connectionist models of learning and memory. *Psychol. Rev.* **102(3)**:419–457.

McCrink, K., and K. Wynn. 2004. Large-number addition and subtraction in infants. *Psychol. Sci.* **15**:776–781.

Melcher, J., and J. W. Schooler. 1996. The misremembrance of wines past: Verbal and perceptual expertise differentially mediate verbal overshadowing of taste. *J. Mem. Lang.* **35**:231–245.

Melcher, J. M., and J. W. Schooler. 2004. Perceptual and conceptual expertise mediate the verbal overshadowing effect in a training paradigm. *Mem. Cogn.* **32(4)**:618–631.

Meltzoff, A. N., and W. Prinz. 2002. The Imitative Mind: Development, Evolution, and Brain Bases. Cambridge: Cambridge Univ. Press.

Mithen, S. J. 1996. The Prehistory of the Mind: The Cognitive Origins of Art, Religion and Science. Cambridge: Cambridge Univ. Press.

Montague, P. R., P. Dayan, and T. J. Sejnowski. 1996. A framework for mesencephalic dopamine systems based on predictive Hebbian learning. *J. Neurosci.* **16**:1936–1947.

Nakamura, K., S. Dehaene, A. Jobert, D. Le Bihan, and S. Kouider. 2005. Subliminal convergence of Kanji and Kana words: Further evidence for functional parcellation of the posterior temporal cortex in visual word perception. *J. Cogn. Neurosci.* **17(6)**:954–968.

Navon, D., and D. Gopher. 1979. On the economy of the human processing system. *Psychol. Rev.* **86**:214–255.

Naya, Y., K. Sakai, and Y. Miyashita. 1996. Activity of primate inferotemporal neurons related to a sought target in pair-association task. *Proc. Natl. Acad. Sci.* **93**:2664–2669.

Nelson, K. 1996. Language in Cognitive Development: Emergence of the Mediated Mind. New York: Cambridge Univ. Press.

Newcombe, N., J. Huttenlocher, and A. Learmonth. 2000. Infants' coding of location in continuous space. *Infant Behav. Dev.* **22(4)**:483–510.

Paulesu, E., J. F. Demonet, F. Fazio, E. McCrory, V. Chanoine et al. 2001. Dyslexia: Cultural diversity and biological unity. *Science* **291(5511)**:2165–2167.

Pepperberg, I. M. 1987. Evidence for conceptual quantitative abilities in the African Grey parrot: Labeling of cardinal sets. *Ethology* **75**:37.

Perfect, T. J., L. J. Hunt, and C. M. Harris. 2002. Verbal overshadowing in voice recognition. *Appl. Cogn. Psychol.* **16**:973–980.

Petersson, K. M., A. Reis, S. Askelof, A. Castro-Caldas, and M. Ingvar. 2000. Language processing modulated by literacy: A network analysis of verbal repetition in literate and illiterate subjects. *J. Cogn. Neurosci.* **12**:364–382.

Pica, P., C. Lemer, V. Izard, and S. Dehaene. 2004. Exact and approximate arithmetic in an Amazonian indigene group. *Science* **306(5695)**:499–503.

Posner, M. I., and C. R. Snyder. 1975. Attention and cognitive control. In: Information Processing and Cognition, ed. R. L. Solso. Hillsdale, NJ: Erlbaum.

Ratcliff, R., and G. McKoon. 1988. A retrieval theory of priming in memory. *Psychol. Rev.* **95**:385–408.

Ratcliff, R., and G. McKoon. 1996. Biases in implicit memory tasks. *J. Exp. Psychol.: Gen.* **125**:403–421.

Ratcliff, R., and G. McKoon. 1997. A counter model for implicit priming in perceptual word identification. *Psychol. Rev.* **104**:319–343.

Rizzolatti, G., and G. Luppino. 2001. The cortical motor system. *Neuron* **31**:889–901.

Sanfey, A. G., J. K. Rilling, J. A. Aronson, L. E. Nystrom, and J. D. Cohen. 2003. The neural basis of economic decision making in the ultimatum game. *Science* **300(5626)**:1755–1757.

Scholl, B. J. 2001. Objects and attention: The state of the art. *Cognition* **80**:1–46.

Schooler, J. W. and T. Y. Engstler-Schooler. 1990. Verbal overshadowing of visual memories: Some things are better left unsaid. *Cogn. Psychol.* **17**:36–71.

Schooler, J. W., S. Ohlsson, and K. Brooks. 1993. Thoughts beyond words: When language overshadows insight. *J. Exp. Psychol.* **122**:166–183.

Shah, P., and A. Miyake. 1996. The separability of working memory resources for spatial thinking and language processing: An individual differences approach. *J. Exp. Psychol.: Gen.* **125(1)**:4–27.

Shallice, T. 1988. From Neuropsychology to Mental Structure. New York: Cambridge Univ. Press.

Shiffrin, R. M., and W. Schneider. 1977. Controlled and automatic human information processing: II. Perceptual learning, automatic attending, and a general theory. *Psychol. Rev.* **84**:127–190.

Spelke, E. S. 2003a. Core knowledge. In: Attention and Performance, vol. 20, Functional Neuroimaging of Visual Cognition, ed. N. Kanwisher and J. Duncan. Oxford: Oxford Univ. Press.

Spelke, E. S. 2003b. What makes us smart? Core knowledge and natural language. In: Language in Mind, ed. D. Gentner and S. Goldin-Meadow. Cambridge, MA: MIT Press.

Squire, L. R. 1987. Memory and Brain. New York: Oxford Univ. Press.

Stanescu, R., P. Pinel, P.-F. van de Moortele, D. LeBihan, L. Cohen et al. 2000. Cerebral bases of calculation processes: Impact of number size on the cerebral circuits for exact and approximative calculation. *Brain*: **123**:2240–2255.

Stewart, L., R. Henson, K. Kempe, V. Walsh, R. Turner et al. 2003. Brain changes after learning to read and play music. *NeuroImage* **20**:71–83.

Tomasello, M. 1999. The Cultural Origins of Human Cognition. Cambridge, MA: Harvard Univ. Press.

Valenza, E., I. Leo, L. Gava, and F. Simion. 2006. Perceptual completion in newborn human infants. *Child Dev.* **77(6)**:1815–1821.

Vinckier, F., S. Dehaene, A. Jobert, J. P. Dubus, M. Sigman et al. 2007. Hierarchical coding of letter strings in the ventral stream: Dissecting the inner organization of the visual word-form system. *Neuron* **55(1)**:143–156.

Vohs, K. D., and J. W. Schooler. 2007. The Value of Believing in Free Will: Encouraging a Belief in Determinism Increases Cheating." *Psychol. Sci.*, in press.

Wicker, B., C. Keysers, J. Plailly, J. P. Royer, V. Gallese et al. 2003. Both of us disgusted in my insula: The common neural basis of seeing and feeling disgust. *Neuron* **40(3)**:655–664.

Wilson, T. D., and J. W. Schooler. 1991. Thinking too much: Introspection can reduce the quality of preferences and decisions. *J. Pers. Soc. Psychol.* **60**:181–192.

Wynn, K. 1992. Children's acquisition of the number words and the counting system. *Cogn. Psychol.* **24**:220–251.

Xu, F., and E. S. Spelke. 2000. Large number discrimination in 6-month-old infants. *Cognition* **74**:B1–B11.

12

How Evolution Outwits Bounded Rationality

The Efficient Interaction of Automatic and Deliberate Processes in Decision Making and Implications for Institutions

Andreas Glöckner

Max Planck Institute for Research on Collective Goods, 53113 Bonn, Germany

Abstract

Classic behavioral decision research has intensively explored deliberate processes in decision making. Accordingly, individuals are viewed as bounded rational actors who, because of cognitive limitations, use simple heuristics that are successful in certain environments. In this chapter, it is postulated that human cognitive capacity is less severely limited than has previously been assumed. When automatic processes are considered, one finds that cognitive capacity is not a binding constraint for many decision problems. The general parallel constraint satisfaction (PCS) approach is outlined, which aims at describing these automatic processes, and evidence supporting this approach is summarized. It is further argued, that in order to describe decision making comprehensively, models must account for the interaction between automatic and deliberate processes. The PCS rule is delineated which specifies this interaction. The model shifts the bounds of rationality considerably and has further evolutionary advantages. Implications for the efficient design of institutions are outlined. Finally, the German legal system is reviewed in terms of its ability to support efficient decision making by implementing many of the prescriptions derived from the PCS rule without explicit knowledge about the underlying processes.

Introduction

One of the most intriguing psychological phenomena is the human ability to make decisions in a complex and uncertain world. Decision experts, such as managers and lawyers, must often make determinations based on myriad pieces of probabilistic and incomplete information. In the tradition of the bounded rationality approach (H. A. Simon 1955), it has been repeatedly argued that fast and frugal heuristics, which are based on simple decision rules and which ignore information, offer one important way for humans to reach solutions to complex decision tasks (Gigerenzer 2006). In this chapter, I summarize theoretical models and empirical findings that suggest an extended perspective; namely, individuals are able to integrate multitudinous information by relying partially on intuitive automatic processes. Specifically, I argue that individuals make use of automatic parallel constraint satisfaction (PCS) processes that have developed through evolution on the basis of perceptual processes. PCS processes can be mathematically simulated using connectionist networks. Both accounts will be discussed in light of recent evidence. Thereafter I describe the PCS rule (Glöckner and Betsch 2008), a hierarchical network model that integrates both approaches and takes into account the interaction between automatic and deliberate processes in decision making. I outline the evolutionary advantage of such a model and discuss the implications this can have for the development and improvement of institutions.

Theories in Behavioral Decision Research

In classic behavioral decision research, two major approaches can be distinguished. First, there are modifications of rational choice theory (RCT) that hold to the general assumption that information is integrated in a *weighted compensatory* manner. For example, prospect theory (Kahneman and Tversky 1979) assumes that individuals select the option with the higher subjective expected utility, which is calculated as the weighted sum of subjective utilities and subjective probabilities. Transformation functions from objective values and probabilities to subjective ones have been specified in light of empirically observed systematic deviations from RCT. Second, following the fundamental critique of H. A. Simon (1955) that such complex computations might overload human cognitive capacity, several heuristic models have been developed which postulate that individuals apply simple integration rules, thereby ignoring most information. Currently, the most influential model of this *bounded rationality approach* is the adaptive toolbox model (Gigerenzer, Todd et al. 1999). It assumes a set of fast and frugal heuristics that are applied adaptively and lead to very accurate decisions by exploiting the structure of the environment. The prototypical fast and frugal heuristic is Take the Best, in which only the most valid piece of information is inspected. If this information favors one option, it is instantly selected; only when this is not the case is the second-most valid piece of information inspected, and so on. The recently developed priority heuristic extended this concept to classic gambling decision tasks (Brandstätter et al. 2006). There is controversy over which approach is more appropriate (e.g., Brandstätter et al. 2006; Glöckner and Betsch, submitted). In the shadow of this conflict and the debates within both approaches, a third idea rooted in cognitive (Schneider and Shiffrin 1977) and social psychology (Bargh and Chartrand 1999; Petty and Cacioppo 1986) has been discussed, albeit less intensively, in behavioral decision research for many years: the *dual-processing approach* (for an overview, see Kahneman and Frederick 2002). According to this approach, individuals use both a deliberate and an intuitive system to make decisions. In contrast to the controlled deliberate system, in which information is consciously integrated according to certain rules and in a sequential manner, the intuitive system relies on automatic, unconscious processing of information.[1] The field of behavioral decision research is still in the early stages of investigating and building theories on processes of the intuitive system, and has not yet sufficiently considered findings from cognitive and social psychology. Even less is known about the interaction between the deliberate and automatic systems. Prominent general approaches that have the potential to explain processes of the intuitive system are cognition- and affect-based memory storage and retrieval models (Anderson and Lebiere 1998; Busemeyer and Townsend 1993; Damasio 1994; Dougherty et al. 1999; Ratcliff et al. 1999; Slovic et al. 2002), as well as PCS models. The former postulates that automatic processes of storage in and retrieval from long-term memory are utilized in decision making. PCS models assume that automatic processes of maximizing consistency between information in temporarily activated networks drive our decision processes.

The PCS Approach to Decision Making

Many cognitive operations function without deliberate control. Behavioral research provides a multitude of empirical findings evidencing the power of the unconscious automatic system. For instance, in the course of adaptive learning, organisms automatically record fundamental aspects of the empirical world, such as the frequency (Hasher and Zacks 1984) and value (Betsch, Plessner et al. 2001) of events or objects. It has been demonstrated repeatedly that automatic processes overrule even deliberately formed intentions: individuals act against their intentions and fall back into routines if they have to make decisions under time pressure (Betsch et al. 2004); they are unable to prevent stereotypes and prejudices from being automatically activated (Devine 1989); and the deliberate intention not to think about an object actually increases the likelihood that it will come to mind (Wegner 1994).

Automatic processes are essential for making sense of a world that provides incomplete information. Automatic processes of perception and social

---

[1] Kahneman and Frederick (2002) use the terms *automatic*, *process opaque* (unconscious), and *parallel* to describe process characteristics of the intuitive system. Note that these characteristics are not independent, nor do they perfectly coincide.

perception enable individuals to recognize objects and social constellations immediately, even if only a small fraction of the total information is available. Research in classic Gestalt psychology (Koffka 1922) provides persuasive demonstrations of these unconscious mechanisms. For example, when presented with an image of changing figure-ground relationships (e.g., the "Rubinian vase"), individuals perceive either a vase or two faces on the basis of exactly the same information. By shifting the focus of attention, perception may flip to the opposite interpretation. Conceptually, a myriad of conflicting information is unconsciously integrated in one consistent interpretation (e.g., vase). In this process, the interpretation of information is modified. Information that speaks against the dominant interpretation (e.g., an object that shades a part of the figure) is suppressed, whereas information that supports the dominant interpretation (e.g., a characteristic shape) is accentuated.

The PCS approach to decision making is based on the same principle (Read et al. 1997; Holyoak and D. Simon 1999). As soon as individuals are confronted with a decision task, automatic processes are initiated which work to form a consistent mental representation of the task. In the process, information supporting the emerging mental representation is accepted while conflicting information is devaluated. Conceptually, automatic processes weigh interpretations of information against each other by taking into account the complex constellation of the information. The best interpretation wins the competition, and conflicting information is eliminated as far as possible. Individuals are not aware of these processes; they are only aware of the results.

Connectionist Implementation of PCS Processes

Connectionist networks allow us to model PCS processes for complex decision tasks. Initially, PCS networks were introduced in psychology to model processes of word perception (McClelland and Rumelhart 1981). Later it was argued that the underlying organizing principle of maximizing consistency among pieces of information is fundamental to a wide range of psychological phenomena, such as social perception (Read and Miller 1998), analogical mapping (Holyoak and Thagard 1989), the evaluation of explanations (Thagard 1989), dissonance reduction (Shultz and Lepper 1996), impression formation (Kunda and Thagard 1996), the selection of plans (Thagard and Millgram 1995), legal decision making (Holyoak and D. Simon 1999; Thagard 2003; D. Simon 2004), preferential choice (D. Simon et al. 2004), and probabilistic decisions (Glöckner 2006, 2007; Glöckner and Betsch 2008).

For pragmatic reasons, let us focus on simple probabilistic decision tasks that have been used predominantly to investigate fast and frugal heuristics (Gigerenzer, Todd et al. 1999). One prominent example is the city-size task: when presented with two cities, a person should select the one which has the larger population based on different probabilistic information. Conceptually, a decision has to be made about a distal criterion (i.e., population of the city) on the basis of proximal probabilistic *cues* (e.g., whether it is the capital of its state) with dichotomous *cue values* (i.e., yes or no) that differ in *cue validity* (i.e., the conditional likelihood that the option is better on the criterion, given a positive or negative cue value).

Connectionist models provide different possibilities to model such probabilistic decision tasks. Fitting connectionist models a posteriori to empirical data provides only weak support for them because of the many degrees of freedom in the models. Thus, I propose a modeling approach that reduces degrees of freedom by specifying the structure of the network a priori. This general structure of a connectionist network for probabilistic decision tasks is delineated in Figure 12.1 and can be used in systematic simulations to derive testable predictions that enable the PCS approach to be differentiated empirically from other models (Glöckner 2006).

In the suggested network, cues and options are represented by nodes, which may have different levels of activation, a. Nodes are interconnected by links that have a certain strength, represented by weights, w. All links are bidirectional and can be excitatory ($w > 0$) or inhibitory ($w < 0$). Options and cues are connected by links that represent cue values. Positive predictions of a cue about an option are represented by excitatory links, whereas negative predictions are represented by inhibitory links. Options are interconnected by strong inhibitory links, because only one option can be chosen. Cues are connected with a general validity node, which is used to activate the network and has a constant activation of 1. The strength of the links w_V represents the initial subjective cue validities that result from learning experience or explicitly provided information.

The connectionist network captures the logical constraints of the decision problem, as represented in the temporarily activated mental representation. In this structure, some elements support each other (e.g., cues and options for which the former make a positive prediction) while others conflict (e.g., cues and options for which the former make a negative prediction). The activation of each node can be interpreted as a subjective judgment of the goodness of the underlying concept (i.e., the attractiveness of the options and the subjective validity of the cues). Note that there is an important distinction between the initial validity of cues, which are represented by the links w_V, and the perceived validity of cues, which are represented by the activation of the nodes a_C. The former are stable constraints in the network, whereas the latter, which will be referred to as *resulting cue validities,* are results of the PCS processes.

As soon as the network is constructed, PCS processes are initiated and alter the activation of nodes until a solution with a high level of consistency is found. Mathematically, the process can be captured by an iterative updating

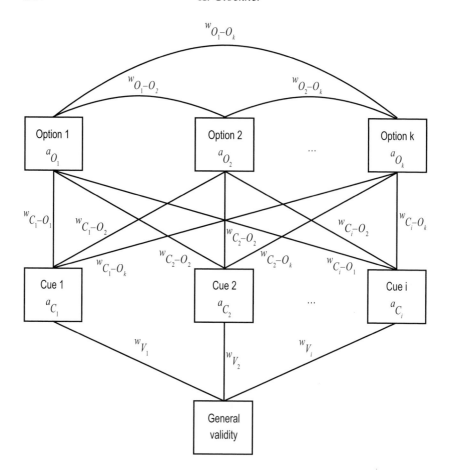

Figure 12.1   General structure of the PCS network for probabilistic decision tasks. Boxes represent nodes. The activation, *a*, of the nodes is modified within the PCS process. Lines represent links between nodes that are all bidirectional and can be inhibitory or excitatory. Links have different weights, *w*, and are fixed constraints in the network that result from learning or from explicitly provided information.

algorithm, which simulates spreading activation in the network (McClelland and Rumelhart 1981):

$$a_i(t+1) = a_i(t)(1 - decay) + \begin{cases} if\ input_i(t) < 0 & input_i(t)\big(a_i(t) - floor\big) \\ if\ input_i(t) \geq 0 & input_i(t)\big(ceiling - a_i(t)\big) \end{cases} \quad (1)$$

The activation a_i at time $t + 1$ is computed by the activation of the node at time *t*, multiplied by the decay factor plus the incoming activation for this node, $input_i(t)$, multiplied by a scaling factor. The scaling factor limits the activation of the nodes to the range –1 to +1 and leads to an S-shaped activation function.

The *input$_i$(t)* to node i is computed as the sum of the activation of all other nodes multiplied by the weight of the connection with node i:

$$input_i(t) = \sum_{j=1 \to n} w_{ij} a_j(t). \tag{2}$$

The updating algorithm maximizes the consistency (i.e., the degree of organization) in the network and minimizes contradiction or energy. The energy can be computed by:

$$Energy(t) = -\sum_i \sum_j w_{ij} a_i a_j, \tag{3}$$

where all weights w_{ij} are multiplied by the activations of the pair of nodes they connect and the resulting products are combined (Read et al. 1997). This means, for instance, that positive connections between positively activated elements increase the level of consistency, whereas negative connections between positively activated concepts decrease it (cf. Heider 1958). The iterative updating algorithm operates to maximize consistency. After a number of iterations, a state of maximal consistency under the given constraints is usually found and activations reach asymptotic levels. The option with the highest activation is selected. The number of iterations an algorithm needs to find the stable solution can be interpreted as the decision time predicted by the model.

In contrast to memory storage and retrieval models, the PCS approach does not describe long-term learning processes of relations in the network. PCS processes simulate ad hoc interpretations of the available evidence, based on constraints that result from learning or from the information that has been provided. Only the interpretation of the evidence is temporarily changed to form a consistent mental representation.

Predictions

Based on theoretical considerations and systematic simulations (Glöckner 2006; Holyoak and D. Simon 1999), five distinct predictions of the PCS approach can be derived:

1. *High computational capacity*: Individuals are able to integrate quickly a multitude of information by relying on automatic processes.
2. *Coherence shifts*: The decision process is inherently constructivist. Subjective cue validities are changed in the decision process to fit the emerging representation of the decision task, resulting in coherence shifts (D. Simon 2004): cues that point away from the favored option are devalued and cues that support the favored option are strengthened. Thus, resulting cue validities depend on the structure of the decision task and differ from initial cue validities.

3. *Approximation of weighted compensatory models*: Choices roughly approximate the weighted compensatory integration of cue values and cue validities.

4. *Decision time differences*: Decision time increases with a decrease in the initial consistency between the pieces of information. If all cues point toward the same option, consistency is high and decision time is short. If almost equally strong sets of cues favor different options, consistency is low and decision time is long.

5. *Confidence judgment differences*: The subjective confidence in a choice is higher in decision tasks when the consistency among pieces of information that cannot be resolved in the PCS process is low. If a highly consistent solution is found, confidence is high; if the resulting interpretation is still rather inconsistent, confidence in the decision is low.

Note that this set of qualitative predictions differs from that of most other decision-making models and thus allows for empirical testing against these models. Most decision-making models, including RCT, the adaptive toolbox, as well as memory storage and retrieval models, rely on the assumption that decision making is based on *unidirectional reasoning*: they assume that individuals select information from a given set and integrate it using certain algorithms to make a decision. Information is merely put into different algorithms; the information itself is not changed in the process. In contrast, the PCS approach suggests that decision making is based on *bidirectional reasoning* (Holyoak and D. Simon 1999): in a holistic process, the constellation of information and options is considered, and options and evidence are weighed jointly. Thus, individuals should not only reason from information to options, they should also infer the validity of cues from the informational constellation in a kind of automatic backward reasoning.

According to the adaptive toolbox model and the bounded rationality approach, individuals should not be able to integrate information quickly in a weighted compensatory manner because human cognitive capacity is too limited. Decision times should not be sensitive to the fact that different pieces of information convey conflicting evidence; only the number of computational steps needed to apply the heuristic should matter (Brandstätter et al. 2006); and confidence judgments should depend solely on the validity of the cue that differentiates between options (Gigerenzer et al. 1991).

Summary of Empirical Evidence

Coherence Shifts

The most comprehensive empirical work on coherence shifts in decision making has been done by Dan Simon and colleagues (Holyoak and D. Simon 1999; D. Simon et al. 2004; D. Simon 2004). For part of their experiments, participants were presented with complex legal cases and asked to judge the subjective validity of the evidence before and after the decision was made. They were able to demonstrate strong coherence shifts (i.e., differences in the ratings of the evidence before and after the decision). The participants, however, were not aware of these shifts, and the ensuing decision was "experienced as rationally warranted by the inherent values of the variables, rather than by an inflated perception imposed by the cognitive system" (D. Simon 2004, p. 545). Interestingly, Simon was able to show that PCS processes not only influence information directly involved in the decision, but also beliefs and background knowledge. Motivation and attitudes influenced the direction of coherence shifts. In line with the assumption that PCS processes are based on temporarily activated networks, it could be shown that coherence shifts are of a transitory nature and disappear after a certain time. Using different material, Glöckner, Betsch, and Schindler (submitted) found that coherence shifts are instantly initiated as soon as a decision task is perceived, even without a decision being made at all. Furthermore, it could be shown that coherence shifts occur in city-size decision tasks. As predicted by the PCS approach, coherence shifts seem to be a stable and general phenomenon that can be observed in a broad range of decision tasks.

Fast Compensatory Information Integration

Bröder (2003) extensively investigated individual decision strategies in probabilistic decision tasks and found that some of the participants searched for information and selected options in accordance with the predictions of fast and frugal heuristics. Furthermore, corresponding to the predictions of the adaptive toolbox model, he found that individuals adapted their behavior to the structure of the environment. However, he concluded that "a [weighted] compensatory strategy may be something like a default strategy that is applied at the beginning of the procedure" (Bröder 2003, p. 617). Considering the fundamental bounded rationality argument (i.e., that human cognitive capacity is limited), this finding seems surprising. Why should individuals use a complex strategy as a default strategy when it could easily overload their cognitive capacity?

To investigate the decision strategies in the city-size decision tasks further, I conducted several experiments (Glöckner 2006). All information was presented simultaneously to measure a person's computational capacity, without limiting information search by the research method (Figure 12.2). Participants were instructed to make good decisions and to proceed as quickly as possible.

A maximum likelihood analysis of the individual choice patterns revealed that, for the majority of participants, choice patterns were most likely produced by the weighted compensatory integration of cue values and cue validities. The average decision time was under three seconds. Thus, in line with the predictions of the PCS approach, individuals are indeed able to integrate quickly

	City A	City B
State Capital	+	−
University	+	+
1st League Soccer Team	−	+
Art Gallery	+	−
Airport	−	+
Cathedral	−	+

Figure 12.2   Example for a city-size decision task.

multitudinous information in a weighted compensatory manner.[2] These findings converge with those by Bröder (2003), indicating that this kind of information integration seems to be the default strategy if no available feedback indicates that a different strategy should be used.

Decision Time and Confidence Judgments

To test the predictions concerning decision times and confidence judgments, Glöckner and Hodges (submitted) conducted a series of experiments on memory-based decisions. University students in the United States were given information about German cities and were asked thereafter to make a memory-based decision as to which city is larger (cf. Hastie and Park 1986). Monetary incentives for correct decisions were used to assure high motivation. Consistency was varied between decision tasks (see Figure 12.3). For participants that estimated the cue "first division soccer team" as the least valid one, consistency was lower in the decision task depicted on the left than in the decision task on the right. According to fast and frugal heuristics (i.e., Take the Best or the equal weight heuristic), decision times should not differ between the two decision tasks because the number of computational steps that are necessary to select an option does not differ between decision tasks. According to the PCS approach, in the decision task on the left, decision time should be higher and confidence judgments should be lower than in the decision task on the right. The PCS predictions could be supported empirically, and the findings could be replicated using different decision tasks, including online tasks and different materials.

To summarize, the predictions of the PCS approach are well supported empirically. Individuals are able to integrate quickly multitudinous information in a weighted compensatory manner and even seem to use this as a default strategy. The interpretation of information is changed in the decision process,

---

[2] This finding is robust and could be replicated in studies using the city-size decision tasks (Glöckner 2007), purchasing decisions based on probabilistic information and classic gambling tasks (Glöckner and Betsch, submitted).

	Wiesbaden	Freiburg
State Capital	+	–
University	–	+
1st League Soccer	–	+

	Dresden	Leverkusen
State Capital	+	–
University	+	–
1st League Soccer	–	+

Figure 12.3 Decision tasks with less consistency (left-hand side) and more consistency (right-hand side).

and decision times and confidence judgments are systematically influenced by the level of consistency in decision tasks.[3]

What about Bounded Rationality?

Obviously, these findings conflict with the bounded rationality approach and, more specifically, with the adaptive toolbox model. Could the reported findings be explained by the fact that decision tasks induced the usage of decision strategies other than fast and frugal heuristics? Could the PCS approach be understood as just another tool in the adaptive toolbox? To address these questions, it is worthwhile to recapitulate the three fundamental premises of the adaptive toolbox approach (Gigerenzer 2001).

First, the research approach proposed by Gigerenzer and colleagues aims to "understand how actual humans (or ants, bees, chimpanzees, etc.) make decisions, as opposed to heavenly beings equipped with practically unlimited time, knowledge, memory, and other infinite resources" (Gigerenzer 2001, p. 38). Decisions rules should be *psychologically plausible* (i.e., they should be based on the actual cognitive repertoire of a species), since they rely on simple search as well as stopping and decision rules. In light of the PCS findings reported above, the adaptive toolbox underestimates the human ability for information integration. As postulated by the PCS approach and demonstrated by empirical evidence, parallel automatic processes that allow multitudinous information to be quickly integrated in a complex way are a part of humans' cognitive repertoire. Consequently, PCS processes seem to be psychologically plausible without relying on simple search and stopping and decision rules. In contrast to the prevailing view, as soon as automatic processes are considered, the mathematical complexity of the algorithm leading to a decision (i.e., the number of elementary information processes; Payne et al. 1988) fails to provide a valid measure of the effort to solve a decision task. According to the findings reported above (Glöckner 2006), people are able to make decisions

---

[3] It should be noted that the PCS approach can be understood as a generalization of the most prominent model for jury decision making: the story-telling model (Pennington and Hastie 1992). That model is empirically well supported, and part of the evidence (cf. Hastie and Wittenbrink 2006; Hastie this volume) lends additional support to the PCS approach.

based on complex algorithms almost instantly that would otherwise take computers several seconds to compute.

Second, the "adaptive toolbox offers a collection of heuristics that are specialized rather than domain general as would be the case in subjective expected utility (SEU)" (Gigerenzer 2001, p. 38). Thus, Gigerenzer argues that the structure of the domain induces the application of different decision algorithms. Although the evidence does not yet allow for final conclusions, the findings reported above indicate that PCS processes are rather general because they are automatically initiated as soon as a decision task is perceived. Individuals are not aware of them and often cannot avoid them. The PCS mechanism itself is always the same, but the structure of the temporarily activated network is adapted to the specific decision task; that is, it reflects the subjective perception of the specific content, learning experiences, and general knowledge.

Third, according to the adaptive toolbox, the structure of the environment has to be taken into account when exploring the efficiency of decision strategies. Heuristics are claimed to be successful because they are domain specific; that is, they adapt to the structure of the environment. In comprehensive simulations of real-world data, it has been shown that there are domains in which fast and frugal heuristics lead to very accurate decisions (e.g., in city-size decision tasks: Gigerenzer and Goldstein 1996). Thus, the domains used in the PCS experiments reported above have to be closely investigated before premature conclusions are drawn. However, a predominant usage of compensatory strategies was observed precisely in the city-size domain. Why did participants not behave adaptively to the environment? Upon closer inspection of the simulation data reported in Gigerenzer and Goldstein (1996) one sees a possible answer: on average, the performance advantage of the Take the Best heuristic over weighted compensatory models in cross prediction was 3 percent. Although people have powerful mechanisms of frequency learning, it would take them far more than 100 learning trials with perfect feedback to learn this advantage. Real life does not usually provide such a perfect and highly repetitive learning environment. Consequently, it is rather unlikely that such a small difference will be learned.

Furthermore, when one abstracts from the process of information integration and considers only choices, one often overlooks that fast and frugal heuristics are always a special case of weighted compensatory decision strategies (Bergert and Nosofsky 2007; Lee and Cummins 2004). Fast and frugal heuristics (i.e., Take the Best and equal weight heuristic) can always be perfectly modeled through weighted compensatory strategies. Thus, for purely mathematical reasons, fast and frugal heuristics can never be better than weighted compensatory models at predicting choices, except when nonoptimal weights are used (as may be the case in cross prediction because of overfitting).

In summary, the materials used in the experiments make it very unlikely that the findings can be simply explained by the fact that the decision tasks hindered the application of fast and frugal heuristics and induced the usage of more complex strategies. Furthermore, the PCS approach cannot be seen as just another fast and frugal heuristic because it conflicts with basic premises of the adaptive toolbox approach: the PCS approach is not based on simple rules for information integration; it does not ignore the majority of information (i.e., it is not frugal); and it does not appear to be domain specific but is instead domain general. Below, I summarize ways in which the adaptive toolbox approach and the PCS approach can be integrated into a more general model.

Toward an Integrative Interactionist Approach

As argued above, the majority of decision-making models view the decision process as a simple unidirectional process: information required for the task is searched or retrieved and integrated to derive a decision. The underlying processes are often considered to be deliberate; some more recent models assume automatic processes. Most models consider either deliberate or automatic processes, but not the interaction between them. Based on the observation that patterns of information search differ systematically, models based on the bounded rationality approach, in particular, lead us to conclude that individuals have a set of decision strategies from which they can select, in contrast to just one universal decision strategy (see, however, Lee and Cummins 2004).

The PCS Rule and its Evolutionary Advantage

Based on the general PCS approach, Glöckner and Betsch (2008) suggest that the PCS rule be viewed as an alternative integrative model for decision making (Figure 12.4). They postulate that automatic PCS processes form the computational core of decision making and that deliberate processes merely supervise or modify the network on which these automatic processes act. A dual-level network architecture is assumed: in the primary network, evidence and options are weighed in their complex constellation; in the secondary network, if necessary, deliberate strategies are weighed that support consistency maximizing in the primary network and allow for quick adaptations.

The Primary Network

As soon as individuals are confronted with a decision task, automatic processes of information search and retrieval take place and lead to the construction of a temporarily activated network (cf. Figure 12.1). Within the network, PCS processes are initiated that serve to maximize consistency by changing the activation level of the contained elements. The architecture of the network provides the constraints under which the quest for consistency evolves. Thus, the final level of consistency is bounded by the network structure. If the level of consistency in the network (C) exceeds a certain threshold (θ), PCS processes are

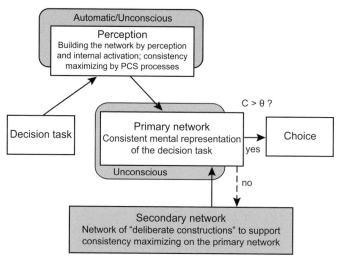

Figure 12.4 Schematic process model of the PCS rule.

terminated and the option with the highest activation is chosen. The network of options and information is referred to as the *primary network*.

Primary networks also capture the automatic processes of behavioral selection in animals, and should thus be considered the older part of decision-making processes in evolutionary terms. Parallel to processes of object perception, information is weighed in its complex constellation; the dominant interpretation is automatically detected and accentuated. This may explain the finding that even sticklebacks have the computational capacity to select mating partners by integrating trait information in a complex compensatory manner (Künzler and Bakker 2001; see also Glimcher et al. 2005). For human decision making, the operations of the primary network lead to the often described phenomenon of "intuition"; that is, which option should be selected is instantly "seen." No deliberation is necessary to reach this insight, and no deliberation appears necessary to validate it. The level of awareness of the resulting mental representation can, however, differ. In some cases, individuals are totally aware of the consistent mental representation and are able to explicate it. In others, only a vague feeling is perceived.

The Secondary Network

If the level of consistency C in the primary network is below the threshold, a secondary network is formed that is instrumental to the primary network. In the secondary network, deliberate strategies are weighed against each other to support consistency maximizing in the primary network. Glöckner and Betsch (2008) postulate that deliberate processes cannot directly influence automatic PCS processes; they can only modify the network on which PCS processes act.

For instance, deliberate processes may be used to include additional information in the network or to change its structure. These deliberate processes, which aim to modify the primary network, are referred to as *deliberate constructions*. They are also assumed to be weighed and selected based on PCS processes. The deliberate construction that is most activated is then implemented. It is reasonable to assume that, if repeatedly trained, deliberate constructions will become automatic (cf. Anderson and Lebiere 1998).

There are two main reasons for a low level of consistency. First, insufficient information is included in the network or the network is nearly empty. In this case, deliberate processes of information search and production are used to add information to the network. Second, the degree of contradiction in the network can be so high that it cannot be sufficiently resolved by PCS processes. To avoid a long period in which one is incapable of action, deliberate processes can temporarily modify the structure of the network or additionally activate or inhibit elements to increase consistency. This mechanism can also be used to simulate different interpretations of the data that could not be reached by mere automatic processes (cf. Bischof 1987; Hastie and Wittenbrink 2006). The reason for this may be that the PCS algorithm is caught in a local maximum of consistency, thereby overlooking a global maximum (Read et al. 1997).

In contrast to lower animals, humans have developed the ability to supervise and manipulate deliberately the powerful but inflexible automatic processes of the primary network (Betsch 2005). Glöckner and Betsch (2008) assume that the relations between elements in the primary network are determined mainly by slow learning processes. Thus, changes in these relations usually take a long time, and quick adaptations to environmental change are impossible (Betsch et al. 2001, 2004). The evolutionary advantage of the additional deliberate system is that it facilitates faster behavioral adaptations and allows for directed information search, qualified information production, and simulations to find the global maxima. However, without the automatic system, the deliberate system would be computationally overloaded on a chronic basis.

Integrating Fast and Frugal Heuristics and the PCS Rule

One of the essential findings of the adaptive toolbox research program is that individuals adapt their decision strategy and, in particular, their search for information to the environmental structure. Simply stated, if individuals receive repeated feedback that the usage of less valid cues is not useful in a certain environment, they will focus, after sufficient learning trials, on the most important cue (Bröder 2003; Rieskamp 2006; Rieskamp and Otto 2006). It is important to differentiate between two classes of situations: those in which information is instantly accessible and those in which it is not (Glöckner and Betsch, submitted). When it is not, which is predominantly the case in experimental research, the primary network is nearly empty at the onset, and consistency is low. Thus, the secondary network is formed to support processes that maximize consistency. Repeated feedback reinforces the deliberate construction "look up information for the most important cue only," and, after sufficient trials, individuals change from a default deliberate-construction strategy (e.g., "look up all information along options") to the alternative deliberate-construction strategy. From this point in time, the primary network consists only of the options and the information for the most important cue. Consequently, choice predictions align with that of the Take the Best heuristic. From such a perspective, the Take the Best heuristic (as well as other fast and frugal heuristics) can be understood as one of many deliberate-construction strategies that are possible elements of the secondary network. However, in each case the decision is based ultimately on the resulting activation in the primary network.

In situations in which information is accessible immediately, the primary network is instantly constructed. Individuals will make decisions based on the network. However, from repeated feedback, the structure of the environment will be learned. Thus, in a noncompensatory environment (i.e., an environment in which the most valid cue is stronger than all the remaining cues taken together), after sufficient learning trials, the dominance of the initial validity of the most valid cue will become more pronounced. As a result, its influence on the decision will decrease, although the lower valid cue information will not be ignored. Over time, this also leads to choices that align with the predictions of the Take the Best heuristic.

In summary, I suggest that the adaptive learning processes highlighted by the adaptive toolbox model are important in decision making; however, they should be integrated into the PCS rule: changes in the relations between elements in the primary network as well as the relations between specific deliberate constructions for certain decision tasks in the secondary network are learned from feedback. Further research will be needed to differentiate and test this hypothesis empirically.

The PCS Rule and Institutions

Work on the PCS rule is still in its early stages, and I wish to emphasize that the model must be further specified and empirically tested. However, it provides a fruitful starting point for rethinking issues relevant to the development and design of institutions. Jointly considering cognitive processes and the structure of institutions facilitates learning from and for institutions (cf. Engel and Weber, submitted). We must assume that institutions are shaped similarly to humans by evolutionary forces and learning mechanisms to optimize their structure over time (Hodgson 1988). If the PCS rule is a valid model, indirect evidence in support of it can be derived by investigating whether successful institutions align with its predictions. Some of the major hypotheses concerning the structure of efficient institutions, according to the PCS rule, are presented.

Predictions of the PCS Rule for the Design of Efficient Institutions

1. Individual decisions are good as long as the structure of the primary network represents the structure of the environment. Efficient institutions support the construction of representative primary networks.

2. The structure of the primary network is influenced by unconscious motivational and emotional factors. Institutions have been developed to reduce the influence of these factors as well as to increase the objectivity of the network.

3. PCS mechanisms artificially increase the consistency of information by eliminating contrary information, which naturally leads to overconfidence. Efficient institutions reduce overconfidence by forcing individuals or groups to consider alternative interpretations.

4. Decision making in diverse groups is problematic because members can form different but fairly stable interpretations of the situation. PCS processes increase divergences in the interpretation of information, which makes them more resistant to change. Institutions have been established to ensure that groups nevertheless reach decisions in time without disintegrating.

5. Decisions based on automatic PCS processes are hard to communicate and justify, because parts of the mental representation of the decision might be unconscious. Institutions provide rules that make decisions easier to communicate and which facilitate an increase in the level of acceptance of the decision.

6. Institutions increase the consistency of decisions over time by providing a set of explicit rules for deliberate constructions (secondary network). As a result, certain important information is always included in the primary network; this stabilizes the general structure, which in turn increases consistency over time.

7. Efficient institutions accommodate and utilize PCS processes. The structure of the environment should be analyzed, and decision makers should be provided with the results. These results can facilitate the construction of more adequate mental representations. However, it is not necessary to provide decision makers with overly simple decision rules because they can manage complexity.

8. PCS processes enhance the efficiency of social interaction in organizations. If institutions ensure that the fundamental goals of the organizations are always included in the primary network, individual decisions will be automatically aligned to the organizational goals, thus eliminating the necessity of specifying a complete set of behavioral rules for all situations.

9. Effective institutions make use of the error detection capabilities of PCS processes and leave room for exploring feelings of mismatch. The conscious part of the mental representation does not equate to the whole representation and might overlook important facts that exert unconsciously an influence.

10. Efficient institutions make use of trained expert decision makers. Expert decision makers are able to manage larger informational networks than lay people. Expert decision makers learn to include automatically a large set of important elements in the network.

11. Efficient institutions establish revision units that (a) test the decision-making process to ensure that all relevant information has been included and (b) provide learning feedback for deliberate constructions as well as for the structure of the primary network.

The German Legal System and the PCS Rule

Successful institutions can be used to test the predictions of the PCS rule. It is my assumption that such institutions have already implemented part of the mechanisms prescribed by the PCS rule, through the process of institutional evolution and learning. Using the German legal system, let us proceed to examine the predictions of the PCS rule for institutions.

Construction of Representative Primary Networks

One of the aims of modern legal systems (e.g. current systems in Anglo-American countries and Germany) is that in decisions, all relevant evidence should be taken into account according to its level of importance (for a discussion of different models, see Jackson 1996). One specific example for this principle in German law is that the German Federal Supreme Court prohibits explicitly the application of simple, schematic rules (i.e., heuristics) in expert assessments of the trustworthiness of eyewitness reports (Decision of the Federal Supreme Court [BGH] July, 30 1999, Az.1 StR 618/98). In line with the predictions 1, 6, and 7, this court decision specifies a set of valid cues (*Realkennzeichen*) which must be considered during the assessment. With this prescription, the institution ensures that these cues are included in the primary network and supports the construction of representative primary networks by the judge. On a more general level, the principle of exhaustive consideration of relevant evidence is a fundamental requirement imposed by the German code of criminal procedure (Schoreit 2003; StPO §261). This code also obligates judges to take into account not only the formal evidence of the case, but also the holistic impressions and insights that arise during the trial (*Gesamteindruck der Hauptverhandlung*; Schoreit 2003).

*Ensuring Objectivity and the Requirement to
Consider Alternative Interpretations*

Another basic aim of modern legal systems is that decisions should be reached objectively. This can be supported through a process of considering alternate interpretations (cf. predictions 2 and 3), which reduces subjective biases in judgments of the evidence caused by coherence shifts (D. Simon (2004). The different roles of prosecutors and defenders are designed to ensure that all relevant information is available in the primary network and that different interpretations can be considered. This availability allows a neutral judge to weigh interpretations against each other, in order to reach a global rather than local maximum of consistency. Likewise, the German code of criminal procedure obligates judges to consider all plausible alternative assessments (or interpretations) of the evidence (Schoreit 2003). Consideration of evidence is invalid if only one of various equally plausible interpretations is taken into account (Schoreit 2003).

Decision Rules in Multiple-judge Courts

Legal institutions have implemented voting rules to enable decision making even if different stable interpretations of the case have been formed by judges in multiple-judge courts (cf. prediction 4). It is not always necessary to convince all judges to agree on one interpretation; majority rules are often applied. This is the case, for example, with the German Federal Constitutional Court. Furthermore, decisions of this court are used as a basis in further legal argumentations (cf. prediction 5).

Installing Revision Units

In the German legal system, appellate courts function as revision units. The German code of criminal procedure requires that decisions be revised if they are found invalid as a result of procedural violations. An example of this would be if it can be proved that relevant aspects or alternative interpretations of the evidence were not considered in the first procedure (Schoreit 2003; cf. predictions 1 and 11).

Use of Expert Decision Makers

Taking a somewhat broader perspective, German legal doctrine can be interpreted as providing a large set of features that have to be regarded as a complex constellation in legal cases. When thinking about a case, experienced lawyers (because of their training) automatically and unconsciously include many (or hopefully all) of the relevant aspects in their primary network, whereas law students use deliberate-construction strategies to include them in a sequential manner (cf. predictions 8 and 10). Furthermore, within defined parameters, German law allows judges to exercise leeway in their judgment, thus allowing them to act on their impressions, which result from automatic PCS processes (cf. prediction 9).

In summary, supporting evidence for the PCS rule can be found when analyzing the German legal system. Many of the predictions for efficient institutions have already been implemented. However, a systematic investigation is needed to strengthen this argument and to inspire a purpose-driven improvement of the institution of German law as well as of other institutions, if necessary.

Conclusions and Outlook

The PCS rule is a complex model, which presently should be considered a work in progress. To strengthen the model, the secondary network will need to be specified further and empirical tests will need to be performed on the inter-action between the networks. Nevertheless, evidence already supports clearly the central claim: individuals are capable of quickly integrating a great deal of information in decision making. Based on this finding, some recommendations for institutions that have been derived from the bounded rationality approach should be reconsidered; others are highlighted even more. As argued by Giger-enzer (2001), it is very important to understand the environmental structure of decision tasks in order to enhance the quality of decisions. However, according to the PCS rule, institutions should try to support individuals to construct more adequate mental representations of the decision task (cf. Gigerenzer and Hof-frage 1995). In some decisions, this might be accomplished by instructing in-dividuals to include only the most valid information in the network; however, in complex decision tasks, this will not likely be the case.

Can the PCS Rule Account for Biases in Decision Making?

By taking a positive perspective in this chapter, my intent was to call attention to the astonishingly rich human cognitive capabilities for decision making (cf. Engel this volume). This stands in contrast to the more prominent views that individuals are poor decision makers who often show biases in decision mak-ing (Kahneman et al. 1982) or that the cognitive capacity of humans is severely limited but adaptive selection of simplifying strategies nevertheless leads to good decisions (Gigerenzer, Todd et al. 1999). Glöckner and Betsch (2008) propose the PCS rule as a descriptive model for decision making; it should also be able to predict when decisions go astray. Thus, it should be able to account for the multitude of evidence showing deviations from rationality in decisions and, in fact, it is able to do so. According to the PCS rule, all deviations from optimal decisions are essentially caused by the fact that the mental representa-tion of the decision task (i.e., the primary network) represents the real structure of the decision task inaccurately. Thus, in contrast to the heuristics and biases program (Kahneman et al. 1982), the PCS rule does not assume that different heuristics lead to certain biases but that one single mechanism accounts for all of them. Systematic misperceptions can be caused by all of the factors that have been repeatedly discussed in the literature, such as framing, anchoring, salience, status quo, mental accounting (for an overview, see Baron 2000).

More research will be needed for a systematic empirical investigation of the influence of these factors on mental representations.

How Does the PCS Rule Connect to Neuroscience Research?

In addition to investigating the PCS rule from a psychological and an institutional perspective, it is necessary to connect the model to recent research in neuroscience. The PCS rule is based on a connectionist network and is at a medium level of abstraction. It opens the opportunity to connect findings and models on the neuronal level with findings and models on the behavioral level. Until now, empirical research on the PCS rule has focused entirely on the behavioral level. However, the PCS rule bears a high resemblance to nonlinear neuroscientific models as advocated by Singer (2003). I argue that the proposed processes of synchronization and binding describe the nonlinear integration processes of the PCS rule on the neuronal implementation level. From such a perspective, the PCS rule is a model that reduces the complexity of neuronal implementations but retains the basic underlying mechanism and allows for deriving testable predictions for human decisions in complex decision tasks.[4]

The PCS model also shares some structural similarities with the global neuronal workspace model proposed by Dehaene et al. (2006), which has been successfully used to integrate a wide range of neuroscience findings concerning conscious, preconscious, and subliminal processing. An important difference between both models that should be addressed in future research concerns the question of whether a single network or a hierarchical two-level network model is more appropriate for representing complex decision tasks.

The close relation of the PCS rule to models of perception might allow a comparison of patterns of activation using neuroimaging techniques, taking into account recent neuroscientific findings on perception and perceptual decision making (Heekeren et al. 2004; Summerfield et al. 2006).

Is Decision Making Based on Linear or Nonlinear Information Integration?

In behavioral decision research as well as in neuroscience, there has been much debate as to whether information integration in perception and decision making is based on a linear aggregation of evidence or on a nonlinear integration process. Gold and Shadlen (2007; see also Shadlen et al. this volume) report findings that support linear evidence accumulation models, which have been also proposed in behavioral decision research (Busemeyer and Townsend 1993;

---

[4] Wagar and Thagard (2004) suggest a subsymbolic network that more closely resembles neurons than the PCS rule does and which aims to copy relevant areas in the brain. However, I argue that the symbolic representations used in the PCS rule (in contrast to the subsymbolic ones used by Wagar and Thagard 2004) are sufficient to capture the major mechanisms of decision making.

Ratcliff et al. 1999). In this chapter, I have summarized behavioral findings in support of the nonlinear PCS rule that are coherent with neuroscientific models of synchronization and binding (Singer 2003). Although these findings cannot be easily explained by linear models, the debate between approaches can be expected to continue. However, I would like to highlight two very general points. First, mathematically, linear models are partial models of nonlinear models. Thus, nonlinear models can usually account for all findings of linear models, but not the other way around. Second, it is not possible to differentiate between linear and nonlinear models in simple decision tasks (which are, for practical reasons, commonly used in neuroscience research on apes) because in such tasks, the predictions of both classes of models converge. A differentiation is only possible in complex decision tasks that allow for nonlinear effects.

Evolution, Cognitive Limitations, and the Bounded Rationality Perspective on Decision Making

Evolution has equipped animals and human beings with powerful automatic mechanisms to integrate large amounts of information. According to the PCS rule, humans have developed the additional ability of being able to supervise and manipulate deliberately the primary network. Although the deliberate processes are rather limited in their computational capacity, they allow for better and faster adaptations by providing further information and temporarily changing the network so as to find quickly a consistent solution and a global maximum of consistency.

The title of this paper was intentionally provocative in promising to explain how evolution "outwits" bounded rationality. It refers to *bounded rationality* in two respects: first, in the narrow sense as limits in capacity for cognitive reasoning; second, in a broader sense as a prominent school of thought in decision research. With the PCS rule, Betsch and I have proposed a decision-making model based on the assumption that decision-making mechanisms have developed phylogenetically from perceptual processes. The model breaks with the assumption that decision making is mainly driven by deliberate reasoning and is sometimes influenced by automatic/unconscious processes or that there are two systems for decision making between which people can switch. In contrast, it postulates that the core processes of decision making are automatic processes that resemble processes of perception. In phylogenesis, these processes have been supplemented by deliberate processes that provided further evolutionary advantages.

With respect to the narrow meaning of bounded rationality, nobody would seriously doubt that there are limits to cognitive capacity. However, I argue that humans have developed capabilities to use automatic and deliberate processes efficiently so that their cognitive capacity is sufficient to solve even highly complex real-world problems, such as legal and managerial decisions.

In this sense, evolution has found a way to shift the "bounds of rationality" dramatically. As for the meaning of bounded rationality as a school of thought in decision making, evolution appears to be way ahead of scientific endeavors: while decision researchers are still focusing on deliberate decision strategies and arguing about the boundaries of rationality, evolution has long taken care of the problem by endowing humans (and animals) with powerful computational capabilities. This chapter has attempted to catch up with the fascinating inventor called evolution as well as to direct our queries toward other long known but unfortunately sometimes forgotten possibilities:

> My first empirical proposition is that there is a complete lack of evidence that, in actual choice situations of any complexity, these [expected utility] computations can be, or are in fact, performed...but we cannot, of course, rule out the possibility that the unconscious is a better decision maker than the conscious (H. A. Simon 1955, p. 104).

Acknowledgments

I am very grateful to Tilmann Betsch, Christoph Engel, Jeffrey Rachlinski, Gerd Gigerenzer, Jeffrey Stevens, Arthur Robson and Robert Kurzban for providing detailed advice on earlier drafts that helped to strengthen this manuscript. I thank Stefan Magen and Melanie Bitter for comments on the parts of the manuscript concerning the German legal system. Finally, I would like to thank Jörn Lüdemann, Stephan Tontrup, Indra Spiecker gen. Döhmann, Alexander Morell and Martin Beckenkamp for helpful discussions of the work.

References

Anderson, J. R., and C. Lebiere. 1998. The Atomic Components of Thought. Mahwah, NJ: Lawrence Erlbaum.
Bargh, J. A., and T. L. Chartrand. 1999. The unbearable automaticity of being. *Am. Psych.* **54**:462–479.
Baron, J. 2000. Thinking and Deciding. Cambridge, MA: Cambridge Univ. Press.
Bergert, F. B., and R. M. Nosofsky. 2007. A response-time approach to comparing generalized rational and take-the-best models of decision making. *J. Exp. Psychol.: Learn. Mem. Cogn.* **33**:107–129.
Betsch, T. 2005. Preference theory: An affect-based approach to recurrent decision making. In: The Routines of Decision Making, ed. T. Betsch and S. Haberstroh, pp. 39–66. Mahwah, NJ: Lawrence Erlbaum.
Betsch, T., S. Haberstroh, A. Glöckner, T. Haar, and K. Fiedler. 2001. The effects of routine strength on information acquisition and adaptation in recurrent decision making. *Org. Behav. Hum. Dec. Proc.* **84**:23–53.
Betsch, T., S. Haberstroh, B. Molter, and A. Glöckner. 2004. Oops-I did it again: When prior knowledge overrules intentions. *Org. Behav. Hum. Dec. Proc.* **93**:62–74.

Betsch, T., H. Plessner, C. Schwieren, and R. Gütig. 2001. I like it but I don't know why: A value-account approach to implicit attitude formation. *Pers. Soc. Psychol. Bull.* **27**:242–253.

Bischof, N. 1987. On the phylogenesis of human cognition. *Schweiz. Zeitschr. für Psychol.* **46**:77–90.

Brandstätter, E., G. Gigerenzer, and R. Hertwig. 2006. The priority heuristic: Making choices without trade-offs. *Psychol. Rev.* **113**:409–432.

Bröder, A. 2003. Decision making with the "adaptive toolbox": Influence of environmental structure, intelligence, and working memory load. *J. Exp. Psychol.: Learn. Mem. Cogn.* **29**:611–625.

Busemeyer, J. R., and J. T. Townsend. 1993. Decision field theory: A dynamic cognitive approach to decision making in an uncertain environment. *Psychol. Rev.* **100**:432–459.

Damasio, A. R. 1994. Descartes' Error: Emotion, Reason, and the Human Brain. New York: Avon Books.

Dehaene, S., J. P. Changeux, L. Naccache, J. Sackur, and C. Sergent. 2006. Conscious, preconscious, and subliminal processing: A testable taxonomy. *Trends Cogn. Sci.* **10**:204–211.

Devine, P. G. 1989. Stereotypes and prejudice: Their automatic and controlled components. *J. Pers. Soc. Psychol.* **56**:5–18.

Dougherty, M. R. P., C. F. Gettys, and E. E. Ogden. 1999. MINERVA-DM: A memory process model for judgments of likelihood. *Psychol. Rev.* **106**:180–209.

Gigerenzer, G. 2001. The adaptive toolbox. In: Bounded Rationality: The Adaptive Toolbox, ed. G. Gigerenzer and R. Selten, pp. 37–50. Cambridge, MA: MIT Press.

Gigerenzer, G. 2006. Heuristics. In: Heuristics and the Law, ed. G. Gigerenzer and C. Engel, pp. 17–44. Cambridge, MA: MIT Press.

Gigerenzer, G., and D. G. Goldstein. 1996. Reasoning the fast and frugal way: Models of bounded rationality. *Psychol. Rev.* **103**:650–669.

Gigerenzer, G., and U. Hoffrage. 1995. How to improve Bayesian reasoning without instruction: Frequency formats. *Psychol. Rev.* **102**:684–704.

Gigerenzer, G., U. Hoffrage, and H. Kleinbölting. 1991. Probabilistic mental models: A Brunswikian theory of confidence. *Psychol. Rev.* **98**: 506–528.

Gigerenzer, G., P. M. Todd, and the ABC Research Group. 1999. Simple Heuristics That Make Us Smart. New York: Oxford Univ. Press.

Glimcher, P. W., M. C. Dorris, and H. M. Bayer. 2005. Physiological utility theory and the neuroeconomics of choice. *Games Econ. Behav.* **52**:213–256.

Glöckner, A. 2006. Automatische Prozesse bei Entscheidungen. Hamburg: Kovac.

Glöckner, A. 2008. Does intuition beat fast and frugal heuristics? A systematic empirical analysis. In: Intuition in Judgment and Decision Making, ed. H. Plessner, C. Betsch, and T. Betsch, pp. 309–325. Mahwah, NJ: Lawrence Erlbaum.

Glöckner, A., and T. Betsch. 2008. Modelling option and strategy choices with connectionist networks: Towards an integrative model of automatic and deliberate decision making. *J. Judg. Dec. Mak.*, in press.

Gold, J. I., and M. N. Shadlen. 2007. The neural basis of decision making. *Ann. Rev. Neurosci.* **50**:535–574.

Hasher, L., and R. T. Zacks. 1984. Automatic processing of fundamental information: The case of frequency of occurrence. *Am. Psychol.* **12**:1372–1388.

Hastie, R., and B. Park. 1986. The relationship between memory and judgment depends on whether the judgment task is memory-based or on-line. *Psychol. Rev.* **93**:258–268.

Hastie, R., and B. Wittenbrink. 2006. Heuristics for applying laws to facts. In: Heuristics and the Law, ed. G. Gigerenzer and C. Engel, pp. 259–280. Cambridge, MA: MIT Press.

Heider, F. 1958. The Psychology of Interpersonal Relations. New York: Wiley.

Heekeren, H. R., S. Marrett, P. A. Bandettini, and L. G. Ungerleider. 2004. A general mechanism for perceptual decision making in the brain. *Nature* **431**:859–862.

Hodgson, G. M. 1988. Economics and Institutions: A Manifesto for a Modern Institutional Economics. Cambridge, UK: Polity Press.

Holyoak, K. J., and D. Simon. 1999. Bidirectional reasoning in decision making by constraint satisfaction. *J. Exp. Psychol.: Gen.* **128**: 3–31.

Holyoak, K. J., and P. Thagard. 1989. Analogical mapping by constraint satisfaction. *Cogn. Sci.* **13**:295–355.

Jackson, J. D. 1996. Analyzing the new evidence scholarship: Towards a new conception of the law of evidence. *Oxford J. Leg. Stud.* **16**:309–328.

Kahneman, D., and S. Frederick. 2002. Representativeness revisited: Attribute substitution in intuitive judgment. In: Heuristics and Biases: The Psychology of Intuitive Judgment, ed. T. Gilovich, D. Griffin, and D. Kahneman, pp. 49–81. New York: Cambridge Univ. Press.

Kahneman, D., P. Slovic, and A. Tversky, eds. 1982. Judgment under Uncertainty: Heuristics and Biases. Cambridge, MA: Cambridge Univ. Press.

Kahneman, D., and A. Tversky. 1979. Prospect theory: An analysis of decision under risk. *Econometrica* **47**:263–292.

Koffka, K. 1922. Perception: An introduction to the Gestalt-Theorie. *Psych. Bull.* **10**:531–585.

Kunda, Z., and P. Thagard. 1996. Forming impressions from stereotypes, traits, and behaviors: A parallel constraint satisfaction theory. *Psychol. Rev.* **103**:284–308.

Künzler, R., and C. M. Bakker. 2001. Female preferences for single and combined traits in computer animated stickleback males. *Behav. Ecol.* **12**:681–685.

Lee, M. D., and T. D. R. Cummins. 2004. Evidence accumulation in decision making: Unifying the "Take the Best" and the "rational" models. *Psychon. Bull. Rev.* **11**:343–352.

McClelland, J. L., and D. E. Rumelhart. 1981. An interactive model of context effects in letter perception. Part 1. An account of basic findings. *Psychol. Rev.* **88**:375–407.

Payne, J. W., J. R. Bettman, and E. J. Johnson. 1988. Adaptive strategy selection in decision making. *J. Exp. Psychol.: Learn. Mem. Cogn.* **14**:534–552.

Pennington, N., and R. Hastie. 1992. Explaining the evidence: Tests of the story model for juror decision making. *J. Pers. Soc. Psychol.* **62**:189–206.

Petty, R. E., and J. T. Cacioppo. 1986. The elaboration likelihood model of persuasion. *Adv. Exp. Soc. Psychol.* **19**:123–205.

Ratcliff, R., T. Van Zandt, and G. McKoon. 1999. Connectionist and diffusion models of reaction time. *Psychol. Rev.* **106**:261–300.

Read, S. J., and L. C. Miller. 1998. On the dynamic construction of meaning: An interactive activation and competition model of social perception. In: Connectionist Models of Social Reasoning and Social Behavior, ed. S. J. Read and L. C. Miller, pp. 27–70. Mahwah, NJ: Lawrence Erlbaum.

Read, S. J., E. J. Vanman, and L. C. Miller. 1997. Connectionism and Gestalt principles: (Re)Introducing cognitive dynamics to social psychology. *Pers. Soc. Psychol. Rev.* **1**:26–53.

Rieskamp, J. 2006. Perspectives of probabilistic inferences: Reinforcement learning and an adaptive network compared. *J. Exp. Psychol.: Learn. Mem. Cogn.* **32**:1355–1370.

Rieskamp, J., and P. E. Otto. 2006. SSL: A theory of how people learn to select strategies. *J. Exp. Psychol.: Gen.* **135**:207–236.

Schneider, W., and R. M. Shiffrin. 1977. Controlled and automatic human information processing: I. Detection, search, and attention. *Psychol. Rev.* **84**:1–66.

Schoreit, A. 2003. StPO § 261 / Freie Beweiswürdigung [Free judgment of the evidence]. In: Karlsruher Kommentar zur Strafprozessordnung und zum Gerichtsverfassungsgesetz mit Einführungsgesetz, ed. G. Pfeiffer. München: C. H. Beck.

Shultz, T. R., and M. R. Lepper. 1996. Cognitive dissonance reduction as constraint satisfaction. *Psychol. Rev.* **103**:219–240.

Simon, D. 2004. A third view of the black box: Cognitive coherence in legal decision making. *Univ. Chicago Law Rev.* **71**:511–586.

Simon, D., D. C. Krawczyk., and K. J. Holyoak. 2004. Construction of preferences by constraint satisfaction. *Psychol. Sci.* **15**:331–336.

Simon, H. A. 1955. A behavioral model of rational choice. *Qtly. J. Econ.* **69**:99–118.

Singer, W. 2003. Synchronizing, binding and expectancy. In: The Handbook of Brain Theory and Neuronal Networks, ed. M. A. Arbib, pp. 1136–1143. Cambridge, MA: MIT Press.

Slovic, P., M. Finucane, E. Peters, and D. G. McGregor. 2002. The affect heuristic. In: Heuristics and Biases: The Psychology of Intuitive Judgment, ed. T. Gilovich, D. Griffin, and D. Kahneman, pp. 397–420. New York: Cambridge Univ. Press.

Summerfield, C., T. Egner, M. Greene, E. Koechlin, J. Mangels et al. 2006. Predictive codes for forthcoming perception in the frontal cortex. *Science* **314**:1311–1314.

Thagard, P. 1989. Explanatory coherence. *Behav. Brain Sci.* **12**:435–467.

Thagard, P. 2003. Why wasn't O.J. convicted? Emotional coherence in legal inference. *Cogn. Emot.* **17**:361–383.

Thagard, P., and E. Millgram. 1995. Inference to the best plan: A coherence theory of decision. In: Goal-Driven Learning, ed. A. Ram and D. B. Leake, pp. 439–454. Cambridge, MA: MIT Press.

Wagar, B. M., and P. Thagard. 2004. Spiking Phineas Gage: A neurocomputational theory of cognitive–affective integration in decision making. *Psychol. Rev.* **111**:67–79.

Wegner, D. 1994. Ironic processes of mental control. *Psychol. Rev.* **101**:34–52.

13

The Evolutionary Biology of Decision Making

Jeffrey R. Stevens

Center for Adaptive Behavior and Cognition, Max Planck
Institute for Human Development, 14195 Berlin, Germany

Abstract

Evolutionary and psychological approaches to decision making remain largely separate endeavors. Each offers necessary techniques and perspectives which, when integrated, will aid the study of decision making in both humans and nonhuman animals. The evolutionary focus on selection pressures highlights the goals of decisions and the conditions under which different selection processes likely influence decision making. An evolutionary view also suggests that fully rational decision processes do not likely exist in nature. The psychological view proposes that cognition is hierarchically built on lower-level processes. Evolutionary approaches to decision making have not considered the cognitive building blocks necessary to implement decision strategies, thereby making most evolutionary models of behavior psychologically implausible. The synthesis of evolutionary and psychological constraints will generate more plausible models of decision making.

Introduction

A hungry female chimpanzee spies a termite mound and quickly fashions a branch into a long twig. She then uncovers a tunnel in the mound and inserts her twig. Soon, she extracts the twig, revealing a dozen wriggling termites clinging on tightly. The expert angler carefully plucks off and consumes each insect. As she repeats the process, she depletes the soldier termites arriving to defend their nest. When should she leave this hole to either excavate another tunnel or seek a new mound altogether? What cognitive process does she use to make this decision? What cognitive building blocks does she need to implement this process? Of the various processes possible, why does she use this one? This foraging situation raises these and numerous other questions for biologists and psychologists interested in decision making in both humans and nonhuman animals.

Tinbergen (1963) posited four levels of analysis for why a behavior exists: the phylogenetic, functional, developmental, and mechanistic levels. Evolutionary biologists focus primarily on why behavioral decisions exist from a functional perspective. For example, what benefit exists for leaving the termite hole now versus in ten minutes? Psychologists, by contrast, explore the mechanistic level, concentrating typically on cognitive mechanisms involved in decision making. For instance, what information does the chimpanzee use to decide when to leave, and how does she acquire this information? Regrettably, the functional and mechanistic studies of decision making have remained largely separate endeavors, with many behavioral biologists and psychologists reluctant to cross disciplinary boundaries. Yet, the emergence of cognitive ecology and evolutionary psychology as fields demonstrates a recent push to integrate behavioral function and mechanism across species (see, e.g., Barkow et al. 1992; Dukas 1998; Hammerstein and Hagen 2005; Kacelnik 2006). This integration should be taken seriously when models of cognitive mechanisms and evolutionary outcomes are constructed. Here, I propose ways in which an evolutionary analysis can aid psychologists and ways in which a psychological analysis can aid evolutionary biologists in studying human and nonhuman animal decision making.

Evolutionary theory offers well-developed models of how a process of selection influences a characteristic or trait over time. I begin by briefly reviewing an evolutionary approach of decision making. Then I explore different selection processes and how they can influence a decision mechanism. Considering the kinds of pressures acting on decisions can help evaluate the feasibility of their mechanisms. Psychologists often characterize the cognitive building blocks or psychological capacities (such as memory capacities, learning structures, and attentional abilities) required for higher-level behavior. Cognitive building blocks are often absent from evolutionary models of behavior, leaving the models unconstrained and incomplete. Combining selective pressures and cognitive building blocks will lead to more plausible evolutionary and psychological models of decision making.

Natural Selection and Decision Making

Natural selection is a process by which biological evolution occurs; it results when heritable variation in a trait has differential influences on fitness. We can define fitness as the expected number of descendents produced by an individual, usually measured as survival and reproduction. Individuals that produce more descendents in future generations have higher fitness. A heritable behavior that gives even a slight advantage in survival to one individual relative to others will propagate over evolutionary time, resulting in more genes for that advantageous behavior in the population. Thus, natural selection favors traits resulting in higher survival and reproduction. With a constant environment and enough genetic variation and time, this type of process results in organisms reaching fitness optima. Many biologists tend to focus on this end state and thereby consider natural selection an optimizing process. Inevitably, a process that favors an increase in fitness results in reaching an optimum, but natural selection as a process does not optimize globally to adapt organisms perfectly to their environments. Instead, natural selection "optimizes under constraints," and a number of factors can constrain the evolution of behavior. First, the fitness payoffs of a behavior must trade off both the benefits and the costs. For instance, a foraging rule that extends the time an animal stays in a patch of food might increase an individual's overall food intake, resulting in a fitness advantage over an individual with a shorter patch exploitation time. This rule, however, has consequences outside of the foraging domain that may balance (or exceed) the benefits of longer foraging times. For instance, foraging in a patch for longer time intervals may increase exposure to predators, potentially offsetting the benefits of higher food intake. Natural selection optimizes total net fitness across all domains of an organism's survival and reproduction, thereby constraining optimization in any single domain. Second, natural selection does not act as a designer, creating traits de novo. Rather, it acts as a tinkerer, building on previous traits and accumulating change. The evolutionary history of an organism sets the starting point and thereby constrains potential evolutionary trajectories (see McElreath et al., this volume). Thus, natural selection optimizes behavior given trade-offs with other behaviors and existing evolutionary building blocks.

Many behavioral biologists accept the assumption of natural selection as an optimizing (under constraints) process and use mathematical optimization techniques as a tool to predict end-state behavior given a set of environmental parameters. Numerous behavioral domains use optimization techniques, especially foraging theory (Stephens and Krebs 1986). The termite fishing example highlights one of the classic models of optimal foraging: the patch model. When in a patch of food, foragers receive a particular rate of gain; that is, a particular amount of food per unit time spent foraging. As the forager continues to consume food, the patch may deplete, thereby diminishing the returns to staying in the patch. Thus, foragers must decide when to leave and travel to a new patch versus stay and continue to deplete the current patch. Optimization theory predicts that in some circumstances foragers should leave a patch when the intake rate at that patch drops below the average intake rate at the remaining patches (Charnov 1976). This optimal policy suggests that longer travel times between patches should result in longer patch residence times. Experimental and field data qualitatively support predictions derived from the optimal policy, but the data do not necessarily provide a good quantitative fit. Including more realistic assumptions about the role of physiological state, predation risk, and alternative activities provides a better account of the data (Nonacs 2001).

Assuming that organisms make optimal decisions, what cognitive process do they use? Optimality theorists readily admit the infeasibility of animals using optimal decision processes to arrive at optimal outcomes: animals do not calculate a range of expected fitness consequences and apply calculus to find the optimum. Instead, optimality theorists suggest that natural selection acts as the optimizing selection process, generating decision processes that result in approximately optimal outcomes (Stephens and Krebs 1986; Smith and Winterhalder 1992; Houston and McNamara 1999). Therefore, animals that use decision processes or strategies approaching the optimum outcome transfer more genes to future generations. This focus on strategies is important because natural selection selects for decision processes not the behavior per se, since only the decision process is heritable.

An evolutionary perspective emphasizes three important components of a decision: the decision processes, outcomes, and selection processes. To understand how natural selection can act on decisions, we must first map out the components of the decision mechanism.

The Anatomy of a Decision

Decisions—broadly defined here as the results of an evaluation of possible options—can take a variety of forms, including both inferences and preferences. *Inferences* go beyond the information given to make predictions about the state of the world; for instance, knowing the color of a fruit, can a decision maker infer its ripeness and sugar content? In contrast, *preferences* rank the desirability of options; for instance, would a decision maker prefer to receive a small food item now or a large food item tomorrow? This distinction has not been widely acknowledged (cf. Gigerenzer and Todd 1999), yet it could have important implications for the evolution of decision making.

Figure 13.1 illustrates the primary components of a decision mechanism. This description of a decision is silent on whether each component acts at a conscious or subconscious level, and most of the components can act at either level. Many decisions begin with a goal or task, such as foraging for food. The decision mechanism then gathers and processes information to reach a decision, which may result in an action and a payoff outcome.

Information

A decision maker must first search for information about possible decision options, although some information may be readily available for processing. The search for information can occur at an internal or external level (Fiedler and Juslin 2006). Internal search often refers to searching through memory for relevant information about options, whereas external search refers to perceiving information in the physical and social environment. In our foraging example, the chimpanzee may retrieve internally from memory information on

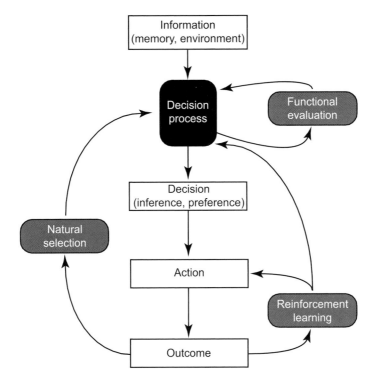

Figure 13.1 The decision mechanism and selection processes. The decision mechanism begins when information from either the internal or external environment feeds into the decision process. The decision process then generates a decision, which possibly leads to an action and outcome. Selection pressures such as natural selection, reinforcement learning, and functional evaluation can alter the decision mechanism by providing feedback about the realized or possible outcomes. Note that reinforcement learning can either influence action directly (learning a behavior) or can influence the decision process (learning a strategy).

the intake rates at other termite mounds and may track externally the gain and foraging time at the current mound when deciding when to leave.

Decision Process

In the decision process, a mechanism processes and integrates information to make a decision. Although other perspectives exist, I focus here on two general views of the decision-making process: unbounded rationality and bounded rationality.

Historically, many models of decision making have been based on the "economic man" perspective, in which decision makers can access all information relevant to a decision and arrive at optimal inferences via rules of logic and statistics (e.g., Bayes's rule, linear regression) or exhibit optimal preferences via rules of probability (e.g., expected utilities). An unboundedly rational decision maker uses all information available to arrive at the decision producing an optimal outcome. Proponents of unbounded rationality focus on the optimal outcomes and skirt claims about optimal processes by stating that agents behave "as if" they are rational. Nevertheless, any claims of unbounded rationality require that agents possess sophisticated mental inference or preference functions that, when supplied with all relevant information, output the optimal decision. Deviations from the norms of linear regression, Bayes's rule, or expected utility are considered normatively "irrational" (but not necessarily unsophisticated) behavior.

An alternative to the omniscience and unlimited computational power required of economic man is a perspective emphasizing a more realistic view of tools available to decision makers. The bounded rationality approach advocates a plausible notion of the capacities of and constraints on the mind, as well as the interaction of the mind and the decision-making environment (Simon 1956; Gigerenzer and Selten 2001). This bounded rationality approach implies a set of computationally simple heuristics that use only partial information to make good, robust decisions that apply to specific decision-making environments (Payne et al. 1993; Gigerenzer et al. 1999). Rather than having general-purpose statistical devices requiring extensive information and complicated computations, decision makers often succeed by using simple heuristics adapted specifically to their environment. The simple heuristics approach makes explicit predictions about the decision process, the outcomes, and the conditions under which heuristics will work.

Decisions, Actions, and Outcomes

The decision process, of course, results in a decision: either an inference or a preference. Though I distinguish between inferences and preferences as separate entities, they can interact such that inferences can feed into preference decisions and vice versa. However, as internal constructs, inference and preference decisions are invisible to selection pressures such as natural selection and reinforcement learning. A decision maker must translate a decision into action (even if the action is not to act) to experience external consequences (Rachlin 1989). A decision process that generates a decision not connected to an action cannot be selected for via natural selection or learning.

In summary, the decision mechanism inputs information from the internal and external environment into a decision process, which generates a decision. The decision maker chooses an action based on this decision and receives an outcome. Stopping here, however, raises the question: How do we know whether a decision is good or bad? An evolutionary analysis provides an answer.

Selection Criteria and Processes

To determine whether a decision is good or bad, a selection process must evaluate the outcome relative to some criterion. Hammond (2000, 2007) described two types of selection criteria: correspondence and coherence. *Correspondence* refers to the degree to which decisions achieve empirical accuracy; that is, whether they reflect the true state of the world. For instance, we can evaluate an inference about how fruit color relates to sugar content based on how well this inference corresponds with the true relationship between color and sugar content. Alternatively, *coherence* refers to following norms, usually rational norms such as Bayesian reasoning and expected utility theory. An inference about fruit color and sugar content cannot only correspond to the state of the world; it can also cohere to a Bayesian analysis of an individual's prior experience with color and sugar content.

Inferences and preferences differ in which types of criteria apply to them. Both criteria can apply to inferences: how accurately they correspond to the state of the world and how consistently they cohere to a norm (as demonstrated by the fruit color/sugar example). Preferences, however, have no correspondence criteria, since they simply reflect an internal ranking and therefore rely only on coherence criteria. When deciding between a smaller, sooner versus larger, later reward, for example, there is no "correct" choice based on the state of the world. Rather, the choice depends on the relevant norm: Are you maximizing expected utility or minimizing the time to your next reward? The lack of a universal criterion makes matching a decision to a coherence criterion quite difficult. Most studies of inference assess whether performance coheres to predictions of logical analysis. For example, in the Wason selection task (Figure 13.2; see also Schooler, this volume), most subjects violate logical analysis of the situation. However, the pattern of data fits the assumption that decision makers are maximizing information gain rather than following logic (Oaksford and Chater 1994). Additionally, when the situation is framed as a social contract rather than an abstract logic problem, subjects provide the logically correct solution much more often, possibly triggering an evolved cheater detection mechanism (Cosmides and Tooby 1992; Gigerenzer and Hug 1992). Given that multiple coherence criteria exist and different criteria seem to govern behavior in different contexts, it may prove difficult to predict a priori which coherence criterion is relevant to a particular decision.

Selection processes evaluate how well outcomes match the selective criteria, and different selection processes require different criteria. As one class of processes, Skinner (1981) proposed selection by consequences—processes which select or reject behaviors based on their realized outcomes. The selection-by-consequences view emphasizes that the process of selection works on previous consequences. In decision making, two selection processes clearly use selection by consequences (natural selection and reinforcement learning), whereas a third (functional evaluation) does not. This is not an exhaustive list

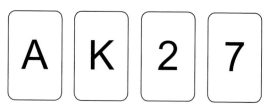

Figure 13.2   Wason selection task. Subjects must decide which of four cards to turn over to test the rule: if there is a vowel on one side, then there is an even number on the other. This is logically equivalent to the rule *if p, then q*. Most subjects choose A or A and 2. The logically correct solution is A and 7; that is, following the rules of logic, subjects should investigate *p* and *not-q*.

of selection processes for human or other animals, but it offers a starting point for exploring feedback mechanisms that shape decisions.

Natural Selection

Natural selection provides the ultimate example of selection by consequences. When an individual with specific inferences and preferences produces more offspring than other individuals, the genes influencing those inferences and preferences will proliferate in the population. Specifically, natural selection favors genes for decision processes that result in good decisions, actions, and outcomes from a fitness perspective. Note that with natural selection no direct pressure exists for accuracy or correspondence per se, just pressure to produce descendents. Accuracy is only valuable when tied to fitness. For instance, it makes no sense evolutionarily for a strict carnivore to make inferences about fruit color and sugar content, because it faces no fitness consequences for making the inference. Similarly, selection cannot act at the decision stage alone because without behavior, no differential fitness exists. Inferences and preferences without action have no consequences upon which selection can act. Even if an action is taken, selection does not act on the action itself because multiple decision processes can yield the same action. Natural selection can only act on heritable decision processes that generate actions and produce outcomes.

   The slow pace at which natural selection can track a changing environment means that genetically coding all decision mechanisms would leave organisms poorly adapted to their environment. Dawkins (1976) pointed out that our brains are not slaves to our genes; they allow us to process information and execute actions flexibly. Dawkins compared our genes to policy makers and our brains to executives. Stanovich (2004) described decisions under direct influence of genes as "short-leashed" and more flexible behavior controlled by brains rather than genes as "long-leashed." Natural selection has equipped decision makers with longer-leashed decision mechanisms by creating other selection processes that respond more flexibly to the environment: reinforcement learning and functional evaluation.

Reinforcement Learning

Learning, of course, does not require evolutionary time or the differential survival of individuals. Instead, over the lifetime of an individual (or potentially much shorter time periods), actions yielding good outcomes occur more often than actions yielding poor outcomes (Skinner 1938). Therefore, learning selects based on the coherence criteria of reinforcer maximization. Why then is one outcome more reinforcing than another? Because natural selection built learning mechanisms to allow flexible decision making, the value of reinforcement is tied directly to evolutionarily relevant commodities. More food, water, and sex, along with less pain, typically result in higher fitness, though not always. A mechanism exploiting this correlation will tend to serve the organism well; substituting reinforcer maximization as a proxy for fitness maximization allows a more flexible proximate mechanism to achieve a good evolutionary result.

Some types of learning differ from natural selection in the decision components used. For instance, in operant conditioning, a response is associated with a reinforcer; this maps onto the action and outcome components of Figure 13.1. Therefore, operant conditioning does not influence the decision process itself but simply the frequency of an action given its outcome. In contrast, Rieskamp and Otto (2006) suggested that reinforcement learning can also work at the level of the decision process or strategy. Decision makers can learn to implement different decision processes based on feedback from the outcomes received. Reinforcement learning can then adapt either actions or the decision process itself to the reinforcement contingencies in the environment.

Functional Evaluation

Natural selection favors appropriate decision processes over evolutionary time, and reinforcement learning selects behavior over the lifetime. Both processes select actions based on previously experienced outcomes. Perhaps natural selection has allowed even more flexibility in decision making by further lengthening the leash. Novel decision-making environments may arise, making hardwired rules obsolete and trial-and-error learning too costly or slow. Perhaps natural selection has generated a selection process that selects not on previous outcomes but on behavior to achieve a desired end state or goal. Using this selection process—here termed functional evaluation—a decision maker mentally evaluates the decision options available and chooses the one with the potential to maximize the relevant selection criterion. Instead of maximizing fitness or reinforcer value, functional evaluation assesses potential actions and outcomes relative to a decision goal.

Because functional evaluation considers the fit between outcomes and the selective criteria directly, selection is embedded completely within the decision process phase of the decision mechanism. Unlike natural selection and learning, functional evaluation selection occurs before making an action. Actions do not die out and are not reinforced, but can be entertained mentally and compared to the decision goal. Functional evaluation requires an internal representation of the coherence criteria, such as a mental utility function. Also, unlike natural selection and learning, there exists no single selective criterion for functional evaluation. Individuals can maximize utility, predictive accuracy, sampling opportunities, or many other criteria. There is no single criterion because decision makers face multiple decision goals simultaneously.

Functional evaluation should not be confused with a decision process. It does not refer to the conscious processing of information. In fact, functional evaluation can occur at either the conscious or subconscious level. It simply refers to the selection process in which outcomes are evaluated before they are experienced.

Optimal Processes and Outcomes

The "anatomical" classification of decision making emphasizes two processes at work: the selection process and the decision process. Recall that the selection process evaluates the outcomes with the correspondence or coherence criteria, whereas the decision process gathers and processes information to arrive at a decision. In natural selection, the selection process works directly on the decision process, which then generates the decision outcome. This hierarchy helps assess which (if any) aspects of decision making are optimal. I contend that an optimal selection process is required to create an optimal decision process, which is required to produce universally optimal outcomes. I define optimal outcomes as the best possible payoffs, optimal decision processes as processes that *always* produce optimal outcomes, and optimal selection processes as processes that *always* produce optimal decision processes.

As previously stated, natural selection is not an unboundedly optimal selection process, rather it optimizes under constraints. Because natural selection optimizes under constraints, it cannot produce universally optimal decision processes and therefore cannot yield optimal outcomes across all decision-making domains. It can nevertheless result in optimal outcomes for specific circumstances. To take an example from foraging, natural selection will not generate a mechanism that obtains all information about all possible foraging opportunities, trades the lost opportunity for other fitness-enhancing endeavors, and then calculates the optimal foraging choice. This would represent a universally optimal decision process that always yields the best fitness outcomes. Yet, a mechanism may evolve that can sample from two foraging patches and choose the one that yields the highest intake rate, resulting in an optimal outcome. The difference lies in the scale: optimality can evolve at small scales for particular circumstances but not at large scales across all domains. As Houston et al. (2007, p. 1532) explain: "We cannot expect natural selection, having no foresight, to shape organisms to act rationally in all circumstances, but only in those circumstances which it encounters in its natural setting."

The limitations of natural selection's optimization under constraints not only influence the decision process and outcomes, but also trickle down into the other selection processes. Because both reinforcement learning and functional evaluation selection mechanisms result from evolution by natural selection, they cannot be unboundedly optimal selection processes; no evolved selection or decision process can be unboundedly optimal. A selection process would have to emerge outside of natural selection to be truly optimal.

In summary, the selection process view makes two contributions to the study of decision making. First, it requires an analysis of the pressures that shape decision making. Natural selection, reinforcement learning, and functional evaluation influence the decision mechanism. Natural selection and reinforcement learning select decision processes or actions based on previous realized consequences, whereas functional evaluation selects decisions in the absence of direct feedback from an outcome.

Second, the selection perspective suggests that the constrained optimization of natural selection will limit the degree of optimality for evolved selection processes and decision processes. It seems implausible for a constrained optimization selection process to generate a universally optimal decision process following a rational norm. Instead, natural selection likely creates decision processes that increase fitness rather than cohere to the rules of logic and probability theory (Hammond 2007). Therefore, the frequent labeling of behaviors as "irrational," "anomalies," or "biases" assumes a particular perspective of rational norms. A broader, evolutionary perspective, however, cautions against using these labels, emphasizing instead an understanding of the decision goals, selection pressures, and decision-making environment.

The Evolution of the Decision Process

Given that natural selection cannot generate universally optimal decisions, what kinds of decision processes are feasible? As mentioned previously, many studies of decision making assume, at least implicitly, unbounded rationality and thereby imply an implausibly omniscient, temporally unconstrained, and computationally unlimited decision maker. There are, however, examples in which agents seem to make unboundedly rational decisions (Glimcher 2003; Glöckner, this volume). These decisions, however, occur in specific circumstances, and the generality of their application remains unexplored. Moreover, even if organisms possess the ability to use higher-order cognitive skills like optimal decision making, they do not necessarily do so when simpler abilities will suffice. For instance, cotton-top tamarins (*Saguinus oedipus*) use simpler, amount-based mechanisms when discriminating different quantities of food, even though they can use more sophisticated, number-based mechanisms in other situations (Stevens et al. 2007).

A more computationally and evolutionarily plausible perspective is the bounded rationality approach, which assumes that decision makers use simple heuristics and satisficing rules to make decisions with minimal information over short time periods (reviewed in Hutchinson and Gigerenzer 2005). Although many behavioral biologists ignore the process of decision making, they work under the assumption that animals do not use optimal decision processes. Instead, biologists often assume that animals use rules of thumb (heuristics) that approach optimal outcomes.

Evolving Simple Heuristics

The simple heuristics approach emphasizes the presence of rules for ordering information search, stopping search, and making a decision (Gigerenzer et al. 1999). These heuristics require little computation and use minimal information to make decisions. The rules of thumb approach in biology has coincidentally focused on the fast and frugal nature of rules of thumb without explicitly considering the search, stop, and decision rules of the heuristics.

Animals use rules of thumb in a number of important decision-making contexts, ranging from navigation to nest construction (Marsh 2002; Hutchinson and Gigerenzer 2005). Rules of thumb are particularly well studied in optimal foraging (Stephens and Krebs 1986), which may seem like a rather unlikely area for their application given the intense focus on optimization models. Biologists, however, distinguish between optimal outcomes and feasible mechanisms that can approach those outcomes.

Biologists have investigated the use of simple rules in the patch choice model of foraging described in the termite fishing example. Recall that in this scenario, foraging chimpanzees must decide when to leave a patch and move on to another. The optimal policy recommends leaving when the intake rate at the current patch equals the average intake rate for the remaining patches under this policy. Calculating or estimating this average intake rate in the environment (including travel times) is not computationally trivial. A number of researchers have proposed simple patch-leaving rules that avoid some of the complicated computations (reviewed in Stephens and Krebs 1986). For instance, rather than comparing the current intake rate to the average rate, animals may just leave a patch when the current intake rate drops below a critical threshold. Other simpler rules even dispense with the requirement of directly monitoring the current intake rate and instead estimate this rate indirectly. Animals using these rules may leave after consuming a certain number of prey items (fixed number rule), after a certain time period after arriving at a patch (fixed time rule), or after a certain time period of unsuccessful foraging (giving-up time rule). Empirical evidence suggests that different animal species use these various rules in different foraging situations (Stephens and Krebs 1986; van Alphen et al. 2003; Wajnberg et al. 2003).

The use of simple rules and heuristics by nonhuman animals is not terribly surprising. This perspective, however, has stimulated more controversy when applied to human decision making (see Todd and Gigerenzer 2000 and subsequent commentaries). Do humans use simple heuristics for important decisions? Gigerenzer and colleagues have argued that in certain environments heuristics can achieve good outcomes. Given that the human brain has been built by evolution through natural selection, we can infer that the costs of decision computations weigh heavily in the evolution of decision processes and that processes with simple decision rules tend to prevail over complex computations when yielding similar outcomes.

Evolving Satisficing Rules

When using another mechanism of bounded rationality—satisficing—decision makers search through options and select the first one that surpasses some threshold or aspiration level (Simon 1956). Economists and psychologists frequently investigate satisficing in decision making from the individual to the institutional level. Biologists, however, have not warmed to the concept of satisficing. Skepticism in biology derives from at least two sources (Stephens and Krebs 1986; Smith and Winterhalder 1992). First, satisficing theory provides no a priori justifications for how thresholds are set: What is "good enough"? Second, if natural selection is an optimizing process, then satisficing is not evolutionarily stable. An individual who optimizes and consistently exceeds another individual's decision threshold (e.g., makes better than "good enough" decisions) will have higher fitness, and this optimizing trait will spread relative to the satisficing trait. Stephens and Krebs (1986) suggested that if the effect of performance on fitness is a step function, a satisficing rule could evolve, but they argue that this rigid function is uncommon in nature. Instead, it is likely that fitness increases continuously with performance.

Despite skepticism towards satisficing, some biologists champion it as a reasonable decision process (Janetos and Cole 1981; Ward 1992), and recent theoretical investigations have modeled satisficing strategies in foraging and mate choice contexts (Todd and Miller 1999; Carmel and Ben-Haim 2005). In these cases, satisficing can produce nearly optimal outcomes with appropriate thresholds, depending on the costs of information acquisition and the level of environmental variation. Additionally, these satisficing mechanisms yield decisions that are more robust to uncertainty (Todd and Gigerenzer 2000; Carmel and Ben-Haim 2005), yielding better than "good enough" results.

Using limited information and simplified decision rules can produce optimal or near optimal outcomes, and thus heuristics and satisficing can offer plausible processes for decision making. These decision processes act independently of the selection process. Heuristics and satisficing can be genetically hardwired, subject directly to natural selection; they can be learned based on reinforcer value; or they can be functionally evaluated relative to a decision goal.

Evolving the Mechanisms for Decision Making

An evolutionary perspective can clarify the role of selection pressures and limit the set of plausible decision processes. Thus far, however, the evolutionary perspective has largely ignored the cognitive building blocks needed to implement decisions. For instance, the rational-actor approach in game theory assumes that all individuals have perfect knowledge of all other individuals' knowledge and beliefs, meaning that I know that you know that I know that you know and on and on. This implies that game theoretic decision making requires the cognitive building block of theory of mind (McCabe and Smith 2000; Hedden and Zhang 2002; McCabe and Singer, this volume), so decision makers can represent the knowledge and beliefs of other agents. The building block approach allows us to predict which types of decision makers utilize which types of decision processes: organisms lacking specific cognitive abilities cannot implement certain decision processes. My colleagues and I have explored this idea in the realm of animal cooperative interactions (Stevens and Hauser 2004; Stevens, Cushman et al. 2005).

A Case Study in Cooperation

One of the most-studied games in biology is the Prisoner's Dilemma (Figure 13.3), a game in which individuals can either cooperate or defect. Cooperation maximizes the total payoff to everyone involved in the interaction (mutual cooperation provides higher benefits than mutual defection); however, any individual receives higher personal payoffs by defecting, resulting in a sizable temptation to cheat. Unilateral cooperation is not evolutionarily stable in this game; therefore, cooperation is altruistic because cooperators pay a fitness cost by foregoing the temptation to cheat. The possibility of altruistic cooperation in the Prisoner's Dilemma intrigues biologists, because the presence of altruistic behavior violates the standard principles of natural selection. A defector will have a higher payoff than an altruist and therefore will contribute more genes to the next generation. Biologists have proposed a number of solutions to the Prisoner's Dilemma that may allow cooperation to exist, including kin selection, reciprocal altruism, punishment, and reputation formation (Dugatkin 1997). Reciprocal altruism, in which individuals pay a short-term cost of cooperation for the future benefit of a social partner's reciprocated cooperation (Trivers 1971), has probably gained the most attention. Axelrod and Hamilton (1981) investigated an evolutionary strategy for reciprocal altruism called Tit-for-Tat (TFT), in which a player begins by cooperating and copies the opponent's previous behavior. TFT can outperform pure defection when individuals repeatedly engage in a Prisoner's Dilemma with the same partners (although TFT is not evolutionarily stable; Selten and Hammerstein 1984; Boyd and Lorberbaum 1987). Therefore, a rule such as TFT can, in theory, maintain cooperation in the face of defection in the Prisoner's Dilemma. Yet, despite

	Cooperate	Defect
Cooperate	R	S
Defect	T	P

Figure 13.3   Prisoner's Dilemma payoff matrix. In the Prisoner's Dilemma, players must decide to cooperate or defect, and the payoffs are ranked such that $T > R > P > S$. Mutual cooperation pays more than mutual defection ($R > P$), but defection always pays more than cooperation for an individual ($T > R$ and $P > S$).

theoretical evidence supporting the viability of reciprocal altruism, it is not well supported by empirical evidence in animals (Clements and Stephens 1995; Noë and Hammerstein 1995; Pusey and Packer 1997; Hammerstein 2003).

Why is reciprocal altruism rare in animals when TFT is such a simple heuristic? Perhaps, despite numerous theoretical investigations of TFT, no models have included the cognitive building blocks required to implement reciprocal strategies (Hammerstein 2003; Stevens and Hauser 2004; Stevens, Cushman et al. 2005). When Trivers (1971) first introduced the concept of reciprocal altruism, he outlined necessary prerequisites, including one cognitive building block: the ability to detect cheaters (individual recognition). This single requirement does not likely capture the cognitive sophistication required for utilizing reciprocal strategies. In particular, the delay between the cost of a cooperative act and the benefit of reciprocated cooperation introduces a number of cognitive challenges. Minimally, this delay interacts with memory, inhibitory control, and impulsivity processes.

Memory

Limitations in memory decay, interference, and capacity can constrain the frequency of reciprocal altruism. Models of forgetting predict exponential or power functions (Wixted 2004) that decay rapidly over time. Therefore, longer time intervals between cooperative acts may make reciprocal altruism more difficult. Even with short time delays between cooperative interactions, previous memories can interfere with recall, and every potential new partner increases the computational load of tracking debts owed and favors given. Tracking reciprocal obligations with multiple individuals may place a computationally intensive burden on memory systems.

Inhibitory Control

Reciprocal interactions begin with an inhibitory problem: Can an individual inhibit the choice of the large benefit (the temptation to defect)? Animals often fail to inhibit their preferences for larger rewards. In the reversed-contingency task, subjects must reach toward the smaller of two visible rewards to receive the larger reward (Boysen and Berntson 1995). Numerous primate species tested in this paradigm failed repeatedly to learn the contingency, because they could not inhibit their response to choose the larger of two options: the inhibitory system appears to be too weak. Subjects can learn to solve this task, but the solution requires hundreds to thousands of trials, correction procedures, or symbolic representation of the quantities (Boysen et al. 1996; Silberberg and Fujita 1996; Murray et al. 2005). This strong preference for larger rewards suggests that choosing altruistic actions (those providing smaller benefits when a larger benefit is available) may also prove difficult. Therefore, strong inhibitory control capacities are required to implement reciprocal strategies.

Self-control

Reciprocal altruism not only requires choosing a smaller benefit but also waiting for the reciprocated benefit, thus, requiring self-control. In reality, however, animals behave quite impulsively. When given a choice between a smaller, immediate reward and a larger, delayed reward, animals show a strong preference for immediacy (Mazur 1987). For instance, when offered a choice between an immediate option and a delayed option, marmoset monkeys (*Callithrix jacchus*) refuse to wait more than 20 seconds for three times as much food (Stevens, Hallinan et al. 2005). Most other species tested so far show a similar lack of self-control, with the exception of the apes, which can wait for minutes instead of seconds (Rosati et al. 2007). This intense preference for immediacy suggests that animals cannot forego the instant benefits of defection in lieu of the delayed benefits from reciprocal cooperation. An operant experiment with blue jays (*Cyanocitta cristata*) demonstrated that some subjects cooperated in a Prisoner's Dilemma more often when they played an opponent using TFT and their impulsivity was experimentally reduced than when playing a defecting opponent or when impulsivity was not reduced (Stephens et al. 2002). Reciprocal altruism requires patience.

A simple heuristic like TFT may be easy for humans to implement, but it requires cognitive building blocks—such as high memory capacity, inhibitory control, and patience—beyond the abilities of many animal species. This perspective raises the question: Are cognitive building blocks constraints on the evolution of behavior or are they evolutionary adaptations tuned for specific decision contexts? For instance, researchers often refer to memory as a constraint, emphasizing memory capacities and loads. Psychologists have begun exploring the adaptive nature of memory, showing how memory processes may track the usefulness of information in the environment (Anderson and Schooler 1991 and Schooler, this volume). Yet, building blocks such as memory may be adaptive only in a specific context. It remains unclear under what conditions they constrain or facilitate higher-level decision making.

Conclusion

A truly integrative study of decision making must synthesize evolutionary and psychological approaches. Though the emerging fields of cognitive ecology and evolutionary psychology have begun this integration, much work remains. Considering the selective pressures on decisions refines which kinds of correspondence and coherence criteria are feasible for decisions. Natural selection does not favor coherence to rational norms, but increases fitness relative to others in the population. Considering selection also emphasizes that natural selection is a process of optimization under constraints. Because a constrained optimization process cannot generate a universally optimal process, unboundedly optimal decision mechanisms cannot exist in nature. Therefore, studying decision making with an eye on evolution can aid in understanding the goals of decision and thereby explain (or dispel) notions of irrational choice. Despite the advantages of accounting for natural selection in decision making, an entirely evolutionary, outcome-based approach overlooks the limitations that cognitive abilities impose on decision processes; certain cognitive building blocks must exist to implement decision processes. Many decisions can be made with a set of simple building blocks, whereas some require more sophisticated cognitive abilities. Thus, a complete understanding of decision making rests on the appropriate integration of ultimate goals and evolutionary pressures with the psychological mechanisms of choice.

Acknowledgments

I am especially grateful to Peter Carruthers, Gerd Gigerenzer, Peter Hammerstein, John Hutchinson, and David Stephens for comments on an early version of the chapter and for thought-provoking discussions about evolution and cognition.

References

Anderson, J. R., and L. J. Schooler. 1991. Reflections of the environment in memory. *Psychol. Sci.* **2**:396–408.

Axelrod, R., and W. D. Hamilton. 1981. The evolution of cooperation. *Science* **211**:1390–1396.

Barkow, J. H., L. Cosmides, and J. Tooby. 1992. The Adapted Mind: Evolutionary Psychology and the Generation of Culture. New York: Oxford Univ. Press.

Boyd, R., and J. P. Lorberbaum. 1987. No pure strategy is evolutionarily stable in the repeated Prisoner's Dilemma game. *Nature* **327**:58–59.

Boysen, S. T., and G. G. Berntson. 1995. Responses to quantity: Perceptual versus cognitive mechanisms in chimpanzees (*Pan troglodytes*). *J. Exp. Psych.: Anim. Behav.* **21**:82–86.

Boysen, S. T., G. G. Berntson, M. B. Hannan, and J. T. Cacioppo. 1996. Quantity-based interference and symbolic representations in chimpanzees (*Pan troglodytes*). *J. Exp. Psych.: Anim. Behav.* **22**:76–86.

Carmel, Y., and Y. Ben-Haim. 2005. Info-gap robust-satisficing model of foraging behavior: Do foragers optimize or satisfice? *Am. Nat.* **166**:633–641.

Charnov, E. L. 1976. Optimal foraging: The marginal value theorem. *Theor. Pop. Biol.* **9**:129–136.

Clements, K. C., and D. W. Stephens. 1995. Testing models of non-kin cooperation: Mutualism and the Prisoner's Dilemma. *Anim. Behav.* **50**:527–535.

Cosmides, L., and J. Tooby. 1992. Cognitive adaptations for social exchange. In: The Adapted Mind: Evolutionary Psychology and the Generation of Culture, ed. J H. Barkow, L. Cosmides, and J. Tooby, pp. 163–228. Oxford: Oxford Univ. Press.

Dawkins, R. 1976. The Selfish Gene. Oxford: Oxford Univ. Press.

Dugatkin, L. A. 1997. Cooperation among Animals: An Evolutionary Perspective. New York: Oxford Univ. Press.

Dukas, R. 1998. Cognitive Ecology: The Evolutionary Ecology of Information Processing and Decision Making. Chicago: Univ. Chicago Press.

Fiedler, K., and P. Juslin. 2006. Taking the interface between mind and environment seriously. In: Information Sampling and Adaptive Cognition, ed. K. Fiedler and P. Juslin, pp. 3–29. Cambridge: Cambridge Univ. Press.

Gigerenzer, G., and K. Hug. 1992. Domain-specific reasoning: Social contracts, cheating, and perspective change. *Cognition* **43**:127–171.

Gigerenzer, G., and R. Selten. 2001. Bounded Rationality: The Adaptive Toolbox. Cambridge, MA: MIT Press.

Gigerenzer, G., and P. M. Todd. 1999. Fast and frugal heuristics: The adaptive toolbox. In: Simple Heuristics That Make Us Smart, ed. G. Gigerenzer, P. M. Todd, and the ABC Research Group, pp. 3–34. Oxford: Oxford Univ. Press.

Gigerenzer, G., P. M. Todd, and the ABC Research Group. 1999. Simple Heuristics That Make Us Smart. Oxford: Oxford Univ. Press.

Glimcher, P. W. 2003. Decisions, Uncertainty, and the Brain. Cambridge, MA: MIT Press.

Hammerstein, P. 2003. Why is reciprocity so rare in social animals? A protestant appeal. In: Genetic and Cultural Evolution of Cooperation, ed. P. Hammerstein, pp. 83–94. Cambridge, MA: MIT Press.

Hammerstein, P., and E. H. Hagen. 2005. The second wave of evolutionary economics in biology. *Trends Ecol. Evol.* **20**:604–609.

Hammond, K. R. 2000. Coherence and correspondence theories in judgment and decision making. In: Judgment and Decision Making: An Interdisciplinary Reader, ed. T. Connolly, H. R. Arkes, and K. R. Hammond, pp. 53–65. Cambridge: Cambridge Univ. Press.

Hammond, K. R. 2007. Beyond Rationality: The Search for Wisdom in a Troubled Time. Oxford: Oxford Univ Press.

Hedden, T., and J. Zhang. 2002. What do you think I think you think? Strategic reasoning in matrix games. *Cognition* **85**:1–36.

Houston, A. I., and J. M. McNamara. 1999. Models of Adaptive Behaviour: An Approach Based on State. Cambridge: Cambridge Univ. Press.

Houston, A. I., J. M. McNamara, and M. D. Steer. 2007. Do we expect natural selection to produce rational behaviour? *Phil. Trans. Roy. Soc. Lond. B* **362**:1531–1543.

Hutchinson, J. M. C., and G. Gigerenzer. 2005. Simple heuristics and rules of thumb: Where psychologists and behavioural biologists might meet. *Behav. Proc.* **69**:97–124.

Janetos, A. C., and B. J. Cole. 1981. Imperfectly optimal animals. *Behav. Ecol. Sociobiol.* **9**:203–209.

Kacelnik, A. 2006. Meanings of rationality. In: Rational Animals?, ed. S. Hurley and M. Nudds, pp. 87–106. Oxford: Oxford Univ. Press.

Marsh, B. 2002. Do animals use heuristics? *J. Bioecon.* **4**:49–56.

Mazur, J. E. 1987. An adjusting procedure for studying delayed reinforcement. In: Quantitative Analyses of Behavior: The Effect of Delay and of Intervening Events on Reinforcement Value, ed. M. L. Commons, J. E. Mazur, J. A. Nevin et al., pp. 55–73. Hillsdale, NJ: Lawrence Erlbaum.

McCabe, K. A., and V. L. Smith. 2000. A comparison of naive and sophisticated subject behavior with game theoretic predictions. *Proc. Natl. Acad. Sci.* **97**:3777–3781.

Murray, E. A., J. D. Kralik, and S. P. Wise. 2005. Learning to inhibit prepotent responses: Successful performance by rhesus macaques, *Macaca mulatta*, on the reversed-contingency task. *Anim. Behav.* **69**:991–998.

Noë, R., and P. Hammerstein. 1995. Biological markets. *Trends Ecol. Evol.* **10**:336–339.

Nonacs, P. 2001. State dependent behavior and the Marginal Value Theorem. *Behav. Ecol.* **12**:71–83.

Oaksford, M., and N. Chater. 1994. A rational analysis of the selection task as optimal data selection. *Psychol. Rev.* **101**:608–631.

Payne, J. W., J. R. Bettman, and E. J. Johnson. 1993. The Adaptive Decision Maker. Cambridge: Cambridge Univ. Press.

Pusey, A. E., and C. Packer. 1997. The ecology of relationships. In: Behavioural Ecology: An Evolutionary Approach, ed. J. R. Krebs and N. B. Davies, pp. 254–283. Oxford: Blackwell Science.

Rachlin, H. 1989. Judgment, Decision, and Choice: A Cognitive/Behavioral Synthesis. New York: W. H. Freeman.

Rieskamp, J., and P. E. Otto. 2006. SSL: A theory of how people learn to select strategies. *J. Exp. Psychol.: Gen.* **135**:207–236.

Rosati, A. G., J. R. Stevens, B. Hare, and M. D. Hauser. 2007. The evolutionary origins of human patience: Temporal preferences in chimpanzees, bonobos, and adult humans. *Curr. Biol.* **17**:1663–1668.

Selten, R., and P. Hammerstein. 1984. Gaps in Harley's argument on evolutionarily stable learning rules and in the logic of "tit for tat." *Behav. Brain Sci.* **7**:115–116.

Silberberg, A., and K. Fujita. 1996. Pointing at smaller food amounts in an analogue of Boysen and Berntson's (1995) procedure. *J. Exp. Anal. Behav.* **66**:143–147.

Simon, H. A. 1956. Rational choice and the structure of the environment. *Psychol. Rev.* **63**:129–138.

Skinner, B. F. 1938. The Behavior of Organisms: An Experimental Analysis. Englewood Cliffs, NJ: Prentice Hall.

Skinner, B. F. 1981. Selection by consequences. *Science* **213**:501–504.

Smith, E. A., and B. Winterhalder. 1992. Natural selection and decision making. In: Evolutionary Ecology and Human Behavior, ed. E. A. Smith and B. Winterhalder, pp. 25–60. New Brunswick, NJ: Transaction Press.

Stanovich, K. E. 2004. The Robot's Rebellion: Finding Meaning in the Age of Darwin. Chicago: Univ. Chicago Press.

Stephens, D. W., and J. R. Krebs. 1986. Foraging Theory. Princeton: Princeton Univ. Press.

Stephens, D. W., C. M. McLinn, and J. R. Stevens. 2002. Discounting and reciprocity in an iterated Prisoner's Dilemma. *Science* **298**:2216–2218.

Stevens, J. R., F. A. Cushman, and M. D. Hauser. 2005. Evolving the psychological mechanisms for cooperation. *Ann. Rev. Ecol. Evol. Syst.* **36**:499–518.

J. R. Stevens

Stevens, J. R., E. V. Hallinan, and M. D. Hauser. 2005. The ecology and evolution of patience in two New World monkeys. *Biol. Lett.* **1**:223–226.

Stevens, J. R., and M. D. Hauser. 2004. Why be nice? Psychological constraints on the evolution of cooperation. *Trends Cog. Sci.* **8**:60–65.

Stevens, J. R., J. N. Wood, and M. D. Hauser. 2007. When quantity trumps number: Discrimination experiments in cotton-top tamarins (*Saguinus oedipus*) and common marmosets (*Callithrix jacchus*). *Anim. Cog.* **10**:429–437.

Tinbergen, N. 1963. On aims and methods of ethology. *Z. Tierpsychol.* **20**:410–433.

Todd, P. M., and G. Gigerenzer. 2000. Précis of Simple Heuristics That Make Us Smart. *Behav. Brain Sci.* **23**:727–741.

Todd, P. M., and G. F. Miller. 1999. From pride and prejudice to persuasion: Satisficing in mate search. In: Simple Heuristics That Make Us Smart, ed. G. Gigerenzer, P. M. Todd, and the ABC Research Group, pp. 287–308. Oxford: Oxford Univ. Press.

Trivers, R. L. 1971. The evolution of reciprocal altruism. *Qtly. Rev. Biol.* **46**:35–57.

van Alphen, J. J. M., C. Bernstein, and G. Driessen. 2003. Information acquisition and time allocation in insect parasitoids. *Trends Ecol. Evol.* **18**:81–87.

Wajnberg, E., P. A. Gonsard, E. Tabone, C. Curty, N. Lezcano et al. 2003. A comparative analysis of patch-leaving decision rules in a parasitoid family. *J. Anim. Ecol.* **72**:618–626.

Ward, D. 1992. The role of satisficing in foraging theory. *Oikos* **63**:312–317.

Wixted, J. T. 2004. The psychology and neuroscience of forgetting. *Ann. Rev. Psych.* **55**:235–269.

14

Gene–Culture Coevolution and the Evolution of Social Institutions

Robert Boyd[1] and Peter J. Richerson[2]

[1]Department of Anthropology, University of California,
Los Angeles, CA 90064, U.S.A.
[2]Department of Environmental Science and Policy, University
of California, Davis, CA 95616, U.S.A.

Abstract

Social institutions are the laws, informal rules, and conventions that give durable structure to social interactions within a population. Such institutions are typically not designed consciously, are heritable at the population level, are frequently but not always
group beneficial, and are often symbolically marked. Conceptualizing social institutions
as one of multiple possible stable cultural equilibrium allows a straightforward explanation of their properties. The evolution of institutions is partly driven by both the deliberate and intuitive decisions of individuals and collectivities. The innate components of
human psychology coevolved in response to a culturally evolved, institutional environment and reflect a prosocial tendency of choices we make about institutional forms.

Introduction

The idea of social institutions has a long history in the social sciences and, accordingly, has been widely used in ways that only partially overlap. Sometimes
the term refers to ideal types, such as religion or the family. Other times, scholars use it to refer to particular organizations: General Motors or the University
of California. Still other times it is used to denote informal norms like Nuer
bride price rules or the ways that Genovese and Mahgrebi traders financed
long-distance trade in the Mediterranean.

Our intention here is not to make a proper scholarly review of the concept.
Instead, we adopt the definition offered by Samuel Bowles in his recent book,
Microeconomics, Behavior, Institutions, and Evolution (2004). According to

Bowles (2004, p. 47), "Institutions are the laws, informal rules, and conventions that give durable structure to social interactions in a population."

Human societies vary on a vast range of culturally transmitted attributes that affect how people behave. People in different populations may have diverse beliefs about the state of the world. Most Americans believe that disease is caused by tiny, invisible organisms, whereas people in some other cultures believe that disease is caused by the actions of malevolent neighbors. People's knowledge of technology can also vary between different populations. Californian agriculture of the 1980s was different from that in the 1880s because mechanical traction and more rapid transportation changed the economics of various crops. Peoples can also differ in their understanding of symbols, their norms about action, and many other concepts. From this long list, Bowles's definition of social institutions focuses on cultural variants that specify how people behave when they interact with others. This includes formal law, but also informal norms and conventions.

Institutions play a key role in shaping human behavior in all human societies. It is obvious that social institutions have played a fundamental role in regulating people's behavior in urbanized, state-level societies over the last few thousand years of human history. Explicit laws, systems of governance, and nongovernmental institutions (e.g., churches, firms, and universities) were central to their organization. However, social institutions also play a crucial role in even the simplest human society. Land tenure, marriage, food sharing, and governance are regulated by culturally transmitted rules. Some institutions in small-scale societies rival those of state-level societies in complexity. For example, among hunter gatherers living in northern and western Australia, marriage and identity were regulated by "eight section" systems so complex that they have baffled generations of anthropology students.

In this chapter, we sketch a theory of the evolution of social institutions. We begin by proposing several stylized facts about institutions which such a theory should explain. We then argue that a theory in which social institutions are conceptualized as alternative, stable equilibria of a cultural evolutionary process can account for these facts. Finally, we contend that the cultural evolution of social institutions over the last half a million years created novel social environments that led to the genetic evolution of new social adaptations in our species.

Institutions illustrate how the processes of cultural evolution economize on information and decision-making costs. In essence, cultural evolution leverages individual decision making by allowing individuals to acquire complex codes for behavior, mainly by the relatively cheap process of imitation. Of course, if everyone always imitated, cultural traditions could be made adaptive only by the painful process of natural selection. Culture is adaptive in certain kinds of variable environments because it can enlist human decision-making capacities as evolutionary forces that shape institutions and other traditions. Some human decisions are made using fast, low-cost, relatively automatic, and often unconscious heuristics. If past genetic or cultural evolution has shaped this sort of decision making to be adaptive on average, even weak, error-prone heuristics can act as forces that cumulatively build cultural adaptations when they are integrated over many individuals and appreciable spans of time.

Cultural evolution can also amortize slow, costly deliberate, conscious decisions over many individuals. In law, for example, legislators, lawyers, and judges expend much effort crafting legislation and interpreting it. To the extent that they are successful, the entire society benefits. Most of us do not need to participate in the costly process of legal decision making; we merely need to know something of the laws that apply to us. Indeed, to the extent that everyday mores and the formal law coevolve, individuals can acquire useful behaviors economically by quite unconsciously imitating the behavior they see around them. In this way, culture is analogous to habit formation in individuals. Variants that were invented by deliberate reasoning and carried to dominance by formal collective decision making may be acquired by subsequent generations through unreflective imitation.

Six Stylized Facts about Social Institutions

The social world is both complex and diverse. Any real social system is immensely complicated. Moreover, systems differ widely from place to place as well as throughout time. This means that the answer to any interesting question inevitably depends on a host of historical and contextual details. Our ability to make formal models of complex, diverse systems is extremely limited, and, as a result, many scholars from diverse disciplines often eschew formal models in favor of rich, contextualized accounts. Practitioners in economics and evolutionary biology, however, take a different approach: they build very simple formal models with the goal of explaining the general features of some phenomenon of interest, and leave the details of particular situations to less formal methods. Economists call the usually-but-not-always-true things that they seek to explain "stylized facts." Here are six stylized facts about human social institutions that we seek to explain:

1. *Social institutions are usually heritable at the population level*; that is, cultural information that causes particular institutions to have the form they do is transmitted through time within populations in such a way that the form of institutions is largely preserved through time. Institutions are not simply a product of the environment and technologies that characterize a particular group. Rather, their form is transmitted from one generation to the next.

   Two types of evidence support this claim. First, what we call "common garden experiments" occur when people from different cultural backgrounds move into the same environment. When these different people maintain their institutions, this provides evidence that the institutions are heritable at the population level. The movement of peoples over the last several hundred years provides numerous examples. For example, Sonya Salamon (1980) compared the farming institutions among Swedish and Yankee settlers of Illinois. The Swedes came to the United States in the middle of the 19th century with institutions governing the transfer of farms from one generation to the next within a family—a practice that differed markedly from that practiced by the Yankees. For example, among the Swedes, parents were expected to vacate the main house and move to a small cottage on the farm when the son took over working the farm, while Yankee parents remained in the house until their death. When Salamon studied the descendants of these people in the 1980s, these differences still existed.

The second kind of evidence is the existence of phylogenetic patterns. Cultural groups that are linguistically similar often have more similar institutions than groups that are more distantly related (Guglielmino et al. 1995; Jorgenson 1980; Mace and Holden 1999), even when one controls for economic or ecological variables. This data indicates that the form of institutions is transmitted in populations from one generation to the next in parallel to lexical and phonological variants that form the basis of genetic linguistic classification. Thus people are plausibly relying on the relatively cheap uptake of traditional institutions by imitation and teaching rather than engaging in the costly rehashing of their form every generation.

2. *Most social institutions are not consciously designed.* In modern societies, institutions like the systems of governance of firms are at least partially designed, or more often result from the competing design aims of multiple interests. However, many institutions, in fact probably most, are not consciously designed, but rather evolve as the result of a variety of evolutionary processes. The mental rules that structure the morpho-syntax of spoken language provide a good example. Grammatical devices begin as lexical items used, often metaphorically, to make some important distinction (e.g., when an action occurred). Then, unconscious choices cause these lexical items to become grammaticized, leading, for example, to a system of verb conjugation that expresses tense (Deutscher 2005). The same applies to many institutions. Even if people wished to operate and change institutions wholly on the basis of deliberate processes, the complexity of institutions would defeat them. Ellickson (1991) gives an interesting example of how informal institutions that apparently evolved in this piecemeal way coexist with the formal law in a modern society. Moreover, in most societies throughout human history, the size of the cultural group that shared an institutional form was much larger than the size of any political decision-making body that could design institutions.

3. *Many social institutions are complicated structures with multiple inter-acting attributes.* Lately, game theorists have taken an interest in social institutions (e.g., Young 1998), modeling them as equilibria of games in which more than one equilibrium is possible. There is much to recommend this approach. However, we wish to point out a possible confusion that needs to be avoided: arguments are often exemplified using very simple binary coordination games, such as the so-called Stag Hunt (e.g., Bowles 2004). Although such simple games may be adequate for didactic purposes, real social institutions, even in simple societies, are complicated structures with many interacting dimensions. A theory of social institutions should be able to explain how such complex institutions arise, how they are maintained, and why they have the properties that they do.

4. *Social institutions often benefit social groups.* Property rights create incentives and reduce transaction costs; legal institutions prevent predatory behavior, help resolve disputes, and maintain contractual relationships. Corporate institutions, like clans and firms, allow the maintenance of productive capital over generations. Marriage rules regulate reproduction, and inheritance systems reduce conflict over intergenerational transfers. The list is long, so long in fact, that sometimes the group functional nature of institutions has been taken as one of their essential features.

5. *Social institutions do not always benefit social groups.* It is easy to think of institutions that seem unlikely to be group beneficial. Take, for example, the Gebusi: a group living in the Fly River region of Papua New Guinea. The Gebusi practice witchcraft and believe that most deaths are due to malevolent magic. Accordingly, deaths are typically followed by an inquest to determine who performed the magic, and when divination methods point to a perpetrator, he is executed by the group. Ethnographer Bruce Knauft (1985) reports that this process was leading to the extinction of the Gebusi. The legalistic formality of the deliberative process by which this maladaptive institution was operated is impressive. On the other hand, the Gebusi seem entirely unaware that the best statistical predictor of witchcraft accusations is unmet obligations to provide marriage partners to other lineages. Although this is a particularly spectacular example, there are many others.

6. *Many social institutions are symbolically marked.* Corporate social institutions, such as clans and nations, are typically associated with symbolic traits that mark both the group and its members. Such markers are arbitrary symbols. The clan's totem, the land crab, could just as well have been a sea turtle, and the tricolor could have been yellow, red, and black. However, the symbols are as much parts of the institution as the more functional rules that regulate behavior. They are endowed with meaning and emotional salience. Such attributes stabilize groups through time but also tend to induce deliberate thinking about them.

The Evolution of Social Institutions

We have argued at length (Richerson and Boyd 2005) that population thinking provides the most natural way of modeling human cultural change and its consequences for cultural variation. Much evidence indicates that the differences between human groups are at least partly due to culturally transmitted beliefs and values. People acquire beliefs about the world, about right and wrong, and what things mean by teaching and imitation from the people with whom they interact. To explain why a group of people have the culturally transmitted beliefs that they do, we need to understand how everyday events cause some beliefs to spread and others to diminish. Some of these processes are psychological: beliefs that are more readily learned or remembered will tend to spread at the expense of those that are less readily learned or remembered. Others have to do with what happens to people with different beliefs: beliefs that lead to long life or high social status are likely to spread at the expense of beliefs that lead to early death or low social status.

The resulting theory, which is sometimes called the theory of gene–culture coevolution, resembles evolutionary game theory. Both theories keep track of the dynamics of the frequencies of different transmitted variants, and evolutionarily stable equilibria of the dynamic system are candidate long-term outcomes of the evolutionary process. The primary difference is that evolutionary game theory assumes that evolutionary dynamics are driven solely by some kind of payoff: fitness when applied to genetic evolution, and utility when applied to social evolution. If the main directional forces in cultural evolution are due to relatively domain-general psychological mechanisms, then gene–culture coevolution will be very similar. However, there is also evidence that cultural change is sometimes affected strongly by narrow, domain-specific psychological mechanisms. For example, Pascal Boyer (2006) has argued that certain kinds of ritual behavior are attractive and memorable because they activate those psychological mechanisms that evolved to protect people against serious risks (e.g., disease and predation).

Institutions Are Social Arrangements with Multiple Stable Equilibria

The six stylized facts about social institutions are consistent with the view that beliefs and values which give rise to a particular social institution constitute one of perhaps many possible evolutionarily stable equilibrium. We illustrate this idea with a very simple "toy" example. Suppose in a particular population there are two cultural variants governing beliefs about inheritance: equal partition among brothers and primogenitor, only the oldest brother inherits. To keep things simple, let us suppose that all families have exactly two sons and that the payoffs associated with each combination of beliefs within a family are:

		Younger son	
		Partition	Primogenitor
Older son	Partition	2, 2	0, 0
	Primogenitor	0, 0	5, 1

When brothers agree, they receive a higher payoff than when they disagree, because disputes are costly. This means that once either system becomes common, people with the more common belief achieve a higher payoff on average, and if the cultural evolution is driven by payoffs (e.g., because people imitate the successful), then both inheritance institutions will be evolutionarily stable.

This conceptualization explains immediately how commonly held social institutions can arise without any group deliberation. Individuals respond myopically to the incentives they experience and, as a result, institutions evolve. It also explains why institutions are heritable at the group level. For traits to be heritable at the group level, two things must be true: (a) there must be stable variation among groups and (b) when groups split, daughter groups must be more similar to each other and the parent. If institutions are multiple stable equilibria, variation among groups will be maintained as long as the rate at which people evolve locally is faster than the effect of mixing of ideas or people among groups. Similarly, cultural variants that are common in the parental group will remain common in the daughter groups.

This simple example leaves out much. First, as evolutionary psychologists have emphasized, humans are not domain-general payoff maximizers. We find it easier to learn and adopt some beliefs rather than others so that payoffs alone are not sufficient to predict outcomes. For example, there is much evidence that people have evolved psychological mechanisms that, under most circumstances, make them averse to mating with close relatives. It might be that brother–sister marriage would be a highly desirable mechanism for preserving property, but that this would not evolve because our evolved psychology makes such marriages unstable. Multiple equilibria might still exist in payoff terms, but the choice-based forces may make some equilibria difficult to achieve or maintain independent of the payoff structure of the game. Second, real institutions are complex structures involving many beliefs. The institution of primogenitor includes rules to apply if there are no sons or if there are illegitimate or adopted sons, to resolve disputes and distribute different kinds of property, to define the rights of the widow, to assess penalties, and so on. The complexity of real social institutions means that they cannot be understood as simple conventions. They evolve cumulatively. Thus, to explain real-world complex institutions, a vast range of different institutions must be evolutionarily stable. Fortunately, this is not much of a problem.

Repeated Interactions Allow a Vast Range of Stable Social Equilibrium

Moralistic punishment can stabilize a very wide range of behaviors. To understand this, consider the following simple example. Imagine a population subdivided into a number of groups. Cultural practices spread between groups because people migrate or ideas are adopted from neighboring groups. Two alternative culturally transmitted moral norms (norm x and norm y) exist in the population, norms that are enforced through moralistic punishment. These could be "must wear a business suit at work" and "must wear a dashiki to work," or "a person owes primary loyalty to their kin" and "a person owes primary loyalty to their group." In groups where one of the two norms is common, people who violate the norm are punished. Suppose that people's innate psychology causes them to be biased in favor of norm y, and therefore y will tend to spread, all other things being equal. Nonetheless, when norm x is sufficiently common, the effects of punishment overcome this bias and people tend to adopt norm x. In such groups, new immigrants whose beliefs differ from the majority (or people who have adopted "foreign" ideas) learn rapidly that their beliefs get them into trouble and thus adopt the prevailing norm. When more norm y believers arrive, they find themselves to be in the minority and learn the local norms rapidly, maintaining norm x despite the fact that it is not the norm that fits best with their evolved psychology.

This kind of mechanism works only when the adaptation occurs rapidly; it is not likely to be an important force in genetic evolution. Normally evolutionary biologists think of selection as being weak and, although there are many exceptions to this rule, it is a useful generalization. For example, if one genotype had a 5% selection advantage over the alternative genotype, this would be thought to be strong selection. Now suppose that a novel group-beneficial genotype has arisen and that it has become common in one local group, where it has a 5% advantage over the genotype that predominates in the population as a whole. For group selection to be important, the novel genotype must remain common long enough to spread by group selection, and this is only possible if the migration rate per generation is substantially less than 5%. Otherwise, the effects of migration will swamp the effects of natural selection. This, however, is not very much migration. The migration rate between neighboring primate groups is on the order of 25% per generation. Although migration rates are notoriously difficult to measure, migration rates are typically high among small local groups that suffer frequent extinction. Migration rates between larger groups are much lower, but so too will be the extinction rate.

Conformist Social Learning Can Also Stabilize Many Equilibria

A conformist bias can also maintain variation among groups. We argue that natural selection can favor a psychological propensity to imitate the common type (Richerson and Boyd 2005, chapter 4). This propensity is an evolutionary force that causes common variants to become more common and rare variants to become rarer. If this effect is strong compared to migration, then variation among groups can be maintained.

As before, think of a number of groups linked by migration. Now, however, assume that two memes affect religious beliefs: "believers" are convinced that moral people are rewarded after death and the wicked suffer horrible punishment for eternity, while "nonbelievers" do not believe in any afterlife. Because they fear the consequences, believers behave better than nonbelievers: more honestly, charitably, and selflessly. As a result, groups in which believers are common are more successful than groups in which nonbelievers are common. People's decision to adopt one cultural variant over the other is only weakly affected by content bias. People do seek comfort, pleasure, and leisure, and this tends to cause them to behave wickedly. However, a desire for comfort also causes thoughtful people to worry about spending an eternity buried in a burning tomb. Since people are uncertain about the existence of an afterlife, they are not strongly biased in favor of one cultural variant or the other. As a result, they are strongly influenced by the cultural variant that is common in their society. People who grow up surrounded by believers, choose to believe, whereas those who grow up among worldly atheists do not.

The difference between moralistic punishment and conformist learning is illustrated by the different answers to the question: Given that people have grown up in a devout Christian society, why do they believe in the tenets of the Christian faith? If cultural variation is maintained primarily through moralistic punishment, those who do not adopt Christian beliefs in a devout Christian society are punished by believers, and people who do not punish such heretics (e.g., by continuing to associate with them) are themselves punished. People adopt the prevalent belief because it yields the highest payoff in readily measurable currencies. If cultural variation is maintained largely by conformist transmission and similar cultural mechanisms, then young people adopt the tenets of Christianity as accurate descriptions of the world because such beliefs are widely held, fit with certain content-based biases, and are difficult for individuals to prove or disprove. (Of course, any mixture of the two effects is also possible; the answer is quantitative not qualitative.)

Conformist transmission can potentiate group selection only if it is strong compared to the opposing content biases, and this can occur only if individuals have difficulty deliberately evaluating the costs and benefits of alternative memes. In some cases this is not very difficult: should you cheat on your taxes or fake illness to avoid military service? The threat of punitive action may be sufficient to keep taxpayers and conscripts honest. However, there are also many beliefs whose effects are hard to judge. Will children turn out better if they are sternly disciplined or lovingly indulged? Is smoking marijuana harmful to one's health? Is academia a promising career option? These are difficult questions to answer, even with all of the information available to us today. For most people at most times and in most places, even more basic questions may be very difficult to answer: Does drinking dirty water cause disease? Can people affect the weather by appealing to the supernatural? The consequences of such difficult choices often have a profound effect on people's behavior and their welfare.

Heritable Variation between
Groups + Intergroup Conflict = Group Selection

With this background, we can now explain why social institutions are sometimes group beneficial. In the *Origin of Species*, Darwin famously argued that three conditions are necessary for adaptation by natural selection:

1. There must be a "struggle for existence" so that not all individuals survive and reproduce.
2. There must be variation so that some types are more likely to survive and reproduce than others.
3. The variation must be heritable so that the offspring of survivors resemble their parents.

Darwin usually focused on individuals, but the multilevel selection approach tells us that the same three postulates apply to *any* reproducing entity: molecules, genes, or cultural groups. Only the first two conditions are satisfied by most other kinds of animal groups. For example, vervet monkey groups compete with one another and groups vary in their ability to survive and grow. However, the causes of group-level variation in competitive ability are not heritable, so there is no cumulative adaptation.

Richard Sosis's (2000) study of the survival of religious communes in the U.S. shows how selection among institutions can give rise to the evolution of group beneficial ones. Sosis collected a sample of 200 communes formed during the 19th and 20th centuries. Of these, 88 were religious; the rest were based on secular ideologies (e.g., Fourierism or Owenism). Sosis excluded 20 Hutterite communities from his analysis. As is shown in Figure 14.1, communes based on religious ideology had a much higher survival rate than communes based on secular ideologies, which means that selection among communities acts to increase the frequency of religiously based institutions. At the onset, about half of the communes were religious; after 40 years, almost all of the communes still in existence are religious. Sosis's work suggests that religious communes survive because they have fewer conflicts and more commitment to group goals.

Group Beneficial Cultural Variants Can Spread
Because People Imitate Successful Neighbors

Competition between institutions is not the only mechanism that can lead to the spread of institutions based on group beneficial ideologies; the propensity

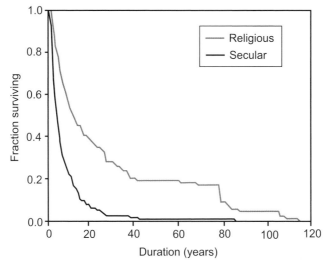

Figure 14.1   Proportion of communes surviving as a function of time since the founding of the commune. The black line traces the development of 112 secular communes and the gray line indicates 88 religious ones (from Sosis 2000).

to imitate the successful can also induce the spread of group beneficial variants. Up to this point, we have focused mainly on what people know about the behavior of members in their own group. Often, people also know something about the norms that regulate behavior in neighboring groups. For example, they know that in a particular firm, employees are discouraged from jumping the chain of command, but that among competitors, the hierarchy is much flatter. Now, suppose different norms are common in neighboring groups and that one set of norms causes people to be more successful. Both theoretical and empirical evidence (Henrich and Gil-White 2001) suggest that people have a strong tendency to imitate the successful. Consequently, behaviors can spread from groups at high payoff equilibria to neighboring groups at lower payoff equilibria because people imitate their more successful neighbors.

One might wonder if this mechanism can really work. It requires enough diffusion between groups so that group beneficial ideas can spread and, at the same time, there cannot be too much diffusion or the necessary variation between groups will not be maintained. Is this combination possible? To answer this question, we constructed a mathematical model of the process, and our results suggest that the process can lead to the spread of group beneficial beliefs over a wide range of conditions (Boyd and Richerson 2002). The model also suggests that such spread can be rapid. Roughly speaking, it takes about twice as long for a group beneficial trait to spread from one group to another as it does for an individually beneficial trait to spread within a group. This process is faster than intergroup competition because it depends on the rate at which individuals imitate new strategies, rather than the rate at which groups become extinct.

The rapid spread of Christianity in the Roman Empire may provide an example of this process. Between the death of Christ and the rule of Constantine, a period of about 260 years, the number of Christians increased from only a handful to somewhere between 6 and 30 million people (depending on whose estimate you accept). This sounds like a huge increase, but it turns out that this is equivalent to a 3–4% annual rate of increase, about the growth rate of the Mormon Church over the last century. According to the sociologist Rodney Stark (1997), many Romans converted to Christianity because they were attracted to what they saw as a better quality of life in the early Christian community. Pagan society had weak traditions of mutual aid, and the poor and sick often went without any help at all. In contrast, in the Christian community, norms of charity and mutual aid created "a miniature welfare state in an empire which for the most part lacked social services. Such mutual aid was particularly important during the several severe epidemics that struck the Roman Empire during the late Imperial period" (Johnson 1976, p. 75, quoted in Stark 1997). Unafflicted pagan Romans refused to help the sick or bury the dead. As a result, some cities devolved into anarchy. In Christian communities, strong norms of mutual aid produced solicitous care of the sick and reduced mortality. Demographic factors were as important as conversion in the growth of Christianity. Mutual aid led to substantially lower mortality rates during epidemics, and a norm against infanticide led to substantially higher fertility among Christianity.

Both mechanisms that lead to the spread of group beneficial beliefs are relatively slow: differential extinction because it depends on the relatively rare group extinctions, and differential diffusion because it depends on the transfer of beliefs among groups. The fact that these selective processes are slow is consistent with the fact that many institutions are not group beneficial. Moreover, social groups are complex and their welfare is affected by many different institutions, so that deleterious institutions may often hitchhike on more successful ones.

Rapid Cultural Adaptation Generates Symbolically Marked Corporate Institutions

Conceptualizing institutions as evolutionary equilibria also explains why corporate institutions are typically symbolically marked. One of the most striking features of human sociality is the symbolic marking of corporate groups. Examples include nations, ethnic groups, clans, guilds, and clubs. Some symbolic markers are seemingly arbitrary traits (e.g., distinctive styles of dress, emblems like flags) whereas others are complex ritual systems accompanied by elaborately rationalized ideologies. It is commonplace that social relations are regulated by norms embedded in a group's sanctified belief system. Even in simple hunting and gathering societies, symbolically marked groups are large. This phenomenon is diverse and impossible to define except in terms of ideal types. Ethnicity grades into class, nation, religion, firm, team, and all the myriad systems of symbolic marking humans use to make intuitive social decisions.

There is considerable evidence that symbolic marking is not simply a by-product of a similar cultural heritage. Children acquire many traits from the same adults, and if cultural boundaries were impermeable, something like species boundaries, this fact would then explain the association between symbolic markers and other traits. However, much evidence shows that ethnic identities are flexible and ethnic boundaries are porous. This argument applies with even more force to corporate groups, such as firms or churches, where membership is not primordial. The movement of people and ideas between groups exists everywhere and will tend to attenuate group differences. Thus, the persistence of differences between institutions requires that other social processes resist the homogenizing effects of migration and the strategic adoption of ethnic identities.

We think that the processes that maintain symbolically marked boundaries are the consequences of rapid cultural adaptation (Richerson and Boyd 2005). The first step in our line of reasoning is to see that symbolic marking is useful because it allows people to identify in-group members. There are two reasons why this would be useful. First, the ability to identify in-group members allows selective imitation. When there is rapid cultural adaptation, the local population becomes a valuable source of information about what is adaptive in the local environment. It is important to imitate locals and to avoid learning from immigrants who bring ideas from elsewhere. Second, the ability to identify in-group members allows selective social interaction. As we have seen, rapid cultural adaptation can preserve differences in moral norms between groups. It is best to interact with people who share the same beliefs about what is right and wrong, what is fair, and what is valuable. Thus, once reliable symbolic markers exist, selection will favor the psychological propensity to imitate and interact selectively with individuals who share the same symbolic markers.

The second, and less obvious, step is to see that these same propensities will also create and maintain variation in symbolic marker traits (McElreath et al. 2003). To understand why, consider the following simple example. Suppose that there are two groups: call them red and blue. In each group, a different social norm is common: call them the red norm and the blue norm. Interactions among people who share the same norm are more successful than interactions among people with different norms. For example, suppose that the norm concerns disputes involving property, and people with shared norms resolve property disputes more easily than people whose norms differ. There are also two neutral, but easily observable marker traits in these groups. Perhaps they are dialect variants. Call them red-speak and blue-speak. Suppose red-speak is relatively more common in the red group, and blue-speak in the blue group. Further suppose that people tend to interact with others who share their dialect. Individuals who have the more common combination of traits, red-norm and red-speak in the red group and blue-norm, blue-speak in the blue group, are most likely to interact with individuals like themselves. Since they share the same norms, they will be relatively successful. Conversely, individuals with the rare combinations will do less well. Then, as long as cultural adaptation leads to the increase of successful strategies, the red-marked individuals will become more common in the red group while the blue-marked individuals will become more common in the blue group. The real world is obviously much more complicated than this. Nonetheless the same logic should hold. As long as people are predisposed to interact with others who look or sound like themselves, and if that predisposition leads to more successful social interaction, then markers will tend to become correlated with social groups.

The same basic logic works for markers that allow people to imitate selectively. People who imitate others with the locally more common marker have a higher probability of acquiring locally advantageous variants. If people imitate both the marker and the behavior of the marked individuals, then individuals with the locally common marker will, on average, be more successful than people with other markers. This will increase the frequency of locally common markers, which in turn means that they become even *better* predictors of who to imitate. If a sharp environmental gradient or a sharp difference in local norms exists, differences in marker traits will continue to get more extreme until the degree of cultural isolation is sufficient to allow the population to optimize the mean behavior.

Tribal Social Instincts Evolved in Social Environments with Culturally Evolved Institutions

We hypothesize that this new social world, created by rapid cultural adaptation, drove the evolution of new, derived social instincts in our lineage. By "social instincts" we mean simply the genetically transmitted components of our social psychology. Cultural evolution created cooperative, symbolically marked residential groups and institutions like descent groups. Such environments favored the evolution of a suite of new social instincts suited to life in such groups:

- A psychology that "expects" life to be structured by moral norms and is designed to learn and internalize such norms.
- New emotions, such as shame and guilt, which increase the chance that norms are followed.
- A psychology with a naive ontology that includes the social world being divided into symbolically marked groups.

Individuals lacking the new social instincts violated prevailing norms more often and experienced adverse selection. They might have suffered ostracism, been denied the benefits of public goods, or lost points in the mating game. Cooperation and group identification in intergroup conflict set up an arms race that drove social evolution to ever-greater extremes of in-group cooperation. Eventually, human populations diverged from societies like those of other living apes and came to resemble the hunter-gatherer societies of the ethnographic record. We think that the evidence suggests that since about 100,000 years ago, most people have lived in tribal-scale societies. These societies are based upon in-group cooperation, where in-groups of a few hundred to a few thousand people are symbolically marked, for example, by language, ritual practices, and dress. These societies are egalitarian, and political power is diffuse. People are quite ready to punish others for transgressions of social norms, even when personal interests are not directly at stake.

Yet why should selection favor new prosocial emotions and intuitive decision-making strategies? People are smart, so should they not just deliberately calculate the best mix of cooperation and defection, given the risk of punishment? We think the answer is that people are not smart enough for evolution to trust them to do the necessary calculations using deliberate reasoning. For example, there is ample evidence that many creatures, including humans, overweight the present in decision making: Most people given the choice between receiving $1000 right now versus $1050 tomorrow, take the immediate offer of $1000. On the other hand, if offered the choice of receiving $1000 in 30 days or $1050 in 31 days, most people choose to wait. However, when 30 days have past, people regret their decision. This bias can cause individuals to make decisions that they later regret because they weigh future costs less in the present than they will weigh the same costs in the future. Now suppose that, as we have hypothesized, cultural evolution leads to a social environment in which noncooperators are subject to punishment by others. In many circumstances the reward for noncooperation will accrue immediately, while the cost of punishment will accrue later, and thus people who overvalue immediate payoffs may fail to cooperate, even though it is in their own interest to do so. If cooperative behavior is generally favored in most social environments, selection may favor genetically transmitted social instincts that predispose people to cooperate and identify within larger social groupings. For example, selection might favor feelings like guilt, which makes defection intrinsically costly, because this would bring the costs of defection into the present where they can be properly compared to the costs of cooperation.

These new tribal social instincts were superimposed onto human psychology without eliminating ancient ones favoring friends and kin. This resulted in an inherent conflict built into human social life. The tribal instincts that support identification and cooperation in large groups are often at odds with selfishness, nepotism, and face-to-face reciprocity. Some people cheat on their taxes, and not everyone pays back the money that they borrow. Not everyone who listens to public radio pays their dues. People feel deep loyalty to their kin and friends, but they are also moved by larger loyalties to clan, tribe, class, caste, and nation. Inevitably, conflicts arise. Families are torn apart by civil war. Parents send their children to war (or not) with painfully mixed emotions. Highly cooperative criminal cabals arise to prey upon the production of public goods of larger-scale institutions. Elites take advantage of key locations in the fabric of society to extract disproportionate private rewards for their work. The list is endless. The point is that humans suffer these pangs of conflict; most other animals are spared such distress because they are motivated mainly by selfishness and nepotism.

Some of our evolutionist friends have complained to us that this story is too complicated. Would it not be simpler to assume that culture is shaped by a psychology adapted to small groups of relatives? Well, perhaps. Interestingly, the same friends believe almost universally an equally complex coevolutionary story about the evolution of the language instinct. The Chomskian principles-and-parameters model of grammar hypothesizes that children have special-purpose psychological mechanisms that allow them to learn rapidly and accurately the grammar of the language they hear spoken around them. These mechanisms contain grammatical principles that constrain the range of possible interpretations that children can make of the sentences they hear. However, sufficient free parameters exist to allow children to acquire the whole range of human languages. These language instincts must have *coevolved* with culturally transmitted languages in much the same way that we hypothesize that the social instincts coevolved with culturally transmitted social norms. Most likely, the language instincts and the tribal social instincts evolved in quite close concert. Initially, languages must have been acquired using mechanisms not specifically adapted for language learning. This combination created a new and useful form of communication. Those individuals prepared innately to learn a little more proto-language, or learn it a little faster, would have a richer and more useful communication system than others not so well endowed. Then selection could favor still more specialized language instincts, which allowed still richer and more useful communication, and so on. We think that human social instincts similarly constrain and bias the kind of societies that we construct, but that very important details are left to be filled in by the local cultural input. When cultural parameters are set, the combination of instincts and culture produces operational social institutions. Human societies everywhere have the same basic flavor, if the comparison is with, for example, other apes. At the same time, the diversity of human social systems is quite spectacular. As with language instincts, social instincts have coevolved with such institutions over the last several hundred thousand years.

Conclusions

If our picture of the evolution of institutions is correct, the reasons why humans exhibit a mixture of more deliberate and more intuitive decision-making strategies are easy to see. If making decisions by formal deliberation (or anything like it) was cheap and accurate, some ur-organism long ago would have evolved something like omniscient rationality, and all subsequent adaptation would have been via phenotypic adjustments of the ur-organism. Photosynthesis optimal in the here and now? Gin up some chloroplasts! Social rules useful? Invent them on the spot!

The rational ur-organism is perhaps barely conceivable, but how would it fare in competition with Darwinian organisms that largely use genes and (in rare instances) culture rather than phenotypic flexibility to adapt to variable environments? Darwinian processes use a distributed blind selection in conjunction with myopic decision making to cause the long-run evolution of very complex adaptations. Although these adaptations can be transmitted genetically or culturally in a relatively inexpensive manner, they are prohibitively expensive to engineer by a single individual using deliberate procedures. The most common "decision" that a Darwinian organism makes is simply to trust the genes and culture it inherits. In the case of genes, decisions play a relatively small role because phenotypic modifications cannot be transmitted (cf. Jablonka and Lamb 2005). While all organisms have mechanisms to adapt as individuals to environmental contingencies, nothing approaching a rational ur-organism has ever evolved.

The problem of the high cost of deliberate decision making is also central to the analysis of cultural evolution. Individuals and groups can invent new cultural variants and choose among existing ones. Both deliberate and unconscious intuitive choices shape cultural evolution. The division of labor between deliberate and intuitive decision making in the cultural evolutionary context is driven by the slower speed and more costly nature of deliberate processes. One of the costs of deliberate processes is errors. Given limited reasoning powers, limited data, and limited time, deliberate reasoning is likely to lead to erroneous choices. Errors are particularly likely when a decision maker tries to improve a complex adaptation. Most changes in such things, even ones that seem reasonable, are liable to degrade the adaptation. Nevertheless, we presumably would not have the capacity for deliberate decision making unless it is sometimes useful. Guthrie (2005, pp. 269–270), following Liebenberg (1990), gives the example of animal tracking by hunters. Successful tracking requires close attention to multiple subtle cues, tapping a store of remembered knowledge of the behavior of the species being tracked, maintaining multiple working hypotheses, and often collaborative discussion with fellow trackers. Guthrie argues that the reasoning that goes into tracking is the same one that we deploy today in science. We suppose that one of the important functions for unconscious intuition is using heuristic rules for calling upon deliberation when it is most likely to be worth the cost of engaging in deliberation.

The institutions that regulate our social life resemble other domains of culture. Human social psychology, we believe, rests on a coevolved complex of genes and institutions. Most people are innately predisposed to follow the rules of the groups to which they belong, and culturally evolved institutions furnish an elaborate set of social rules even in simple societies. Foreign travel highlights the extent to which institutions are unconscious or nearly so. One's everyday social habits often serve poorly in other lands. One suddenly becomes aware of practices that are not even perceived at home. At the same time, other practices are scrutinized under a deliberate decision-making microscope. Every human social group has politics. Ongoing environmental changes will probably destabilize existing institutional equilibria and make other potential equilibria more attractive. Deliberate, collective decision making is a means to escape failing equilibria and to negotiate a path to a superior new one. In these often controversial domains, we are extremely well aware that there are choices to be made. The arts of reason, empirical science, and rhetoric are deployed to persuade others that some change in an institution is necessary or not.

The visibility of politically driven institutional change might suggest that every institutional feature of a society is subject to strong political influences. History, however, teaches us that institutions have deep roots that guide politics via unexamined attitudes, intuitions, and emotions. The historian David Hackett Fischer (1989) describes how the institutional geography of the U.S. was formed by the four original streams of British migration to North America. The endurance of these influences is reflected in the famed Southern Strategy of the Republican Party. Southern conservatives, disproportionately drawn from the Scots–Irish migrants to the U.S., were deliberately targeted as the civil rights legislation disaffected them from their traditional party, the Democrats. The attitudes of the Scots–Irish that this strategy exploited trace back to the Border Counties of England and Scotland and the turbulent life there before the Union of the Scottish and English Crowns in 1607. Nisbett and Cohen (1996) describe the enduring institutional differences between areas of Scots–Irish settlements in the U.S. and the rest of the country.

References

Bowles, S. 2004. Microeconomics, Behavior, Institutions, and Evolution. Oxford: Oxford Univ. Press.

Boyd, R., and P. J. Richerson. 2002. Group beneficial norms can spread rapidly in a structured population. *J. Theor. Biol.* **215**:287–296.

Boyer, P. 2006. Why ritualized behavior? Precaution systems and action-parsing in developmental, pathological and cultural rituals. *Behav. Brain Sci.* **29**:1–56.

Deutscher, G. 2005. The Unfolding of Language. New York: Metropolitan Books.

Ellickson, R. C. 1991. Order Without Law: How Neighbors Settle Disputes. Cambridge, MA: Harvard Univ. Press.

Fischer, D. H. 1989. Albion's Seed: Four British Folkways in America. New York: Oxford Univ. Press.

Guglielmino, C. R., C. Viganotti, B. Hewlett, and L. L. Cavalli-Sforza. 1985. Cultural variation in Africa: Role of mechanisms of transmission and adaptation. *Proc. Natl. Acad. Sci.* **92**:7585–7589.

Guthrie, R. D. 2005. The Nature of Paleolithic Art. Chicago: Chicago Univ. Press.

Henrich, J., and F. J. Gil-White. 2001. The evolution of prestige: Freely conferred deference as a mechanism for enhancing the benefits of cultural transmission. *Evol. Hum. Behav.* **22**:165–196.

Jablonka, E., and M. J. Lamb. 2005. Evolution in Four Dimensions: Genetic, Epigenetic, Behavioral, and Symbolic Variation in the History of Life. Cambridge, MA: MIT Press.

Johnson, P. 1976. A History of Christianity. London: Weidenfeld and Nicolson.

Jorgensen, J. G. 1980. Western Indians: Comparative Environments, Languages, and Cultures of 172 Western American Indian Societies. San Francisco: W. H. Freeman.

Knauft, B. 1985. Good Company and Violence: Sorcery and Social Action in a Lowland New Guinea Society. Berkeley: Univ. California Press.

Liebenberg, L. 1990. The Art of Tracking: Origin of Science. Cape Town: David Philip.

Mace, R., and C. Holden. 1999. Evolutionary ecology and cross-cultural comparison: The case of matrilineality in sub-Saharan Africa. In: Comparative Primate Socioecology, ed. P. C. Lee, pp. 387–405. Cambridge: Cambridge Univ. Press.

McElreath, R., R. Boyd, and P. J. Richerson. 2003. Shared norms and the evolution of ethnic markers. *Curr. Anthro.* **44**:122–129.

Nisbett, R. E., and D. Cohen. 1996. Culture of Honor: The Psychology of Violence in the South (New Directions in Social Psychology). Boulder, CO: Westview Press.

Richerson, P. J., and R. Boyd. 2005. Not by Genes Alone. Chicago: Univ. Chicago Press.

Salamon, S. 1980. Ethnic differences in farm family land transfers. *Rural Soc.* **45**:290–308.

Sosis, R. 2000. Religion and intra-group cooperation: preliminary results of a comparative analysis of utopian communities *Cross-Cult. Res.* **34**:70–87.

Stark, R. 1997. The Rise of Christianity: How the Obscure, Marginal Jesus Movement Became the Dominant Religious Force in the Western World in a Few Centuries. San Francisco: Harper Collins.

Young, P. 1998. Individual Strategy and Social Structure: An Evolutionary Theory of Institutions. Princeton, NJ: Princeton Univ. Press.

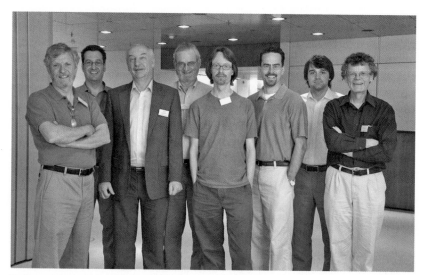

Left to right: Rob Boyd, Stefan Magen, Gerd Gigerenzer, Pete Richerson, Richard McElreath, Jeff Stevens, Andreas Glöckner, Arthur Robson

15

Individual Decision Making and the Evolutionary Roots of Institutions

Richard McElreath, Rapporteur

Robert Boyd, Gerd Gigerenzer, Andreas Glöckner,
Peter Hammerstein, Robert Kurzban, Stefan Magen,
Peter J. Richerson, Arthur Robson, and Jeffrey R. Stevens

Introduction

Humans hunt and kill many different species of animals, but whales are our biggest prey. In the North Atlantic, a male long-finned pilot whale (*Globicephala melaena*), a large relative of the dolphins, can grow as large as 6.5 meters and weigh as much as 2.5 tons. As whales go, these are not particularly large, but there are more than 750,000 pilot whales in the North Atlantic, traveling in groups, "pods," that range from just a few individuals to a thousand or more. Each pod is led by an individual known as the "pilot," who appears to set the course of travel for the rest of the group.

This pilot is both an asset and a weakness to the pod. The average pilot whale will yield about a half ton of meat and blubber, and North Atlantic societies including Ireland, Iceland, and the Shetlands used to manipulate the pilot to drive the entire pod ashore. In the Faroe Islands, a group of 18 grassy rocks due north of Scotland, pilot whale hunts have continued for the last 1200 years, at least. The permanent residents of these islands, the Faroese, previously killed an average of 900 whales each year, yielding about 500 tons of meat and fat that was consumed by local residents. Hunts have declined in recent years. From 2001 to 2005, about 3400 whales were killed, yielding about 890 metric tons of blubber and 990 metric tons of meat.

The whale kill, or *grindadráp* in the Faroese language, begins when a fishing boat spots a pod close enough to a suitable shore, on a suitably clear day. A single boat, or even a small group of fishermen, is not sufficient to trap a pod in a fjord, so the first step is to recruit more vessels. In ancient times, a signal fire was lit atop the boat and elected whale marshalls and sheriffs on the land lit bonfires to signal whale marshalls on neighboring islands. Nowadays, mobile phones have proven to be more efficient. As more boats join the hunt, men gather equipment and station themselves on the beach. The boats enclose the pod in a semicircle, driving them ashore. As the pod follows their pilot onto land, the men there kill each whale with one or two cuts through the spine, using specially sharpened knives. Sometimes the pilot will not be driven to land, in which case—according to custom—the pod must be driven back out to sea and allowed to escape.

Shares called *skinn*, a traditional unit of about 34 kilograms of blubber and 38 kilograms of meat, are distributed via a long-standing system of property rights. Roman numerals are assigned to each whale, and numerals are assigned to those who have rights based upon both residence and participation in the *grindadráp*. *Skinn* are cut from these whales, carried home, and the local sheriff ensures that the beach is clean within 24 hours.

The *grindadráp* is an example of what many call an "institution"—a term that is used in various ways across the human sciences. Sometimes, it indicates modern, formal organizations, like firms and parliaments. Other times it refers to any shared set of understandings, such as "kinship" or "childhood." In this chapter, we use the term to refer to locally stable, widely shared rules that regulate social interaction. This is not a claim about the nature of all things social scientists call "institutions." Rather it is meant to be a practical operationalization of a complex, multifaceted phenomenon.

The *grindadráp*, like many human institutions, recruits and coordinates human labor, regulating each stage of the event. It has evolved over hundreds of years, both changing and remaining stable as population, economy, and technology have evolved in the islands. The details of this story, however, as is the case for most institutions, are poorly understood. Do the regulations defining the *grindadráp* function well, or would alternative regulations do better? If the latter, why have those alternatives not evolved? How did the specific rules come to be, and is there any meaningful fit between the structure of human cognition—both in the physiological details and decision processes—and the structure of the institution? We cannot yet construct a widely believed story to explain the specific design of any reasonably complex institution nor for the diversity of institutional forms among human societies.

Just as many aspects of individual decisions are sometimes called "unconscious" or "automatic," we know that some institutions have evolved through "unconscious," nondeliberative mechanisms. Their function can also be largely nondeliberative, as in the case of some institutions that may structure behavior without requiring any reflection on the part of the participants. On the other hand, political institutions exist for the purpose of bringing deliberative mechanisms to bear on institutions in the hope of changing them for the better. The immense project of building an integrated explanation of institutions—

from individual brains to nations—has only barely begun. In this chapter, we report on our discussions that attempted to sketch the mechanisms that connect individuals to large-scale institutions. We begin with a discussion of current thought on the design of individual decision making. If institutions regulate behavior, then presumably the mechanisms that have evolved to produce individual behavior will be relevant to the broader enterprise of integrating these two scales of explanation. Then we explore ways in which institutions may have evolved, both as a result of individual decision making and as a result of processes distinct from those that govern individual behavior. We approach this topic from two perspectives. Seen one way, unconscious psychological forces constrain the design of institutions, sometimes powerfully. Seen another way, unconscious population-level processes create functional institutional design that few social architects could conceive of with their individual deliberate faculties.

Evolution of Individual Decisions

In the first half of the 20th century, most biologists thought about the evolution of decisions and learning in terms of selection for general intelligence. A number of key experiments, including demonstration of cue-specific learning in rats (Garcia and Koelling 1966), convinced most that the general intelligence approach was mistaken. As biology textbooks now argue, we understand how natural selection designs cognition by understanding the characteristic problems that each different organism faces.

For example, both birds and mammals use some form of association learning to identify and avoid toxic food. Reinforcement, however, is sometimes specific to the nature of the cues. Birds remember the color of distasteful food, whereas rats remember odor, even when the experimenter associates toxicity with only one or the other. If color, rats do not learn to avoid the poison. If odor, birds have a similar problem. A usual interpretation of this result is that birds forage from a distance in daylight, where color is the first available cue, while rats forage in the dark, where color is unavailable or unreliable. Even among different bird species, association learning varies in efficacy, depending upon the ecological details (Balda et al. 1997).

Biologists have come to expect most organisms to be good at ecologically relevant problems, rather than simply to differ in general problem-solving ability. Sometimes this specificity of ability is discovered in animals people tend to regard as rather dim (e.g., birds). Recent experiments by Nicola Clayton and her coworkers show that humans are not the only animals that plan for the future (Raby et al. 2007). It had previously been thought that while humans can represent future needs and act accordingly, provisions for the future observed in other animals resulted from either fixed action patterns or current motivational states. Clayton and her coworkers experimented with the Western Scrub

Jay, a species that caches food. The jays were housed in three rooms, call them A, B, and C. Sometimes they spent the night in room A, while other times in B. Experiments manipulated how they were fed in different rooms in the morning. For example, in one experiment, when they spent the night in A, they received no breakfast. If they slept instead in room B, they did receive breakfast. During the previous afternoon, birds were given an opportunity to cache in either room, and then one of the rooms was chosen at random and they spent the night in that room. The jays cached food preferentially in room A, perhaps anticipating that they would be hungry the next morning. This decision was independent of whether they were hungry or satiated in the afternoon.

Despite cases such as this one, there are reasons to consider that some decision mechanisms may be quite general across behavioral domains. Such a view is more common in the human sciences, and there are different routes to this opinion. First, experiments such as those that illustrate learning differences in birds and rats demonstrate only specificity of cues. The ways in which cues are processed may be quite similar. Some evolutionary psychologists argue that human reasoning comprises many special-purpose cognitive mechanisms (Cosmides and Tooby 1992), and yet some of their favorite examples demonstrate only specificity of cues, not of processing. For example, the Wason selection task shows that people make different selections when the task is framed in one of two ways (they receive alternative cues), but the core information remains unchanged (for further discussion, see chapters by Stevens and Schooler, both this volume). Different cues may activate different processing algorithms. The reasoning employed in either case, however, may be employed routinely in other contexts. The experiments do not address this question.

Another reason to consider some generality of processing is to account for the findings that decision behavior in animals (e.g., Real 1991) and humans (e.g., Kahneman and Tversky 1972) can sometimes be predicted by weighted-additive integration of information. Single-strategy models may also be frugal, in a way, by avoiding the problem of a meta-decision to select between different specific cognitive strategies. Glöckner (this volume) suggests a very general decision model—consistency maximizing by parallel constraint satisfaction—which he thinks can account for many findings in the field. According to the model, decision making is based on mental representations of the decision tasks that are formed by automatic processes. In every decision task, these processes, which have evolved from processes of perception, modify the information and form consistent mental representations (i.e., interpretations). Parts of these mental representations enter awareness and lead to decisions. The amount of information provided as input to the algorithm may vary tremendously, and the sensory modalities in each case may be distinct. However, if the mental representation reflects the structure of the environment properly, it necessarily produces good decisions in all possible contexts. From the perspective of the model, there are no distinct decision strategies; there are only distinct ways of looking for information and structuring the mental representation of the decision task. From such a perspective, any simplifying heuristic is a completely nested model to the network model. Perhaps redundancy of processing, but also variation in input and information structuring could be an efficient adaptive design.

Others, in the bounded rationality tradition of Herbert Simon, criticize the view that there can be any single robust decision algorithm (Gigerenzer et al. 1999). Flexible decision models, just like regression in statistics, can indeed be fit to many contexts. This fitting, however, has drawbacks. First, the parameters have to be fit by some process, whether learning or evolution. If this process takes place over behavioral time (learning), then the goodness of fit will be limited to those contexts sufficiently sampled behaviorally. For complex contexts with many states to sample over, either the organism makes do with a small sample, and risks over-fitting, or pays large costs of learning. Over-fitting occurs when a parameter-rich model is trained on too little information. Unless parameters can be estimated sufficiently well, an organism (just like a statistician) can actually make more accurate predictions by considering less information (Gigerenzer et al. 1999; also, for an accessible introduction to over-fitting, see Forster and Sober 1994). For some learning problems, no cost will be enough, because the problem is combinatorially hard enough that the organism (if not the solar system) will be dead before enough sampling or calculation is completed. If the organism uses a general, parameter-rich mechanism, the organism will be stuck over-fitting. If the fitting process is evolution through natural selection, then the individual's lifespan is not the problem, but individual organisms will not be able to respond to novel contexts adaptively. In long-lived organisms in variable environments, like ourselves, the costs of rigid innate fits might be quite high. This is due to another kind of over-fitting, this time as a result of the nonstationary nature of the environment.

An alternative to models that require a lot of fitting is to have simple heuristics that can be combined and employed in specific contexts (Gigerenzer et al. 1999). These mechanisms avoid over-fitting by having few, if any, adjustable parameters. In out-of-sample prediction tests, such heuristics often win soundly over more information-rich strategies. However, heuristics err on bias, where parameter-rich models err on variance. Their success depends upon being properly selected for the appropriate decision context and information environment. This requires a hierarchy of heuristics, or perhaps "meta-heuristics." This requirement begs additional questions, of course. There is a healthy theoretical and experimental literature comparing simple heuristics to complex learning models (see, e.g., Bröder and Schiffer 2003; Bergert and Nosofsky 2007). We expect this debate over the generality and complexity of decision mechanisms to continue for some time.

Another argument sometimes offered for expecting special-purpose cognitive mechanisms is via the analogy to organs (Tooby and Cosmides 1992). Kidneys, hearts, lungs, and livers are functionally discrete, localized adaptations to different physiological challenges. The discovery of potentially similar localization of function in the brain, with Wernicke's and Broca's language areas, led to speculation that much of the brain exhibited functional specialization, instead of general mechanisms. This is suggestive analogizing, but some evolutionary logic is needed to put this on solid scientific footing. If there are good functional reasons for less-specialized mechanisms, they do appear to evolve. The immune system, for example, contains a broad learning system, that generates variation and selective retention. An alternative would be to have specialized immune modules for different diseases, yet given how pathogens evolve, a learning immune system better fulfills the functional needs of the organism.

Evidence suggests that selection does sometimes favor "general" intelligence. Humans aside, some evidence from the field suggests that brain size in primates and birds is correlated with rather general increases in problem-solving abilities. Reader and Laland (2002) found that field reports of innovation, social learning, and tool use correlated with the species' executive brain size. Sol et al. (2005) found that birds from groups with larger brains established more successfully in novel environments and that they did so by generating novel adaptive behaviors.

How Does Selection Design Mechanism?

There are many ways to make a clock (see Schooler, this volume). Chinese water clocks function by converting a continuous process of pouring water into a periodic process of emptying full buckets. Pendulum clocks use wave momentum, and modern quartz clocks exploit the vibrations of tiny crystals, when exposed to current. The surface "behavior" of each of these mechanisms is similar, yet the details are distinct, and the differences matter for cost and accuracy.

Similarly, evolved decision-making mechanisms can be considered at both algorithmic and implementation levels (Schooler, this volume). The algorithmic level of abstraction refers to the crude grammar of how information (cues) is translated into a decision (or output signal). The implementation level refers to the details of the machinery. These two levels do not map necessarily directly onto one another. For example, both humans and bees can learn by reinforcement, in some contexts. However, the last common ancestor of these species, the urbilaterian, had a very simple brain. Bees and humans likely implement reinforcement using quite different neural architectures. Granted, if we specify algorithms, sufficiently precisely, even very similar information processes will appear different. However, at the level of abstraction of much work in modeling cognition, we suspect this distinction is of value.

This distinction is important for our purposes because there are reasons to believe that natural selection may leave many aspects of implementation unspecified. In the case of protein evolution, a similar phenomenon is well understood. Many different sequences of DNA yield identical, or functionally identical, chains of amino acids (proteins). Neutral mutation can tinker with the sequence harmlessly for long periods of evolutionary time. Eventually, the sequences drift close enough to a change such that the function of the protein is drastically altered. Then one mutation will cause a sudden shift in function, with important consequences. Different lineages, however, will have functionally identical proteins, but very different underlying sequences.

If cognitive evolution bears any resemblance, then it may be quite hard to make good predictions about implementation, given function and algorithm. At the scale of decision mechanisms, we might expect variation in the underlying implementation, because organic evolution is path dependent: there are multiple ways to build an organ or algorithm, and one may be better than all others, but the organism cannot get there from where it is.

Once more is known about the fine structure of cognition, it will turn out that local optima and path dependency broadly stabilize diversity in implementation of decision making, as well.

Implementation Costs

Another reason to be pessimistic about our ability to deduce accurately or infer implementation from algorithms is the difficulty of specifying correctly the costs of alternative implementations. This is not always true: evolutionary biologists who study flight have powerful principles derived from aerodynamics that allow them to make educated guesses at marginal costs of variations in wing shape and muscle attachment. These systems are also conducive to experimentation. Together, this has allowed them to explain variation in wing design among birds, as well as why insect wings are both so different from bird wings and from one another (Alexander 2002; Dudley 2002).

There have been important attempts to quantify costs of alternative decision algorithms, such as the widely cited analyses of Payne, Bettman, and Johnson (1993). In neuroscience, however, we know of no easy—or at least agreed upon—way to infer the differential costs, in evolutionary terms, of alternative implementations. We may be able to make profitable guesses, but these would not be derived from any engineering knowledge of the brain. There are hints, however, that it is possible to estimate some potentially fitness-relevant metabolic costs. In a recent set of studies, Gailliot et al. (2007) provided some evidence about the metabolic costs associated with "hard" mental processes. In particular, they looked at tasks that required "self-control." In one case, subjects were shown a video with words at the bottom of the screen but were instructed to ignore them—a task that requires exercising control over one's attention. First, by measuring blood glucose (sugar) levels pre- and post-task, it was shown that performing this task (relative to a control task with no attentional instructions) led to a relatively greater depletion of glucose. This general result was obtained for a variety of self-control measures. Most interestingly, another study was conducted in which the same task was performed, but this time some subjects ingested a high glucose drink (lemonade) before the test; other subjects were given a placebo drink that contained no sugar, only artificial sweetener. When the subjects were given a subsequent demanding task (a Stroop task), those who had consumed the sugared drink performed better than those who received the placebo control, suggesting that the glucose had "replenished" their ability to do a task with high attentional demands.

These experiments illustrate a possible way of estimating costs, but they also illustrate another concern: the distinction between normal operating costs and capacity costs. An analogy to the power industry is helpful here. Electrical grids that supply cities and states with power must be designed for peak load, not for average load. Thus, examining the grid at some times of the day would suggest that it is over-designed. At peak usage however (hours and seasons), such grids can buckle under the combined drain of, for example, millions of air conditioners. If natural selection has designed nervous systems to cope with similar time-variant demand problems, then we will need to understand how much circuit implementations cost in comparison to one another under several different system conditions, including energy shortage and "peak load."

Yet another kind of cost to consider is opportunity cost. Most people have had the experience of walking or driving the wrong way, in a familiar place, because they had been lost in thought. Different implementations may imply different conflicts among circuits or sensory inputs. To give a simple example, organisms that rely mainly upon a single sense, vision for example, may not be able to afford devoting attention to a single task. Monkeys tend to have quite short attention spans, from the perspective of human researchers, perhaps as a result of an history of selection under predation. With only a single set of eyes, a monkey pays an opportunity cost of increased risk of being eaten if he fixes his eyes only upon the task at hand.

If any of these conjectures—path-dependent local optima or the difficulties of deducing evolutionarily relevant costs—holds, it will be hard to make useful predictions about the cognitive machinery from only the function or algorithm that provides for a decision. This, however, is not necessarily a negative message. We expect progress will be made in time, by appreciating how details matter in organic evolution. Evolutionary biology has made fantastic progress, over the last fifty years, in understanding the evolution of behavior, partly because evolutionary biologists came to appreciate that proximate details (such as how traits are inherited and how sex determination works) have profound effects on ultimate outcomes. It is usually not enough to understand the evolutionary function (how the trait enhances survival or reproduction) in isolation, if we aim to understand the design of behavior. We expect the same principle will hold as we delve more deeply into the structure of cognition.

The Evolution of Deliberative Decisions

Many social scientists and philosophers are interested in a seemingly unique human decision-making capacity: deliberative reasoning. By deliberative reasoning, we mean decision processes accessible to consciousness. Sometimes these processes are represented explicitly in human language. It is possible that the process of deliberative reasoning is different from nondeliberative, "unconscious," decision mechanisms. Conscious reasoning is often thought to take more time than automatic mechanisms, but it is also perceived as more flexible. This is a folk-psychological cluster of concepts, so many scientists and philosphers are suspicious of its value, despite the enthusiasm for the distinction on the part of other scientists and philosophers.

However, philosophers of psychology sometimes invoke a gambit known as the simple correspondence thesis (Fodor 2005). This gambit applies to many domains, but is sometimes directed to theory of mind, the mechanisms that allow people to attribute mental states to and predict the behavior of others. Since our theory of mind mechanisms seem to work (i.e., they do better than chance at predicting behavior), they may correspond partially to the real structure of the mind. To the extent that the deliberative/automatic distinction is widespread in human societies, the simple corresponding thesis leads us to entertain it as a scientific concept, but not to commit to it on any evidential basis. Explaining why some, or any, thought is consciously accessible seems worthwhile.

If deliberative reasoning is a valid concept that describes the structure of human cognition, what evolutionary function might it have been selected to serve? There are no dominant hypotheses. We do note four possibilities, none mutually exclusive.

First, deliberative reasoning, because of its often explicit linguistic nature, may be the mind's press secretary (Kurzban, this volume). Explaining one's mental states and motivations to others can be of great value in social life. In order to encode these states as language, they must be made conscious. Press secretaries sometimes lie, of course, but not always.

A second possibility is that deliberative reasoning facilitates verbal encoding which in turn serves collective decision-making functions. Juries must deliberate to reach a verdict. Judges must write closely argued opinions which will be reviewed by appellate courts and perhaps eventually vetted as a correct interpretation of the law. An executive decision maker confers typically with advisors before making important decisions.

Third, the function of deliberative reasoning may be to "tame" automatic reasoning. That is, deliberative reasoning might function to halt and re-fit trained automatic mechanisms. For example, once a musician has learned to play an instrument, many aspects of performance are automatic, requiring little conscious deliberative effort, if any. In fact, some musicians report that deliberative processes interfere with performance. However, if a musician observes another musician using a better technique, the musician must halt and retrain the automatic system in order to incorporate this new technique.

A fourth option is that explicit deliberative reasoning is related to the manipulation and transmission of complex, socially transmitted behavior—cultural traditions. For example, explaining to a neophyte how a machine or an institution works may facilitate rapid acquisition of knowledge compared to merely observing examples of the object in action.

Cultural Evolution and the Design of Institutions

Most of the previous discussion treats humans as any other animal. In a very real sense, we are just another animal. However, like any other animal, we are unique. In our case, there is substantial evidence that humans are unique among mammals in relying heavily on social learning to acquire large, important aspects of our behavior (Richerson and Boyd 2005). Other animals, such as song birds and some apes, clearly have stable socially transmitted traditions (see Fragaszy and Perry 2003). However, in all cases, these traditions are quite simple—few if any are more complex than what could be invented by an individual in its lifetime—and confined to a narrow range of behavioral domains. Humans, in contrast, acquire extraordinarily complex, locally adapted patterns of behavior in nearly every domain of belief and behavior. Humans occupy every environment on the planet, with the same basic tropical-ape physiology. With less genetic variation than that found between different populations of chimpanzee, humans exhibit a greater range of subsistence type and social organization than all the other primates combined.

Formal evolutionary models of social learning mechanisms suggest that social transmission of this sort is favored in variable environments. Above, we explained that learning is favored when organisms experience different environments on timescales that are neither too short (when learning would be pointless) nor too long (when genetic fixation would suffice). Embedded in the middle of the same spectrum of evolutionary outcomes is a broad range of stochastic contexts in which a heavy reliance on social learning is favored (Aoki et al. 2005; Wakano and Aoki 2006). The insight is that environmental change that is autocorrelated favors social learning, because while variation favors learning, the autocorrelation means there is enough time to build locally adapted cumulative traditions, before the next shift in the environment. The Pleistocene climate record exhibits exactly this sort of environmental stochasticity, and this is the period when human brains expanded and archaeological signs of human "culture" began to appear (Richerson et al. 2005).

Much of the adaptive advantage of culture comes from the way it economizes on cognitive effort. If every individual has to acquire the behaviors necessary to cope with a variable environment for themselves, much of what is learned will have to be relearned by every individual in every generation.

By allowing individuals to imitate other individuals at a much lower cost than learning for oneself, great economies are possible. Accurate imitation also supports the accumulation of innovations to build complex technological and institutional adaptations. The legal code that any competent lawyer can master represents the cumulative wisdom of generations of legal scholarship and practice. No single lawyer, no matter how energetic or brilliant, could do as well. Thus, the population-level properties of culture leverage the costly deliberative decision-making systems. Formal institutions may be largely a product of this process. Cultural evolutionary processes also leverage less costly nondeliberative decision making. If many individuals exercise evolved decision heuristics that are at least accurate on average to bias their acquisition of cultural variants, cultural adaptations will arise without anyone having to invest in costly decision making. As with natural selection, weak biases that are only slightly better than chance at the individual level will act as powerful evolutionary forces when cumulated over many individuals and many generations. Informal institutions may evolve mainly by nondeliberative mechanisms.

The human reliance on social transmission builds complex technology, as well as knowledge that individuals can use to improve their own decision making. However, much of conspicuous cultural variation in our species takes the form of shared rules for behavior. As we said in the introduction, we define institutions as locally stable, widely shared rules that regulate social behavior. While it is possible, and probably true in some cases, that decision mechanisms independent of culture and social learning can stabilize shared patterns of behavior (as in a classic Nash equilibrium), institutions like the *grindadráp*, Roman law, and even the diversity of systems of exchange and property contain substantial amounts of shared rules that suggest social transmission and evolution. All of the knowledge contained in, for example, complex Australian aboriginal age-grade systems—which specify which men control the marriage options of other men, as well as how men move from one age-grade to the next—requires social transmission of explicit knowledge. This begs the questions of how the detailed structure of individual cognition interacts with human institutions, as well as mechanisms by which institutions themselves evolve, both under the influence of individual decision mechanisms, as well as other higher-level mechanisms.

How Does Individual Decision Making Influence Institutions?

When Spanish explorers encountered the highly structured and complex Aztec and Inca empires of the Americas, it was almost as if they were encountering aliens. The last common ancestor of the Spaniards and the Native Americans lived deep in the Pleistocene, long prior to the advent of agriculture. In many ways, their languages and cultures could not have been more different, given the length of separation. Nevertheless, the Spaniards discovered many similar themes in the organization of American societies, themes they quickly exploited.

Amazed at the diversity of human societies and their institutions, we sometimes overlook the incredible convergences. Despite their long separation and independent evolution of agriculture, political hierarchy, construction, architecture, accounting, exchange, and a number of other institutions, the Europeans and Americans found that a broad set of their assumptions about life in their own complex society applied also, with small modification, to life in the other.

It seems likely that a common set of individual psychological processes tend to structure human societies in a limited number of ways. Consider social exchange. Exchange is a key institutional foundation of human economies. Exchange permits individuals to specialize in productive activities that take advantage of their inherent and acquired characteristics, while allowing these individuals to consume a radically different basket of goods.

Human beings may have an inherent proclivity for barter even with unrelated individuals. Charles Darwin was an astute observer of human beings, as well as of the natural world. When the Beagle reached Tierra del Fuego, at the southern tip of South America, Darwin had an opportunity to interact with the locals. He wrote (Darwin 1845, Chapter X):

> Some of the Fuegians plainly showed that they had a fair notion of barter. I gave one man a large nail (a most valuable present) without making any signs for a return; but he immediately picked out two fish, and handed them up on the point of his spear.

Whatever the evolutionary scenario that gives humans widespread prosocial motives such as this, they possibly underwrite similarities in the design of institutions for exchange, the world over. This is not to say that the differences in markets and exchange customs are not significant. However, the fact that the Fuegian, who could not speak a word of English, understood Darwin's gift as an invitation for trade implies that individuals bring a set of characteristically human motives and filters to the table. These motives help structure both explicitly designed institutions as well as institutions that evolve through the nondeliberative action of many individuals. We discussed two interesting cases in which the plausible design of individual decisions, often unconscious, have quite strong effects on social institutions.

Marriage rules illustrate how evolved psychological mechanisms may shape the cultural evolution of institutions. The institution of preferential cousin marriage exists in many societies. In some cases it is thought to function to prevent the kin groups from losing assets through marriage. For example, the institution of patrilateral parallel cousin marriage—men marry their father's brother's daughters—is common in Middle Eastern societies. Many scholars believe that this institution functions, at least in part, to preserve property within the patrilineage (Khuri 1970), a view consistent with an equilibrium selection model of institutional evolution. However, if so, preferential brother sister marriage would be an even better institution for preserving such assets. Yet no ethnographically known society supports an institution of brother sister marriage.

The likely reason is that this solution is precluded by the evolved psychology of sexual desire. There is much evidence that people are not sexually attracted to those with whom they had frequent, close social contact when they were growing up, and that if marriages between brothers and sisters were prescribed, they would likely have low fertility, high rates of infidelity, and high divorce rates (Fessler and Navarrete 2004). Moreover, contemplating sexual relations among brothers and sisters elicits strong feelings of disgust. Both mechanisms appear to preclude the evolution of institutionalized brother sister marriage, even though it might be a good solution to the problem of maintenance of property within the family. While there are rare examples of elites who attempted to institutionalize sibling marriage, these are quite rare and were apparently ephemeral.

Another example comes from certain kinds of ritual. In every culture ever studied, religious ceremonies, changes in life stage, and threatening situations such as death or disease are accompanied by culturally specified behavior. This behavior is often "ritualized," meaning that the actions (a) are compulsory, (b) rigidly conform to a script, (c) are divorced from observable goals, (d) exhibit internal repetition, and (e) share common themes of danger and pollution. Boyer and Lienard (2006) argue that commonness of ritualized behavior can be explained in terms of an evolved "precaution system" present in human psychology. This specialized system was favored by natural selection because it allowed individuals to detect potential, but not yet manifest dangers (e.g., such as contamination, disease, or predation). Boyer and Lienard believe that when this system is working it helps people detect and deal with environmental hazards. When it misfires, it gives rise to Obsessive Compulsive Disorder (OCD). Cultural rituals that activate this system are more attention grabbing, more memorable, and more satisfying, and as a result ceremonial routines that involve ritualized behavior tend to spread and persist to a greater extent than ceremonies that do not activate this system.

If either of the above examples is correct, it would constitute a case where the adaptive design of individual decision making has a strong influence on the design of institutions, and therefore on the decisions individuals make within those institutional contexts.

How Do Institutions Evolve?

However strong unconscious individual forces like attraction to ritualized behavior, many different ritual institutions can and are stabilized in human societies. While the 16th century societies of Europe and the Americas were quite alike in many ways, they were also strikingly different, and these differences had important consequences. European societies have had a huge influence on the Americas, while American societies have had little influence on Europeans. Differences in technology and military organization had tremendous consequences. Therefore understanding why societies evolve different institutions, at different rates, is the other side of theoretical coin.

We recognize four mechanisms operating within human societies that may transform and stabilize institutions, including creating institutional diversity.

1. Long-lived organisms such as humans have many repeat interactions with the same individuals. Game theoretic models strongly suggest that, in any sufficiently repeated game, there are a great many stable points.

2. Literature exists on the algorithmic structure of mechanisms of social and cultural learning (Henrich and McElreath 2003; Laland 2004). One powerful mechanism is conformity, preferentially adopting majority behavior (Boyd and Richerson 1985). Conformity can be a highly adaptive learning heuristic, because it exploits the fact that many adaptive processes make locally successful behavior into common behavior. While classic social-psychological evidence of "conformity" (Asch 1951) does not distinguish between linear (in number of people) forms of social learning and greater-than-linear influence of majority behavior, there is experimental evidence that people possess a conformist tendency, and that it responds to parameters of the environment as predicted by evolutionary theory (McElreath et al. 2005). While exploiting this statistical feature of human environments, conformity also tends to homogenize groups and stabilize variation between groups (Henrich and Boyd 1998).

3. Different kinds of path dependency can stabilize behavior within groups and variation between groups. Coordination payoffs (I do best when I do what you do) can achieve this, even when one equilibrium is more efficient. However, even in the absence of explicitly coordinated payoffs, the path dependency of complex behavior makes it hard to get from local optima to global optima that would homogenize the population. For example, technology tends to evolve in small improvements, not giant leaps (Richerson and Boyd 2005 review the evidence). This means that local improvements in design space may tend to differentiate further groups that started from different initial designs. The evolution of Chinese and European sailing vessels illustrates this point. Chinese vessels began from rafts made from lashed-together bamboo poles, while European vessels began as dugout canoes. The rafts evolved eventually into hulled, masted vessels without a keel—the weight of the forces was supported more evenly across the hull. European boats, in contrast, built a series of "ribs" up from the dugout canoe core, the keel, supporting the forces with a rigid spine. Starting in different directions, the two traditions of sailing technology evolved quite different paths of innovation.

4. Once institutions of hierarchy or command and control have evolved, small groups of individuals within larger groups can dictate rapid changes in social organization. In this case, the motivations and decisions of those in command will have big effects on social evolution.

However, even if a single individual initially calls all the shots, there are good reasons to believe that social evolution will not be easily explicable in terms of individual cognition. The reason is that between-group processes may affect the long-term fates of different institutional variants. Provided that some between-group variation in institutions is stable (and the above four mechanisms suggest reasons for the ethnographic and historical observation of stable institutional variation in human societies) and that this variation has effects on the fates of societies, then institutional forms can spread or vanish through processes not cleanly tied to many types of individual decision mechanisms. Furthermore, the precise way in which an institution affects a society's fate, in the ecology of societies, implies design aspects of the institutions that will persist and spread over time. It makes a difference whether societies succeed because they conquer their neighbors or because they survive droughts. In the first case, we might expect existing societies to be good at defense and warfare but not necessarily prepared for environmental crisis; in the second, those differences in institutions spread because of differential conquest. We can think of four useful distinctions to make, along these lines.

1. Social evolution might proceed by differential extinction. If some social arrangements are more likely to survive environmental calamities, these arrangements might increase in frequency among human societies. Here it is a game of society-versus-environment. How information flows through a society, how quickly it can respond to information, and how it mediates and suppresses internal conflicts might all contribute to survival. Polynesian societies faced periodic typhoons that denuded islands, perhaps selecting strongly for institutions of storage and recovery managed by chiefs.
2. Social evolution might proceed by differential growth. Ammerman and Cavalli-Sforza (1984) and Sokal, Oden, and Wilson (1991) have argued that agriculture spread into Europe mainly through the spread of farmers, not the spread of farming. If some societies replace others demographically because of fecundity, this might lead to the spread of social institutions that encourage population growth. Richerson, Boyd, and Bettinger (2001) argue that agriculture, once present in a region, spread partly because numerically superior farmers could usually defeat foragers in contests over territory.
3. Social evolution might proceed by differential conquest, even when groups are of comparable sizes. In his book about the rise of European world powers, *The Pursuit of Power* (1982), William McNeill argues that competition for control of land and resources between rather small European polities created a ratchet for the development of modern military

institutions, technologies, and goals of elites, and these fueled the later expansive colonial ambitions of European states. Kelly's (1985) synthetic study of the Nuer conquest of the Dinka suggests that institutions do spread by differential conquest, even in traditional societies without professional militaries.

4. Social evolution might proceed by differential influence. Societies sometimes adopt willingly the social arrangements and beliefs of their neighbors. David Boyd (2001) documents the decision-making process through which the Irakia Awa of Papua New Guinea eventually adopted the economic and ritual institutions of their neighbors, the Fore. The Irakia Awa observed that the Fore were better-off, and they set out to imitate them at the institutional level. These transformations might operate without extinction, replacement, conquest, or coercion. Exactly what makes societies favorable in these comparisons matters, of course. If rates of extraction and consumption are what is driving social evolution, then we should not expect societies to be well-equipped to manage their environments.

These four different mechanisms may imply quite different rates of change, as well, and this may help us evaluate the relative importance of each. Soltis et al. (1995) surveyed New Guinea ethnographic history to estimate the rate at which social competition might spread institutions. They concluded that social complexity would spread very slowly, requiring in the order of many hundreds of years, by this mechanism. Differential extinction by environmental failure certainly interacts with direct group competition, but its rate seems unlikely to be more rapid. While internally caused extinctions are known (Diamond 2004), populations have existed at low densities for much of human history, making it hard to exhaust local resources. Islands, such as Easter Island, are possible exceptions. Differential influence might diffuse innovations rather quickly (Boyd and Richerson 2002) because it is limited by the rate of social comparison rather than the rate of tragedy or violent conflict.

References

Alexander, D. E. 2002. Nature's Flyers: Birds, Insects, and the Biomechanics of Flight. Baltimore: Johns Hopkins Univ. Press.

Ammerman A. J., and L. L. Cavalli-Sforza. 1984 The Neolithic Transition and the Genetics of Populations in Europe, pp. 109–113. Princeton: Princeton Univ. Press.

Aoki, K., J. Y. Wakano, and M. W. Feldman. 2005. The emergence of social learning in a temporally changing environment: A theoretical model. *Curr. Anthro.* **46**:334–340.

Asch, S. E. 1951. Effects of group pressure upon the modification and distortion of judgment. In: Groups, Leadership and Men, ed. H. Guetzkow. Pittsburgh: Carnegie Press.

Balda, R. P., A. C. Kamil, and P. A. Bednekoff. 1997. Predicting cognitive capacities from natural histories: Examples from four corvid species. *Curr. Ornithol.* **13**:33–66.

Bergert, F. B., and R. M. Nosofsky. 2007. A response-time approach to comparing generalized rational and take-the-best models of decision making. *J. Exp. Psychol.: Learn. Mem. Cogn* **33(1)**:107–129.

Boyd, D. J. 2001. Life without pigs: Recent subsistence changes among the Irakia Awa, Papua New Guinea. *Hum. Ecol* **29(3)**:259–282.

Boyd, R., and P. J. Richerson. 1985. Culture and the Evolutionary Process. Chicago: Univ of Chicago Press.

Boyd, R., and P. J. Richerson. 2002. Group beneficial norms spread rapidly in a structured population. *J. Th. Biol.* **215**:287–296.

Boyer, P., and P. Leinard. 2006. Why ritualized behavior? Precaution systems and action parsing in developmental, pathological and cultural rituals. *Behav. Brain Sci.* **29**:1–56.

Bröder, A., and S. Schiffer. 2003. "Take The Best" versus simultaneous feature matching: Probabilistic inferences from memory and effects of representation format. *J. Exp. Psychol.: Gen.* **132**:277–293.

Cosmides, L., and J. Tooby. 1992. Cognitive adaptations for social exchange. In: The Adapted Mind, ed. J. Barkow, L. Cosmides, and J. Tooby, pp. 163–228. New York: Oxford Univ. Press.

Darwin, C. 1845. Journal of Researches into the Natural History and Geology of the Various Countries Visited by H.M.S. Beagle. London: John Murray. http://darwin-online.org.uk/content/frameset?itemID=F14andviewtype=sideandpageseq=1

Diamond, J. 2004. Collapse: How Societies Choose to Fail or Succeed. New York: Viking Adult.

Dudley, R. 2002. The Biomechanics of Insect Flight: Form, Function, Evolution. Princeton: Princeton Univ. Press.

Emlen, S. T. 1970. Celestial rotation: Its importance in the development of migratory orientation. *Science* **170**:1198–1201.

Fessler, D. M. T., and C. D. Navarrete. 2004. Third-party attitudes toward sibling incest: Evidence for Westermarck's hypotheses. *Evol. Hum. Behav.* **25**:277–294.

Fodor, J. 2005. The Language of Thought. Cambridge, MA: Harvard Univ Press.

Forster, M., and E. Sober. 1994. How to tell when simpler, more unified, or less ad hoc theories will provide more accurate predictions. *Brit. J. Philos. Sci.* **45**:1–35.

Fragaszy, D. M., and S. Perry, eds. 2003. The Biology of Traditions: Models and Evidence. Cambridge: Cambridge Univ. Press.

Gailliot, M. T., R. F. Baumeister, C. N. DeWall et al. 2007. Self-control relies on glucose as a limited energy source: Willpower is more than a metaphor. *J. Pers. Soc. Psych.* **92(2)**: 325–336.

Garcia, J., and R. A. Koelling. 1966. Relation of cue to consequence in avoidance learning. *Psychon. Sci.* **4**: 123–124.

Gigerenzer, G., P. M. Todd, and the ABC Research Group. 1999. Simple Heuristics That Make Us Smart. Oxford: Oxford Univ. Press.

Henrich, J., and R. Boyd. 1998. The evolution of conformist transmission and the emergence of between-group differences. *Evol. Hum. Behav.* **19**: 215–242.

Henrich, J., and R. McElreath. 2003. The evolution of cultural evolution. *Evol. Anthro.* **12**:123–135.

Kahneman, D., and Tversky, A. 1979. Prospect theory: An analysis of decision under risk. *Econom.* **47**:263–292.

Kelly, R. C. 1985. The Nuer Conquest: The Structure and Development of an Expansionist System. Ann Arbor: Univ. Mich. Press.

Khuri, F. I. 1970. Parallel cousin marriage reconsidered: A middle eastern practice that nullifies the effects of marriage on the intensity of family relationships. *Man* **5**:597–618.

Laland, K. N. 2004. Social learning strategies. *Learn. Behav.* **32(1)**:4–14.

Land, M. F., and D.-E. Nilsson. 2002. Animal Eyes. Oxford: Oxford Univ. Press.

Lohmann, K. J., C. M. F. Lohmann, L. Ehrhart et al. 2004. Geomagnetic map used in sea turtle navigation. *Nature* **428**: 909–910.

McElreath, R., M. Lubell, P. J. Richerson et al. 2005. Applying evolutionary models to the laboratory study of social learning. *Evol. Hum. Behav.* **26**:483–508.

McNeill W. 1982. The Pursuit of Power: Technology, Armed Force, and Society since A.D. 1000. Chicago: Univ. Chicago Press.

Nilsson, D.-E. 1989. Vision optics and evolution. *BioScience* **39(5)**:298-307.

Payne, J. W., J. R. Bettman, and E. J. Johnson. 1993. The Adaptive Decision Maker. Cambridge: Cambridge Univ. Press.

Raby, C. R., D. M. Alexis, A. Dickinson, and N. S. Clayton. 2007. Planning for the future by western scrub-jays. *Nature* **445**:919–921.

Reader, S. M., and K. N. Laland. 2002. Social intelligence, innovation, and enhanced brain size in primates. *Proc. Nat. Acad. Sci.* **99**:4436–4441.

Real, L. A. 1991. Animal choice behavior and the evolution of cognitive architecture. *Science* **253**:980–886.

Richerson, P. J., R. L. Bettinger, and R. Boyd. 2005. Evolution on a restless planet: Were environmental variability and environmental change major drivers of human evolution? In: Handbook of Evolution: Evolution of Living Systems (including Hominids), ed. F. M. Wuketits and F. J. Ayala, vol. 2, pp. 223–242. Weinheim: Wiley-VCH.

Richerson, P. J., and R. Boyd. 2005. Not by Genes Alone. Chicago: Univ. Chicago Press.

Richerson, P. J., R. Boyd, and R. L. Bettinger. 2001. Was agriculture impossible during the Pleistocene but mandatory during the Holocene? A climate change hypothesis. *Am. Antiq.* **66**:387–411.

Sauer, F. 1957. Die Sternenorientierung nächtlich ziehender Grasmücken (*Sylvia atricapilla, borinund curruca*). *Zeitschrift Tierpsychol.* **14**:29–70.

Sokal R. R., N. L. Oden, and C. Wilson. 1991 Genetic evidence for the spread of agriculture in Europe by demic diffusion. *Nature* **351**:143–145.

Sol, D., R. P. Duncan, T. M. Blackburn, P. Cassey, and L. Lefebvre. 2005. Big brains, enhanced cognition, and response of birds to novel environments. *Proc. Nat. Acad. Sci.* **102(15)**:5461–5465.

Soltis, J., R. Boyd, and P. J. Richerson. 1995. Can group-functional behaviors evolve by cultural group selection? An empirical test. *Curr. Anthro.* **63**:473–494.

Tooby, J., and L. Cosmides. 1992. The psychological foundations of culture. In: The Adapted Mind: Evolutionary Psychology and the Generation of Culture, ed. J. Barkow, L. Cosmides, and J. Tooby, pp. 19–136. New York: Oxford Univ. Press.

Wakano, J. Y., and K. Aoki. 2006. A mixed strategy model for the emergence and intensification of social learning in a periodically changing natural environment. *Theor. Pop. Biol.* **70**:486–497.

16

The Neurobiology of Individual Decision Making, Dualism, and Legal Accountability

Paul W. Glimcher

Departments of Neural Science, Economics and Psychology, Center for Neuroeconomics, New York University, New York, NY 10003, U.S.A.

Introduction

Over the course of the last decade there has been an increasing interest in neurobiological analyses of the causes of behavior among many practitioners of criminal law. In some institutional circles this has crystallized as an interest in providing a physical method for classifying the actions of human agents according to preexisting social–legal categories. The impetus driving this search for neurobiological classification tools stems from both the longstanding Western legal requirement that actors be held accountable only for those voluntary actions which are preceded by what is termed a culpable mental state (those for which *mens rea* can be established) and the longstanding legal difficulty in establishing culpable mental state at trial. Thus a pressing question for many legal practitioners is whether existing neurobiological techniques or data can be used to identify the socially defined categories that guide law and punishment.

If neurobiological measurements did suggest a division of the physical causes of behavior into biological categories closely aligned with social categories, then neuroscience might indeed be very useful for making this legal distinction. In contrast, if neurobiological data suggested that (at a physical rather than a social level) no fundamental division of behavior into these categories could be supported, then we would face a social dilemma of sorts. We would have to decide whether the social consensus that supports differential punishment of actors based on their psycho–legal mental state should persist even if there is compelling neurobiological data that the physical causes of real human actions cannot be divided into the category or categories this legal classification imposes.

In this chapter, I suggest that both the modern epistemological views of natural scientists and the available neurobiological evidence indicates that there is no meaningful sense in which the possible states of the brain can be reduced to a standard psycho–legal state. Indeed, our current level of understanding suggests that at an empirical neurobiological level the distinctions employed by the criminal justice system may be nearly meaningless. These data suggest that there is no compelling evidence for a neural partition that uniquely includes either "rational," voluntary, conscious, or for that matter even "unemotional," mental states.[1]

If in the near future these hints from the neural data become certain conclusions, society and its institutions will face an interesting problem. We will have to decide whether to continue to regard socially defined categories of behavior, like the legal notions of rational and irrational, as fundamental to our institutions.

The Law and Neuroscience

The Legal Classes of Behavior: Involuntary, Compelled, or Rational

Nearly all extant Western legal systems reflect a widely held social conviction that whether an actor should be punished for actions that can be attributed to the actor depends on more than whether the agreed upon events contravene legal statute. Indeed, even whether an agreed upon physical event (e.g., "Jill's arm put a knife into Jack,") can or cannot be considered an "action" in the legal sense depends on Jill's mental state when the knife entered Jack's body. Whether Jill is responsible for a crime depends upon a series of behavioral classification judgments which seek, ultimately, to separate actions into those for which an actor should be held responsible and those for which the actor should not be held responsible. In a perhaps overly simplified sense, the goal of these classifications is to establish whether the observed act was the conscious product of a rational mind, or whether it reflected involuntary, unconscious, or automatic processes as defined at a psycho–legal level.

To make these classifications clear (or at least clearer) to psychologists and neurobiologists, consider the example of an individual who enters knowingly an environment in which it is illegal to utter a profanity. In a first example, the actor suffers from a suddenly acquired and quite severe case of Tourette's syndrome and while in the environment swears loudly. A crime? No. The existing legal structure leads us to conclude that this action was "involuntary"; it

---

[1] There may be, however, significant evidence being developed to support the conscious/non-conscious distinction in a manner that separates it from the rational/irrational distinction (Dehaene et al. 2006).

was committed without the "intent" to swear. In the absence of a voluntary action, there is no crime. In a second example, the actor is approached by an individual with a knife and told to swear loudly on pain of death. The actor swears. A crime? In this case there is no doubt (according to standard legal definitions) that the actor swore voluntarily, but he did so under an external compulsion to which a normal person would have yielded. No crime. A third actor steps on an exposed nail and in response to the bolt of pain from his foot swears loudly. A crime? There are two ways to go here that yield the same result. We can conclude that the act was involuntary; the actor could not have done otherwise given the foot pain, so no crime has been committed. Alternatively, we could conclude that the action was the irrational product of the pain. More precisely we could conclude that a normal person experiencing this pain could not be expected to control his vocal behavior rationally. Again, no crime. A final agent enters the same environment and seeing someone he dislikes swears loudly at them. In legal terms this is a voluntary act, and one committed by a rational person. A crime.

To psychologists and neurobiologists, these categories may seem a bit arbitrary, but they provide the tools by which legal professionals categorize behavior into punishable and nonpunishable (or less punishable) categories. In addition, these two main categories (punishable and nonpunishable) are ones to which nearly all humans are committed. To make that clear, consider two cases. Two men return home to find their wives in bed with other men. In the first case the husband, enraged by this act of infidelity and seeing a loaded gun on the table, shoots and kills his wife. In the second case the husband deliberates for two days, then goes to a gun store, purchases a gun, and returns home to kill his wife. In almost all Western legal systems, the first man's rage is at least partly exculpatory because that rage impaired his rationality; it caused him to behave irrationally at the time of the shooting. The second man, however, must assume full responsibility for his actions because of their deliberative character. The absolutely key point then becomes: was the shooting a "rational" act? If, at the time of the shooting, the man was acting "irrationally" (or more precisely was incapable of acting rationally) or "involuntarily," then he is innocent.

So what exactly are these legal categories that determine culpability? Acting "rationally" here has a very specific legal meaning. It does not mean that the man was producing behavior that maximized anything in the economic sense, although the sense of calculation this evokes does suggest rationality of the legal kind. It does not require that he was engaged in explicitly symbolic psychological processing, although the sense of this class of processing is what the legal definition clearly invokes. It does not mean that regions of the frontal cortex were at least potentially in control of his motor system, although again this is a related sense of the word. According to the *Oxford English Dictionary* "rational action" in the legal sense means: exercising (or able to exercise) one's reason in a proper manner; having sound judgment; sensible, sane.

The critical notion that emerges from these notions of culpability is that actors can be in one of two states (although there may be gray areas between these two states): rational with intent to commit a crime or everything else. If you are rational in this sense at the time of the action, you are guilty; otherwise you are innocent, or at least less guilty. This notion of rational intent is closely tied to terms from psychology such as voluntary, conscious, or (to follow a more recent psychological trend) simply *system 2*. It is criminal behavior that rests within this category which Western legal systems tend to punish most severely. When an actor commits a crime while in a rational mental state, then he receives maximal punishment. The man above who deliberated and purchased a gun before killing his wife provides an example of this kind of rational action.

Behaviors for which actors are not criminally responsible (or at least less responsible) are those which lawyers call involuntary or irrational, and these categories are tied to psychological (but not legal) notions of involuntary, nonconscious, automatic, (sometimes) emotional, or simply system 1 behavior. If it can be demonstrated that a specific criminal act engaged an emotional, automatic, or involuntary process that limits or eliminates the agent's ability to act "rationally," then the process itself becomes exculpatory. There are many examples of behavior of this type, and it cannot be overstated that the Western legal tradition places lighter sanctions on actors guilty of crimes that can be attributed to this class of mental state. If, for example, an actor can be shown to be enraged (under some circumstances), this can mitigate against punishment for a crime.

While each of these categories (rational and the super-category of all exculpatory states) constitutes, in a sense, a doctrinal universe of its own, each of them has recently become of interest to neurobiologically minded lawyers. Precisely because lawyers have become interested in the relationship between neurobiological measurements and rational versus exculpatory classes of behavior, these categories are the subject of this review. These categories are often presumed by legal professionals to be particularly tractable to neurobiological analysis, and it is with that in mind that we begin by examining the social, ethical, and physical basis of the rational/exculpatory distinction—why it is that we punish.

Consequentialist vs. Retributivist Justice

One of the most interesting features of judicial systems, and a feature that engages closely the categorization of behavior into rational and involuntary-irrational, is the underlying reason why institutions punish actors who commit illegal acts. Speaking very broadly, reasons for punishment can be classed as either *retributivist* or *consequentialist*. In these simple black and white terms, a consequentialist legal system is one in which punishments serve only to reduce or eliminate crimes. In designing a consequentialist legal code, for example, one need only consider whether a proposed punishment will reduce crime or improve Society. In contrast, a retributivist system seeks to punish actors who commit crimes specifically because their actions deserve punishment in an ethical or moral sense.

One place where this distinction becomes particularly clear might be in a hypothetical discussion of capital punishment. Consider an imaginary Society in which one could chose between imprisoning particularly heinous criminals for life or executing them. Let us further assume that the monetary cost of executing one of these criminals was higher than the monetary cost of life imprisonment. If we observed that the Society executed criminals, what would this tell us? We might draw one of two conclusions. Working from Jeremy Bentham's consequentialist analysis, we might conclude that the rate of murder was probably being reduced by the visible execution of murders. However, what if we had unimpeachable evidence that executing these criminals had no effect on the rate at which these crimes were committed *and* that everyone was aware of this evidence? Under these conditions a perfect consequentialist system would never perform executions, for executions neither decrease crime nor reduce costs. If one observed executions under these conditions, one could conclude that one was studying a retributivist system of justice. Of course real legal systems do not admit such a simple dichotomous analysis. Executions may reduce murders, or at least members of Society might believe that executions reduce murders. On the other hand, it does seem that there may be more than just consequentialist motives at work in many legal systems.

The reason I bring this up is that retributivist systems seem to rely particularly heavily on the voluntary-rational/involuntary-irrational exculpatory super-category distinctions for their existence. To make this clear, consider a legal system that lacked this distinction. Actors commit crimes. Demonstrating that an individual killed someone, a simple finding of fact, would be a complete finding of guilt. Once we determine that fact-finding establishes guilt, then we must decide whether everyone receives the same punishment for the same crime. Without the voluntary-rational/involuntary-irrational distinction there can be only one reason for differential punishment of our different actors: the conclusion that minimizing the risk of future crimes required that different degrees of punishment be meted out to different individuals. If there is a single category of behavior then we punish all actors who commit that externally observable crime in the same way, or we adjust punishment individual-by-individual so as to minimize future crime.

However—and this may not be immediately obvious to natural scientists—this is not what we often observe in the Western legal tradition, particularly in the U.S. tradition. Some actors are punished more severely than others and not because those receiving harsher punishment require a higher level of deterrence. Instead, the force of punishment in these Western laws reflects both our convictions about the actor's culpability for his or her actions and considerations about the positive effects of punishment for Society at large. To make that clear, let us return to the example of the two men who kill their wives. Why do we punish more severely the man who deliberates for two days than the one who kills impulsively while enraged? Certainly not because we want to discourage deliberation when enraged. If we were simply attempting to deter crime, we might even conclude that it was the enraged man who should be punished more severely. We might well hypothesize that only the threat of very severe punishment has a hope of deterring someone in that mental state. In other words, the structure of our punishment system is, if anything, anti-consequentialist. Behaviors that are more automatic would probably be punished more harshly in a consequentialist system. We observe the opposite in our system. People are largely being punished because they deserve it.[2]

Many natural scientists may object to the conclusion that retributivist approaches to justice reflect a social consensus. They may argue instead that retributivism in our culture reflects an antiquated feature of the Western legal tradition, and one that is on the wane. It is important to point out that this is simply not the case. Notions of fairness drive human behavior in a wide variety of situations, many of which have been well studied by social scientists. Consider, for example, the ultimatum game popular in behavioral economics (Blout 1995; Güth et al. 1982; McCabe et al. 2001). Two players in different cities, who have never met and who will never meet, sit at computer monitors. A scientist gives one of these players $10 and asks her to propose a division of that money between the two strangers. The second player can then decide whether to accept the proposed split. If she accepts, the money is divided and both players go home richer. If she rejects the offer, then the experimenter retains the $10, and the players gain nothing. What is interesting about this game is that when the proposer offers the second player $2.50 or less the second player rejects the offer. The result is that rather than going home with $2.50, the second player goes home with nothing. Why does she give up the $2.50?

We might derive a partial answer to this question from examining what happens when the first player is replaced by a computer program which, the second player is informed, plays exactly the same distribution of strategies that real human players employ. Under these conditions, if the computer offers $2.50 the second player almost invariably accepts it. Why?

The standard interpretation of this finding is that players refuse the $2.50 from a human opponent because they perceive the offer to be unfair. They want to punish the proposer by depriving her of $7.50, which the players have determined that she does not deserve. Players will happily spend $2.50 to achieve this goal. When playing a computer, whose actions they see as mechanical and involuntary, they happily accept the $2.50. I think that we have

---

[2] This point (that our legal systems are significantly retributivist in structure) is widely acknowledged in legal circles, although it may be unfamiliar to natural scientists. In developing this point in more detail, the American legal scholar, Owen Jones, has argued that we must be aware of the biological imperatives that drive some classes of crimes when we design criminal codes. This issue was addressed in his famous article, "The Law of Law's Leverage" (Jones 2001).

a clear pattern here. Under conditions ranging from splitting $10 to murder, nearly all people indicate a conviction that actors should be punished when they voluntarily act unjustly. One can speculate about the evolutionary roots of this taste for justice (e.g., Brosnan and deWaal 2003) or this drive for fairness, but there is no escaping the conclusion that it is an essential feature of human behavior today.

Wherefore Neuroscience in Law?

In the preceding sections, I hoped to make two points. The first was that the Western judicial tradition and nearly all members of Western societies possess a preexisting consensus that there is a social distinction between voluntary-rational and an exculpatory super-class of involuntary-irrational behaviors. This is a deeply fixed element in our institutional designs and probably in the evolved biological fabric of our brains. The second point was that our judicial systems are at least partially retributivist in nature. Like the distinction between these two classes of behavior, this reflects a strong social consensus. It is important, however, to note that these two principles interact. We take retribution for actions socially defined as voluntary and rational. For acts socially defined as involuntary, irrational, or compelled we mete out limited punishment—punishment that is often more consequentialist in nature.

The point that we have to keep in mind here is that, in a very real sense, *this works*. We have a working social consensus, so what possible role could neuroscience play in any of this from the point of view of a practicing lawyer or judge? The answer stems from the institutional need to segregate (in particular) voluntary and rational behavior from these other classes of behavior which are deemed exculpatory[3]. This is a fundamental problem with the system as it currently exists, and there is much hope in some legal circles that neuroscientific evidence can be used to segregate voluntary, conscious, and rational acts from involuntary, nonconscious, irrational acts. The reason this is necessary should be immediately obvious: Because we punish voluntary-rational acts more severely, it is in the interest of all defendants to establish that their crimes were committed in an irrational or involuntary mental state. This means that juries and judges are often in the position of trying to decide whether an act was rational. The question in legal circles, then, is: Can neurobiological data, for example from a brain scanner, be used to identify voluntary-rational behavior as the preexisting legal system defines it?

At least logically, the answer to this seems like it should be yes. Imagine that we used our social consensus to label each of one million particularly

---

[3] Currently, there is also great interest in the possibility of using neuroscientific methods to establish issues of liability: "Did she do it?" The rising interest in using brain scanners to identify lying is an example of this interest. Here I am discussing only the issue of responsibility which bears on the voluntary/involuntary distinction. In considering issues of liability, the reader is referred to Wolpe et al. (2005) and Garland and Glimcher (2006).

unambiguous crimes as voluntary-rational or excusable: five hundred thousand in each category. Then imagine that we subjected all one million of these individuals to brain scans. Intuitively, it seems obvious that such an endeavor would yield a portrait of the distinction between voluntary-rational and involuntary-irrational crime at the neural level. But would this really have to work?

To answer that question, consider more mathematically what we are trying to accomplish. During the brain scans, we measure the average activity of each cubic millimeter of brain, or voxel. Imagine that we scanned only three of the cubic millimeters in each individual. Then we could represent the activity of each brain as a trio of measurements, the activity in each of the three voxels, a point on a three-dimensional graph. Now imagine that we do this on 500,000 people guilty of voluntary crimes. The result is a cloud of points, we can imagine them colored red, in this three-dimensional space. Then we do the same thing for the people who committed crimes involuntarily. They produce a second cloud of points, imagine them colored green. Of course in a real brain scan we would observe the activity of about 60,000 voxels simultaneously so these clouds of points would be distributed in a much more complicated (60,000-dimensional) space, but we have good mathematical tools for moving back and forth between these kinds of graphs so the higher dimensional space presents no conceptual barrier that we cannot overcome. Having generated a graph of these one million points, here is the critical question that we want to answer: Can we draw a circle[4] around the voluntary-rational points that includes none (or at least very few) of the exculpatory-state points? That is the critical question.

If the answer is yes, then whenever we want to establish if an actor committed a crime in a culpable mental state, we place her in a brain scanner. If her point falls within the circle, then she is guilty. What this analysis reveals is that for this approach to work, the clouds of points must land in separate places in the 60,000-dimensional space; if the points are all intermingled, then the approach will fail. Now if, for example, conscious rational-voluntary acts (as defined legally) are the specific product of a single brain area; if brain area X, made up of 1000 voxels, was more active when a crime was committed in a culpable mental state than when it was committed in an exculpatory state, causing the two clouds of points to separate, then the method will work. If, on the other hand, there is no coherent logical mapping between the states of these brain voxels and the legal notion of culpable mental state, then this approach is doomed to failure.

Although I have explained this logic for a contemporary brain scanner, it is important to note that what I have explained is true, in principle, for all of the neural (or more generally all physical) measurements we could imagine making. Consider measuring the brain levels of a single neurotransmitter. If

---

4   More formally, we would be searching for a hyperplane in the 60,000-dimensional space after computing and removing the covariance matrix.

culpable crimes are uniquely associated with low levels of this neurotransmitter, then the method will work. If there is a completely overlapping distribution of neurotransmitter levels in the culpable and exculpatory groups, then the method will fail. The same is true for some bigger and better future brain scanner. If there is any feature of the anatomy or physiology of the human brain that can support a partition of behavior into these categories, then neuroscience will be relevant to this problem. If no feature of the natural structure of the brain can support this categorization of action into two domains, then neuroscience will not be of use, and it may even call into question the wisdom of this categorization depending upon your convictions about the relationship between physical and social phenomena.

To proceed, what we have to do next is to understand how likely it is that neuroscientific evidence can support the division of behavior into these two categories. It is certainly true that both philosophy and physiology seemed to support the existence of these two categories up until about a hundred years ago, but that may be changing. So next we turn to both the epistemology and physiology of voluntary-rational action. What we will find is compelling evidence to discard, at the neurobiological level of analysis, the philosophical notion of Free Will. Secondary to that conclusion, we will also find that the available empirical evidence leans against the notion that the socially defined categories of voluntary-rational and involuntary-irrational can be identified neurobiologically. While this second point is admittedly a preliminary empirical conclusion, it will raise some potentially troubling issues.

Neuroscience and the Law

To understand how neuroscientists see the issues of voluntary-rational and exculpatory classes of behavior, it is critical to recognize what it is that neuroscientists are trying to understand when they study the brain. Consider the hotly debated topic of face perception. The human ability to identify familiar faces is astonishing. Show a human a stack of 24 pictures of different peoples' faces for a few seconds each. Wait 15 minutes. Then show the person a stack of 48 faces: the 24 old faces and 24 new faces. The average human can correctly pull out 90% of the faces that they saw (Bruce 1982). The average human cannot do this with pictures of sheep, pictures of cars, or pictures of houses (cf. Kanwisher and Yovel 2006; Gobini and Haxby 2007). Now how does this ability arise at the mechanistic level?

Prior to the research that yielded the neuroscientific evidence on this issue, there were two theories. Theory 1 argued that humans had a highly specialized (and probably anatomically localized) brain system for recognizing human faces: a machine, in our heads, optimized for the recognition of faces and nothing else. In essence, this theory argued that there was a face recognition system and an "everything else" recognition system. It was a two-system view of face recognition. Theory 2 argued that there was only one system for general recognition, but this theory went on to argue that since humans spend so much time recognizing human faces in normal everyday life, this general-purpose system happens to be particularly good at recognizing faces. This theory, in essence, argued that while it is true that we are better at recognizing human faces than houses, this ability arises from the actions of a single system.

Brain imaging weighed in on this issue when it was discovered that if you show a human subject pictures of faces for two minutes and then pictures of houses for two minutes, you see two very different patterns of brain activation (Kanwisher at al. 1997). When humans view faces, a small region in the temporal lobe of the brain, now called the fusiform face area, becomes highly active. This phenomenon is highly reproducible. In fact, the level of activation in this area can be used to determine whether a human subject is looking at a picture of a face or a house even if she refuses to tell you verbally. So what does this mean? First, and unarguably, this means you can tell what a human subject is looking at in this example, but does this also mean that neuroscientists have concluded that the brain can be usefully described as being made of two recognition systems: one for faces and one for other things? The answer to this is much more complicated and far from settled. To resolve that question, one group of neurobiologists trained a small group of humans to become experts at recognizing a class of non-face geometric objects called "greebles" and then asked whether "greeble experts" used the "fusiform face area" when they recognized greebles. Their evidence suggests that this was the case, and so they concluded that either (a) there is a brain area responsible for "expert" recognition and a more general system for "nonexpert" recognition or (b) there is no expert system, but the fusiform face area is active for any recognition problem which is difficult and for which subjects are well trained (Gauthier et al. 1999).

These experiments were followed by a host of other experiments: on car recognition by car experts, studies of patients with damage to the fusiform face area (who cannot recognize faces but can perform normally at many other recognition tasks), recognition of inverted faces (Haxby et al. 2001). In total, literally millions of dollars and hundreds of first-class scientists struggled to resolve this problem. The problem that they wanted to resolve was whether the architecture of the brain could be described as having a face recognition system and an "other-stuff" recognition system in a deep and natural sense. They were asking: Is there an intrinsic distinction in the neural architecture between face and non-face? There may not yet be a consensus on this issue, but at the moment it is probably safe to say that more neuroscientists believe that face recognition is accomplished by a discrete system than feel otherwise. Still, this is an incredibly controversial issue, and the case is far from closed. It does, however, look like faces may be a natural neural category.

Is there a similar neural distinction between voluntary-rational and involuntary-irrational? Can we determine whether there is a meaningful neural category for voluntary-rational behavior? Or at least the possibility of segregating voluntary-rational states from all other brain states? To answer those questions, neurobiologists take two approaches: an epistemological approach that asks whether, in principle, there are reasons to expect such a category and an empirical approach, such as the one described above, for face perception. First, let us turn to the philosophical roots of the voluntary-rational versus involuntary-irrational problem.

Epistemic Beliefs about the Voluntary vs. Involuntary Distinction

Free Will

Prior to the enlightenment, Aristotelian and Platonic notions of the mind dominated scholarly debates about the sources of human action. Aristotle had concluded, largely in *De Anima*, that all living beings possessed souls and that the complexity of these nonphysical objects increased as the mental complexity of living beings increased. Aristotle saw the nonmaterial souls of humans as causal agents uniquely responsible for observed behavior. Although questions were raised during this period about whether souls really occurred in non-human organisms, the notion that a nonmaterial soul was the unique causal agent responsible for human behavior became a widely held idea. During the Reformation, this notion was challenged by emerging Protestant theologians (for example Luther and Calvin) who, working from the ideas of Aquinas and Augustine, developed the doctrine of predestination. This doctrine argued against the classical notion of a causal soul on at least two grounds. First, the doctrine argued that only God could act as a causal agent. Second, and more importantly, the doctrine recognized that making the human soul a causal agent independent of *God's will* or *God's omniscient knowledge* meant that at least some future events would be unknown to God. This set up a conflict between the omniscience of God and the causal independence of the human soul. They resolved this conflict by concluding that although there was a nonmaterial human soul, it was not a causal agent. (This is a theology typically referred to as "double predestination" and is particularly associated with the works of Calvin). Thus according to the early Protestants, human action was the mechanical product of a deterministic soul that reflected a preordained divine program. For these theologians, and a major segment of the European intelligentsia during the Reformation, human actors were, at least at a philosophical level, viewed as entirely deterministic devices.

Within the Catholic Church, this philosophy prompted a heated debate during the 16th and 17th centuries. At that time, a group of scholars centered around the Flemish theologian, Cornelius Jansen, argued that this Protestant notion was logical and compatible with Catholic doctrine. The Jesuits and others close to the Papacy believed, however, that the human soul must be viewed as a causal agent for the notions of moral judgment, especially salvation and damnation, to be meaningful. In the end, the Jesuits triumphed in this debate, and much of Jansen's writings were declared heretical by the middle of the 17th century. The result was that the Catholic Church initially adopted a unitary classical position on the causes of human behavior: The soul of man makes choices that are causally responsible for all actions taken by a person. The choices that the soul makes are unconstrained; man is free to produce any action. God judges all of those actions as just or unjust, and on this basis saves or damns each individual.

For our purposes, I want to draw attention to the fact that neither of these approaches is really compatible, at a deep philosophical level, with the Western retributivist tradition, which rests on two classes of behavior. If all human action is equally predestined, then how can one support different levels of culpability based on mental state? The same question, in reverse, can be asked of the Catholic tradition: If all human action is the product of a unitary voluntary-rational mechanism, then how can we single out some actions as exempt from punishment? The existence of these philosophical traditions, however, had very little impact on the ongoing Western legal tradition. When the city of Geneva became Protestant, it did not abandon Roman law. The law and its psycho–legal consensus were effectively partitioned from these metaphysical conclusions. I mention this because it is a point to which we will have to return later.

In any case, it was the reconciliation of these two models, in the 17th century, that led to the widely held modern metaphysical and empirical conviction that there are at least two independent sources of human action. I turn next to the reconciliation that occurred principally within the Catholic Church.

The Catholic Dualization of Human Action

The history of this dualization began with the surge in anatomical studies conducted during the 1500s, which revealed that the human physical corpus was surprisingly material and much more mechanistic than had been previously supposed. Great European anatomists, like Vesalius, Sylvius, and Fallopius, catalogued the intricacies of human anatomy meticulously (cf. Vesalius 1543/1998). Concurrently, the progenitors of physiology sought to provide clear mechanistic explanations of the functions of these human anatomical components. William Harvey (1628/1995), to take the most prominent example, went so far as to explain that the human heart, which Aristotle (in *De Anima*) had identified as the physical location of the soul, was nothing more than a pump. These scientists, modeling their physiological investigations on the emerging field of mechanics, described simple cause and effect relationships that accounted for the actions of the human body. Basing their understanding of physiology on the clockwork deterministic mechanisms that were being invented every day during this period, they began to perceive the human body as a predictable machine.

Descartes' avowed goal was to provide a philosophical basis for understanding the material interactions that governed the physical world while preserving the Catholic notion that the actions of the human soul were a distinct category of events that could not be deterministically tied to the material events and processes of the corporeal realm. He accomplished this goal by dividing all of human behavior into two exclusive categories. He presumed the first category to be the deterministic product of the physical body—a class of behaviors we now often call *reflexes*. The second category included those actions that could be attributed to the causal force of the human soul. These *voluntary* actions were characterized empirically by being unpredictable, and it was Descartes' conclusion that the causes of these actions lay outside the material world and could not form the subject of physiological inquiry. Descartes thus opened a segment of human behavior for physiological study while reserving to voluntary behavior an extra-physical notion of agency. However, from a legal and ethical point of view, Descartes did something else: for the simple behaviors that he classed as *deterministic reflexes*, there could be no (or at the very least a diminished) moral culpability; for the more complicated and unpredictable behaviors, there was complete moral culpability. The distinction between voluntary and involuntary was reified at both the metaphysical and empirical levels, thus removing a preexisting tension between the law and philosophers (natural and otherwise).

The critical feature of the scientific study of voluntary and involuntary behavior that I am trying to bring out here is a debate about whether the causes of behavior can be usefully described as intrinsically breaking apart along the voluntary-rational and involuntary-irrational (or exculpatory) boundary. Descartes argued that this would be the case: that involuntary behaviors, reflexes, would be shown to have a straightforward physical implementation and that if one could trace a deterministic path through the nervous system that accounted for the behavior then it could be labeled involuntary. The voluntary behaviors, he argued, could not be deterministically accounted for by simple mechanical and deterministic components; these behaviors were the product of what philosophers now term "contra-causal metaphysical libertarian freedom."

One really nice feature of this approach is that it suggests that the neurobiological approach will identify two categories of mechanisms that map directly to the social–legal notion of voluntary-rational/involuntary-irrational. In other words, if neurobiologists persist long enough, then we will have simple and direct neurobiological markers for the voluntary-rational/involuntary-irrational distinction. What is most amazing to many neurobiologists is that by the early 20th century, the courts had begun to settle on this approach.

A particularly clear example of this is a U.S. Supreme Court decision from the early 1900s: Hotema v. the U.S. The case concerns a plaintiff, Solomon Hotema, who was convicted of killing Vina Coleman on April 14, 1899. Hotema plead not guilty by reason of insanity, although this defense failed. In evaluating his insanity plea the court noted:

> A safe and reasonable test is that whenever it shall appear from all the evidence that at the time of committing the act the defendant was sane, and this conclusion is proved to the satisfaction of the jury, taking into consideration all the evidence in the case, beyond a reasonable doubt, he will be held amenable to the law. Whether the insanity be general or partial, whether continuous or periodical, the degree of it must have been sufficiently great to have controlled the will of the accused at the time of the commission of the act. Where reason ceases to have dominion over the mind proved to be diseased, the person reaches a degree of insanity where criminal responsibility ceases and accountability to the law for the purpose of punishment no longer exists.

The decision continues in this vein, citing the lower court's decision:

> The real test, as I understand it, of liability or nonliability rests upon the proposition whether at the time the homicide was committed Hotema had a diseased [186 U.S. 413, 417] brain, and it was not partially diseased or to some extent diseased, but diseased to the extent that he was incapable of forming a criminal intent, and that the disease had so taken charge of his brain and had so impelled it that for the time being his will power, judgment, reflection, and control of his mental faculties were impaired so that the act done was an irresistible and uncontrollable impulse with him at the time he committed the act. If his brain was in this condition, he cannot be punished by law. But if his brain was not in this condition, he can be punished by law, remembering that the burden is upon the government to establish that he was of sound mind, and by that term is not meant that he was of perfectly sound mind, but that he had sufficient mind to know right from wrong, and knowing that the act he was committing at the time he was performing it was a wrongful act in violation of human law, and he could be punished therefore, and that he did not perform the act because he was controlled by irresistible and uncontrollable impulse. In that state of case the defendant could not be excused upon the ground of insanity, and it would be your duty to convict him. But if you find from the evidence, or have a reasonable doubt in regard thereto, that his brain at the time he committed the act was impaired by disease, and the homicide was the product of such disease, and that he was incapable of forming a criminal intent, and that he had no control of his mental faculties and the will power to control his actions, but simply slew Vina Coleman because he was laboring under a delusion which absolutely controlled him, and that his act was one of irresistible impulse, and not of judgment, in that event he would be entitled to an acquittal.

What is clear here is that the court is separating behavior into two possible categories: those which are rational and those which are irrational, involuntary, or exculpatory—a perfectly normal, if in this case somewhat ambiguous, legal thing to do. Rational behaviors are subject to legal sanction; irrational, involuntary, or compelled actions are not. A second feature of the decision is the court's effort to tie the irrational or compelled behavior to the properties of Hotema's brain. Punishing Solomon Hotema reflects a conviction that it was his voluntary-rational self, and not simply an irrational or involuntary action (in this ruling an action linked to his brain), that is responsible for this action.

To be clear, let me stress that this was not the only way that the court could have gone in interpreting the issue of insanity. In other settings the same court stressed the idea that what makes an act insane is the mental (and here I specifically use mental not neural) state of the person at the time of the criminal act. When that occurs, a behavioral criterion is used to identify behavior that lies beyond legal sanction in a very traditional way. What makes this case so interesting are two things. First, the court extended a tradition hundreds of years old when it argued that behavior should be categorized into what are basically voluntary-rational and exculpatory divisions. Second, it did something fairly novel in trying to develop a biological marker for an exculpatory class of behavior.

Beyond Descartes and Hotema: Metaphysical Issues

To understand how these philosophical notions of voluntary and involuntary behavior influence the thoughts of neurobiologists *today*, we have to look beyond Descartes and the Hotema decision at two critical advances in Western scientific thought. The first of these advances is the rise of materialism during the last century and a growing conviction among both scholars and much of the lay public that all phenomena, even all of human behavior, are the exclusive product of purely material events. The second is a recent (and perhaps unexpected) challenge to determinism. This challenge reflects a growing conviction among some scientists that although all of the events that we can observe are the product of the material world, not all of these events are necessarily predictable in principle. Some events reflect irreducible randomness in the physical world.

One of the central, if not *the* central, products of the Enlightenment was the philosophical stance of materialism. The philosophers of the Enlightenment argued against the notion that magical powers (like those implicitly evoked by traditional notions of Free Will: an unmeasurable force that cannot be studied with physical methods but which shapes the universe around us) played a causal role in the physical world. Instead they sought to explain, at a material level, everything about the world. By the late 20th century, this notion had been extended even to the study of human behavior. It is now commonplace to state that the mind is produced entirely by the brain. Essentially all Western scientists now accept the notion that materialism extends unequivocally to the human mind.

If we accept that even human behavior is a material product of the brain, then it seems likely that we have to accept the notion that all of human behavior is deterministic in character. And, if we accept that this is true, then humans are no more causal agents than billiard balls interacting on a pool table. Indeed, this extreme stance argues that humans cannot be seen by biologists as causal agents in any meaningful way, irrespective of whether jurists choose to retain a social consensus that labels some behaviors voluntary or rational. Many modern thinkers, however, find this notion implicitly distasteful and are troubled by the fact that much of human behavior does not seem deterministic. On these grounds, many scholars (including many biologists) dismiss materialist notions that all of behavior obeys simple physical laws. This deterministic conclusion, however, is not necessarily true for reasons that are not always obvious, and I want to take a few paragraphs to explain why. Understanding this last issue is important before we try to understand the current tension between consequentialist and ethical approaches to human behavior, because we have to understand why materialism and determinism are not identical before we try to understand the sources of human behavior.

Prior to the 20th century, it was assumed that all physical objects would obey the laws of physics which were then believed to be fully deterministic. In the early 20th century, however, quantum theory challenged that notion. What quantum theory demonstrated was that under some conditions, physical events are fundamentally unpredictable because they are random[5]. Let me be very clear about this though. This does not mean that some events in the physical world are unpredictable because we do not yet understand them, or because they show a pattern of behavior that is so complicated that they simply appear random to human observers (a mathematical property called "complex non-linear dynamics" or more popularly "chaos theory"). This means that they are unpredictable in a fundamental way, and that this unpredictability follows clear physical laws. There is nothing magical here, just a recognition that fundamentally random processes are one of the processes within the physical domain. The point is that these processes are both fully lawful (in the physical sense) and unpredictable. For a physical scientist there is no conflict or magical thinking implicit or implied by these notions.

So what does the existence of fundamentally random processes in the physical world mean for a philosophical understanding of the causal role of human agents in the physical world? First, it means that an agent could, at least in principle, be unpredictable while being fully material. This distinction is important because it removes a central barrier (for many people) to accepting a material stance with regard to human action. Human action does not appear deterministic, and there is no material reason why it should be deterministic.

---

[5]   In this regard, quantum theory differed in a philosophical way from the work of earlier scientists such as Quetelet, who studied human behavior at the statistical level, or Maxwell and Boltzmann, who studied the statistical behavior of small particles. Although their work rested on a strongly probabilistic foundation, it did not challenge the scientific assumption that physical events were deterministic. In fact, Quetelet was often attacked for suggesting that the statistical regularities in human behavior implied some kind of determinism—a point from which he often tried to distance himself.

Second, it means that the events which follow from the actions of a stochastic actor cannot be predicted completely from the state of the environment or from the state of actor. Unpredictable events are set in motion, *caused,* by the stochastic actions of the actor. It does not mean that any special property that lies outside the physical world, such as the magical force of Free Will, is required. The critical points are:

1. The apparent contradiction between materialism and the notion that humans are fundamentally unpredictable actors is not a contradiction at all. It would only be a contradiction if it were the case that all of human action is deterministic.

2. If we allow humans to incorporate stochasticity (true randomness) into their behavior, we recover the notion that humans can cause unpredictable events *de novo,* but *not* the notion that they can exercise Free Will in any meaningful way, a kind of *will-free agency* (or agency without Free Will).

3. Only if we place the source of human action outside the material domain, beyond the laws of both determinate and indeterminate physics, can we recover *free-willed agency* for human actors.

The problem, of course, is that the last of these possibilities contradicts the materialistic philosophical stance that Western science has taken as axiomatically true for the last century or two. (It is also undeniable that the past two centuries, i.e., the period since the adoption of that axiom, have been very productive for the physical and natural sciences.)

Beyond Descartes and Hotema: Empirical Issues

The Empirical Search for a Voluntary-Rational Boundary

The discussion above reflects a view held by many neurobiologists; namely, that humans do not have Free Will in any deep sense. Still, even in the absence of such a belief, we may well be able to divide behavior into the socially defined categories of voluntary-rational and exculpatory at the neurobiological level. To see how these philosophical insights have influenced the empirical data we use to parse the natural categories of neural function, consider a recent experiment on monkey decision making which was conducted under two sets of conditions: one yielded behavior that could be socially classified as involuntary whereas the second yielded behavior that could be classified as voluntary and rational (Glimcher 2005; Dorris and Glimcher 2004). About four years ago Michael Dorris and I trained both humans and monkeys to perform two tasks. The first was very simple and designed to elicit an involuntary behavior. A central spot of light appeared on a computer monitor in front of the subject. The subject's task was to fixate that light. After a delay, two other lights illuminated (one green and one red) on either side of the fixation spot. After a pause, the central spot then turned red or green and the subject was rewarded for simply looking at the color-matched target as quickly as possible. To make this orienting eye movement as reflexive as possible, we overtrained our subjects on this task. They performed this response literally tens of thousands of times. They did this task until it was as automatic as possible. Then, we traced some of the neural pathways active during this behavior in the monkeys and found that much of the nervous system governing eye movements behaved deterministically under these conditions and accurately foretold the deterministic actions of the monkeys. In particular, we focused on a group of cells in the posterior parietal cortex that behaved deterministically and could, at least in principle, account for the behavior of the monkeys during this automatic and presumably involuntary task.

Next, we trained the same subjects to play a strategic game developed by economists known as "Work or Shirk" or "The Inspection Game" (Fudenberg and Tirole 1991). In this situation, two agents face each other and play a repeated game of strategy in which they have to outwit their opponents in order to maximize their winnings. Importantly, we taught both humans and monkeys to play this game. When we asked the humans if their behavior during the game should be classified as voluntary, they all responded by saying yes. When we compared the behavior of the humans and the monkeys during the game, their behavior was identical. One could not tell the behavior of an individual monkey from the behavior of an individual human. If monkeys are capable of voluntary-rational behavior, then we reasoned that this must be it.

Now the interesting part is what happened when we studied the posterior parietal cortices of these monkeys. Once again we found that the same brain area was active, and that this same single brain area continued to predict the behavior of the monkeys. Only now, these same neurons were behaving stochastically. In other words, we found no evidence for the voluntary/involuntary distinction at a neural level. Instead, we found a single neural machine that could produce (and from which we could predict) both the deterministic and stochastic behavior of our monkeys. From the point of view of these neurons, there was no distinction that we could find between voluntary and involuntary action.

While this is admittedly only one experiment (and I have only provided the very briefest description of that experiment), it does seem to suggest that the voluntary/involuntary distinction may not be a natural category at the neurobiological level. Since that time a number of other experiments in humans have seemed to bear out this conclusions (see the many chapters in this volume for more examples).

For me, this comes as no surprise. The entire Western scientific tradition rests on the axiom that all the phenomena that we observe are the product of events governed by physical law and thus that all phenomena in the universe can, at least in principle, be the subject of scientific inquiry. While I recognize that there are some scholars who would disagree with this axiom, I take it as a starting point. Second, given that starting point, the classical metaphysical notion of Free Will—a causal process not constrained by either the deterministic or the stochastic laws of physics—is untenable at this time and can be rejected. Third, even the notion that the socially defined construct of voluntary behavior will have a clear and meaningful neurobiological substrate seems unlikely. In fact, much of the data presented in this volume seems to suggest that this is now a consensus view. While the brain involves many systems for generating actions, there seems no compelling evidence that the two-system description is of any utility in describing the brain.

Do Neuroscience and Law Collide?

What all of this suggests is that we need to be very careful how we use neurobiological evidence in addressing the question of responsibility. Neurobiological evidence, from its metaphysical stance to the available empirical data, seems to argue against the existence of a voluntary/involuntary distinction at the physiological level. Our legal systems, our (presumably evolved) sense of fairness, our willingness to place justice in the hands of government all rest on this distinction between voluntary-rational and involuntary-irrational-exculpatory behavior at the psycho–legal level. That inconsistency makes reductionist approaches to the law, which seek to map explanations explicitly at these two levels to one another, perilous at best.

As a society we have a consensus that children are less responsible for their acts than adults. At a scientific level, it is easy to see how we can categorize actors into children and adults. We can even use neurobiological evidence to support this categorization in a fairly clear way (although for reasons that will be come clear below, I think that even this is a slippery slope that should be avoided). As a society we have a consensus that people experiencing strong emotional states such as rage are acting less rationally than those in emotionally neutral states and so should be held less responsible for their actions than others. However, where exactly do we draw the line between the two categories of voluntary-rational and exculpatory under these emotional conditions? In the American legal system, we draw the line on this issue by asking if the stimulus that produced the emotional state would have enraged an "ordinary and reasonable person" making it difficult or impossible for him to act rationally. What the many contributions in this volume and the work of neurobiological scholars who are experts on emotion tell us is that this distinction does not correspond to a natural category of neural function.

So what emerges from this discussion, at least for me, is a profound skepticism about the notion that behavior can be meaningfully divided into two useful legal categories by any of the materialistic methods we encounter typically. I am arguing that the common belief that we can divide behavior into voluntary-rational and involuntary-irrational categories on neurobiological grounds and can conclude that involuntary-irrational behaviors lie beyond legal sanction is an artifact of how Descartes chose to engage the issues of Free Will and ethical responsibility in a material world. Conscious or nonconscious (as it is typically used), voluntary or involuntary, mind or brain (the worst of the three when used in this way) are all notions that I believe were originally rooted in ideas about Free Will as a contra-causal mystical force.

Are these ruminations simply the puzzled thoughts of a neurobiologist, or are any of them directly relevant to contemporary legal issues? To answer that question let me turn to studies of serotonin (a neural chemical also called 5-hydroxytraptamine or 5-HT), depression (a psychologically defined state), and violence. This is relevant because a number of legal cases involving violent acts have begun to involve measurements of brain serotonin, and I believe that these cases involve the critical error of trying to map a neurobiological phenomenon onto the voluntary/involuntary distinction—a mapping which I have argued is probably impossible, and certainly premature.

The data we have that motivates this legal use goes like this: We begin with a psychological-level definition of clinical depression and note that individuals meeting these psychological criteria are more prone to violence than the average human. Second, we treat most forms of depression today with drugs that increase brain levels of serotonin. Drugs of this type include the widely known Eli Lilly drug Prozac. Increasing brain levels of serotonin decreases the risk of violence and controls the psychological state of depression in many individuals[6]. Thus we have a clear set of isomorphic relationships at the neurobiological, psychological, and behavioral levels. Given these facts, the goal of some criminal defense lawyers has been to argue, from neurobiological measurements, toward the definition of the defendant's action as involuntary or irrational. This means that the defense argues in violent crimes, typically homicides, that either (a) low brain levels of serotonin are evidence that the defendant could not commit a willfully criminal (or intentional) act because of a diminished capacity for rationality or (b) punishment would be unjust because the low serotonin levels indicate a diminished voluntary component to the crime[7].

The first of these issues, the issue of criminal intent and its relation to the existence of a predisposing brain state, arises principally in defenses during second-degree murder trials. One of the requirements in such a trial is for the prosecution to show that the defendant formed a clear criminal intent that motivated his act. That it was his intention—and here I use a psychological word strongly but not uniquely associated with the idea of the conscious self—to commit homicide. What we find is that recently a number of defendants have

---

[6] Indeed, we even know that decreases in brain serotonin levels increase the risk of both depression and violent acts.

[7] I think that these two arguments are different for reasons that I hope will be clear in the following pages.

argued that the existence of their low brain serotonin levels means that they could not form a true criminal intent, essentially because their behavior can be related to a measurable state of their brain (for an excellent review of this literature and its often circular reasoning, see Farahany and Coleman 2006). In my reading of these cases, the defense in question basically seeks (a) to tie the behavior to the involuntary-irrational class *on the grounds that a brain chemical is involved* and (b) to place the involuntary-irrational behavior (involuntary because it involved a brain chemical) beyond the bounds of legal sanction on ethical grounds. For me this is essentially the Hotema case—antique notions of the relationship between brain and psychology (and Free Will) in a modern legal defense. Although I am sure these revisitations of the Hotema case deserve a more complete treatment, I am going to dismiss these classes of defense as silly now that we know that "caused by the brain" cannot possibly mean exactly the same thing as involuntary (or irrational).

The second of these issues, the more challenging one, involves the use of brain levels of serotonin to mitigate punishment in a more subtle way. In Hill v. Ozmint, an important case carefully reviewed in Farahany and Coleman (2006), David Clayton Hill was convicted of shooting a South Carolina police officer at a car wash. His lawyers made several related arguments during the sentencing phase of his trial, described here in the record of his appeal:

In his IAC claim, Hill maintains that his defense lawyers were ineffective in calling Dr. Edward [**39] Burt to testify during the trial's sentencing phase. At sentencing, Hill's lawyers sought to show that Hill suffered from a genetic condition that caused neurochemical imbalances in his brain. Specifically, they contended that Hill suffered from a genetically based serotonin [*202] deficiency, which resulted in aggressive impulses. After his arrest and incarceration, Hill had been prescribed medication that they believed had successfully curbed these impulses. Thus, according to Hill's lawyers, the death penalty was not warranted because Hill's aggressive behavior was genetic (i.e., beyond his control) and treatable. To this end, Hill's lawyers presented the testimony of Dr. Emil Coccaro, who explained the role of serotonin in brain chemistry, as well as how genetics affects serotonin levels. Next, the defense called Dr. Bernard Albiniak, a forensic psychologist, who had performed a series of spinal taps on Hill to monitor his serotonin levels. Dr. Albiniak opined that Hill suffered from a chronic serotonin deficiency.

Finally, the defense called Hill's psychiatrist, Dr. Edward Burt. Dr. Burt was expected to testify that he had prescribed Prozac to treat Hill's serotonin deficiency, and [**40] that Hill had responded favorably to the medication. Dr. Burt's testimony sought to establish that Hill's serotonin deficiency caused his aggressive behavior, and that a long history of violence and suicide in his family indicated that his aggressive impulses resulted from a genetic condition. Dr. Burt, however, apparently suffered a breakdown while on the witness stand. Thus, while testifying during the trial's sentencing phase, Dr. Burt had difficulty responding to questions, particularly on cross-examination.

While these claims were ultimately rejected, the legal argument raises interesting questions. If the defense had been able to establish that (a) Hill's behavior was causally related to his serotonergic brain chemistry and that (b) this brain state (the level of serotonin) was unusual, would this mitigate his punishment[8]?

My own feeling is that this is a difficult question even for a consequentialist and that it has to be approached carefully. In thinking about it, first we have to be clear that saying Hill had lower than average serotonin levels and that he was more violent than average may be saying the same thing at two different levels of reduction. (At least this is the argument that his lawyers were trying to make.) If this is true, can the argument that he had low serotonin levels (equivalent to saying that he was a violent kind of person—remember that his lawyers are arguing that these are the same thing) be used to mitigate the punishment? To answer that question I think that we have to get a bit more quantitative both in how we define "different" and in how we approach issues of punishment efficacy. Consider the graphs in Figure 16.1. Let me stress that *both are imaginary*; I use them only to illustrate a point. The first plots brain serotonin levels in a population of individuals. Note that serotonin levels can be high or low with a Gaussian distribution centered around a mean level, which I have arbitrarily called 100. Beneath that graph I have included a hypothetical plot of the likelihood that a person at any given serotonin level will commit a violent act. These (*imaginary*) numbers report how much of an increase in the chance of violent behavior is associated with any given level of whole-brain serotonin. People to the left of the graph are, on average, more violent. People on the right are, on average, less violent. How then should we use this data?

One approach, and the one for which Hill's lawyers in effect argued, is that we should set some lower bound on this graph and not punish people below that bound. Where, however, should we set this lower bound? If we believe that there are two categories of violent behavior and that these two categories map to serotonin levels[9], then where shall we find the boundaries between these two categories? At two standard deviations below the mean? At 3? At 5? Where to set that lower limit seems problematic because there does not seem to be anything qualitatively different about a specific group of these people. There do not seem to be two *categories* here in any meaningful physical sense. For reasons like these, it seems almost impossible to argue up from the raw neurobiological data to any conclusion about the natural categories of social responsibility.

---

[8] Let me also put aside, for the purposes of this discussion, the consequentialist notion that Hill should be put away to protect society specifically because his behavior is refractory to punishment. Of course, this is almost certainly a point juries and judges consider, but not a point made in this case.

[9] Something that I have argued is unlikely, but which is in the end an empirical question.

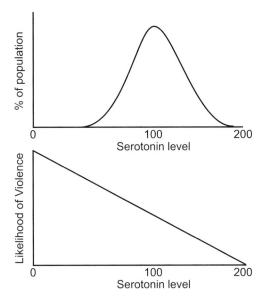

Figure 16.1 Imaginary graphs of (a) brain serotonin levels in a population of individuals and (b) a hypothetical plot of the likelihood that a person at any given serotonin level will commit a violent act.

What we have here is a typical physically continuous variable and that suggests, if anything, that the deterrence effect of punishment may influence the behavior of all of these people in different ways. Imagine we knew (and again I recognize that this is not the case) that different degrees of punishment reduced the likelihood that any given individual would commit a violent act. Of course people on the right of the distribution shown here do not need much incentive to act nonviolently while people on the left do. A rational choice theorist *working from this neurobiological data to a theory of law* might argue that the likelihoods of violence should be matched by a strength-of-punishment function. Indeed, working from the neural data, the logical conclusion would be that punishment should be a continuous function of the convicted criminal's serotonin level. If convicted with a high serotonin level, Hill should get a lighter sentence; that is, his sentence should be inversely proportional to his serotonin level. I think that for almost everyone reading this article, the idea that if Hill was a nonviolent (or equivalently "high serotonin") individual then his crime should go largely unpunished is completely unacceptable.

Let me finish, though, by saying that it is entirely possible (at least in principle) to reason in the other direction. If we found (though I think this highly unlikely) that killers we define on social grounds as not responsible for their actions had particular serotonin levels, then we could begin to use those serotonin levels (be they high or low) to identify these socially categorized individuals. Whether this works is an empirical, rather than a philosophical issue. My own suspicion is that this approach will also fail. Social categories of this type will not yield robustly to neural measurements because the social categories we have are too different from the physical structure of the brain. However, this is a hypothesis that will continue to be tested in the years to come.

Reductionism, Law, and Neuroscience Together?

Over the course of the last decade or two, there have been tremendous steps made towards a reductive synthesis that relates neurobiology, psychology and economics[10]. Each of these disciplines can be seen as a description of the causes of human behavior at differing levels of reduction. Neurobiology seeks to describe the physical processes that generate behavior. Psychology seeks to describe the mental processes that generate this same behavior, and, at a more global level of analysis, economics seeks highly parsimonious models that predict behavior from initial conditions without explicit regard to underlying mechanism.

Beginning in earnest with the introduction of modern brain scanners less than two decades ago, there have been strong linkages created between the neurobiological and psychological levels of analysis. The premise that guides the formation of these links is that psychological theories compatible with the underlying neural architecture are more likely to be robust and extensible than those psychological theories that are incompatible with the underlying physiology. At about the same time economics and psychology began to interact in a similar way, and more recently, a similar set of linkages has begun to emerge between neuroscience and economics. The result of this interdisciplinary activity has been a growing alignment of the models and theories that guide these three disciplines.

One example of that growing alignment seems to be an emerging consensus that the boundary between voluntary-rational and involuntary-irrational-exculpatory behavior (as either a lawyer or a psychologist might define them) is not nearly as clear at the economic, psychological, or neurobiological level as had been previously supposed. This is a fundamental theme that has emerged throughout this Ernst Strüngmann Forum. From the four working groups, the first three discussions challenged repeatedly the distinction between conscious/ voluntary and nonconscious/involuntary. The corresponding chapters convey an emerging empirical consensus at the neurobiological, psychological, and economic levels that one cannot successfully describe behavior as the product of two independent systems (or groups of systems).

---

[10] Note, however, that there is no evidence that economic and psychological levels are about to be reduced completely to neurobiology. Indeed, the history of chemistry and physics suggests that strong reductive relationships will continue to emerge while full reduction will probably remain elusive.

The fourth working group (see Lubell et al., this volume) and its corresponding chapters reveal a different story. At the level of institutions, the notion of a voluntary-rational/exculpatory distinction is more than just alive and well. It seems clear that this distinction and the notion of justice to which it is closely related are necessary components of our institutions. Institutional actors, like courts, serve as proxies for those they govern. People accept the rule of law and grant governments the power to imprison when the actions of those governments align with their own goals.

Summary

We have overwhelming evidence that the Western legal system reflects a widely held conviction among its citizens both that the voluntary/involuntary distinction is meaningful and that punishment for crimes must reflect this distinction. My own opinion is that this distinction has its roots in the classical division of behavior into reflex and voluntary/free-willed categories, a division that was stated so clearly by Descartes and which now permeates so many aspects of Western culture. Regardless of the cultural source of this division of behavior into two categories, it is clear that people have a "taste" for fairness and this taste is rooted irrefutably in distinctions between voluntary and involuntary or irrational behavior. Criminal law, and perhaps institutions in general, implement this division with a complex patchwork of tools. Some behaviors are labeled involuntary, others are labeled compelled, some are described as rational, others as the product of emotional states. What cuts across all of these categories, for me, is that we observe two super-categories: actions for which an actor will be held responsible and actions for which he will not be held responsible. There may be gray areas between these two super-categories, but it is these super-categorical boundaries that do all the work of deciding who will be punished and who will not. Legal systems are, in essence, evolved social systems that both function effectively and rest on this distinction.

A century ago, neurobiological and psychological analyses of behavior reflected a widely held conviction among scholars that the physical and mental roots of action supported the empirical division of behavior into two super-categories. In neurobiology these categories were called reflex and cognition. In psychology these categories have had many names, ranging from involuntary and voluntary to conscious and unconscious. In fairness, neoclassical economics never supported such a distinction—behavior was behavior—although more recently even economics has begun to search for such a distinction. Over the last few decades, however, neurobiologists and psychologists (and now increasingly economists) have become more convinced that this dipartite approach to behavior is critically flawed. Most have become convinced that neither the physical brain nor any really workable psychological descriptions of mind can be made to rest on this dualist approach. If those conclusions are correct, then we simply have to make one of two choices. Either we abandon the hope for a reductive synthesis between institutional design and the neurobiological and psychological roots of behavior, or we abandon the super-categorical boundaries that underlie much of our institutional design.

Over the next several decades it seems unavoidable that descriptions of human behavior at the neural, psychological, and economic levels will become increasingly compatible. It also seems clear that those descriptions will not include a clear voluntary/involuntary distinction at the level of causal agency. Still, *one has to be clear that this is a line of reasoning that, at least today, cannot propagate upwards to the institutional level*. It is my conviction that neurobiology cannot guide law, because these two disciplines rest on differing, and to my mind irreconcilable, foundations. Law is based on social, not scientific, principles, and scientists must make their peace with that fact.

The implications for such a conclusion in law are significant. If these two systems for describing behavior rest on irreconcilable premises, then we simply cannot use neurobiological data to shape deep structural features of institutions. We can, for example, continue to search for neural measurements to identify culpable mental states (despite my personal skepticism about this endeavor) even if those measurements are not reducible to any theory of the brain. We can continue to use psychological theories to inform us about consequentialist issues in the design of punishments. What we cannot do, however, is to argue upwards to notions of responsibility and culpability from neurobiological data. We must continue to be cautious in our aspirations. Brains are exceedingly complicated devices, and it is not at all clear what features constitute the natural categories, or even the system-level descriptions of these devices. Imposing social constructs on our interpretations of these categories is not guaranteed to yield legal clarity. Instead it may only yield injustice. Discussions like those in the Hotema case make that clear.

Acknowledgments

The author is grateful to Stephen Morse, Christoph Engel, and the participants at this Ernst Strüngmann Forum for their comments and assistance.

References

Aristotle. 1987. *De Anima*. Oxford: Penguin Classics.
Blount, S. 1995. When social outcomes aren't fair: The effect of causal attributions on preferences. *Behav. Hum. Dec. Proc.* **63**:131–144.
Brosnan, S. F., and F. B. M. deWaal. 2003. Monkeys reject unequal pay. *Nature* **425**:297–299.
Bruce, V. 1982. Changing faces: Visual and non-visual coding processes in face recognition. *Brit. J. Psychol.* **73**:105–117.

Calvin, J. 1863/1964. *Ioannis Calvini Opera Quae Supersunt Omnia*, ed. J. H. Guilielmus, E. C. Baum, and E. Reuss. Braunschweig.

Dehaene, S., J. P. Changeux, L. Naccache, J. Sackur, and C. Sergent. 2006. Conscious, preconscious, and subliminal processing: A testable taxonomy. *Trends Cogn. Sci.* **10**:204–211.

Descartes, R. 1649/1989. *Passions De L'Ame* [The Passions of the Soul], trans. S. Voss. Indianapolis: Hackett Publ. Co.

Descartes, R. 1664/1972. *L'Homme*, trans. T. S. Hall. Harvard Univ. Press.

Dorris, M. C. and P. W. Glimcher. 2004. Activity in posterior parietal cortex is correlated with the subjective desireability of an action. *Neuron.* **44**:365–378.

Farahany, N. A., and J. E. Coleman. 2006. Genetics and responsibility: To know the criminal from the crime. *Law Contemp. Probs.* **69**:115.

Fudenberg, D., and J. Tirole. 1991. Game Theory. Cambridge, MA: MIT Press.

Garland, B., and P. W. Glimcher. 2006. Cognitive neuroscience and the law. *Curr. Opin. Neurobiol.* **16**:130–134.

Gauthier, I., M. J. Tarr, A. W. Anderson, P. Skudlarski, and J. C. Gore. 1999. Activation of the middle fusiform "face area" increases with expertise in recognizing novel objects. *Nature Neurosci.* **2**:568–573.

Glimcher, P. W. 2005. Indeterminacy in brain and behavior. *Ann. Rev. Psychol.* **56**:25–56.

Gobbini, M. I., and J. V. Haxby. 2007. Neural systems for recognition of familiar faces. *Neuropsychologia* **45**:32–41.

Güth, W., R. Schmittberger, and B. Schwarz. 1982. An experimental analysis of ultimatum bargaining. *J. Econ. Behav. Org.* **3**:367–388.

Harvey, W. C. 1628/1995. *Exercitatio Anatomica de Motu Cordis et Sanguinis in Animalibus* [An Anatomical Disquisition on the Motion of the Heart and Blood in Animals]. New York: Dover Publ.

Haxby, J. V., M. I. Gobbini, M. L. Furey, A. Ishai, J. L. Schouten et al. 2001. Distributed and overlapping representations of faces and objects in ventral temporal cortex. *Science* **293**:2425–2430.

Jones, O. 2001. Time-shifted rationality and the law of law's leverage: Behavioral economics meets behavioral biology. *Northwestern Univ. Law Rev.* **95**:1141–1205.

Kanwisher, N., J. McDermott, and M. Chun. 1997. The fusiform face area: A module in human extrastriate cortex specialized for the perception of faces. *J. Neurosci.* **17**:4302–4311.

Kanwisher, N., and G. Yovel. 2006. The fusiform face area: A cortical region specialized for the perception of faces. *Phil. Trans. Roy. Soc. Lond. B* **361**:2109–2128.

McCabe, K., D. Houser, L. Ryan, V. Smith, and T. Trouard. 2001. A functional imaging study of cooperation in two-person reciprocal exchange. *Proc. Natl. Acad. Sci.* **98**:11,832–11,835.

Vesalius, A. 1543/1998–1999. *De Humani Corpus Fabrica* [On the Fabric of the Human Body], trans. W. F. Richardson and J. B. Carman. Novato, CA: Norman Publ.

Wolpe, P. R., K. R. Foster, and D. D. Langleben. 2005. Emerging neurotechnologies for lie detection: Promises and perils. *Am. J. Bioethics* **5**:39–49.

17

Conscious and Nonconscious Cognitive Processes in Jurors' Decisions

Reid Hastie

Center for Decision Research, Graduate School of Business,
University of Chicago, Chicago, IL 60637, U.S.A.

"…Is there a split between mind and body, and, if so, which is it better to have? … Special consideration is given to a study of consciousness as opposed to unconsciousness, with many helpful hints on how to remain conscious."

—Woody Allen (1967)

Abstract

How should we conceptualize the relationships between conscious and nonconscious processing in some important decisions? This question is addressed in the context of an institutionally significant legal decision—the reasoning processes engaged in by American jurors when rendering verdicts in typical criminal and civil trials. A cognitive–psychological process model for the juror's decision task is outlined and some of the behavioral evidence for the validity of that interpretation is presented. Thereafter, a discussion of the roles of conscious and nonconscious processes is provided within that framework.

Introduction

The juror's decision is an active, constructive comprehension process in which evidence is selected, organized, elaborated, and interpreted during the course of the trial to create a summary mental model, in the juror's mind, of what happened in the events under dispute. This theoretical framework is called the "Story Model" because in most cases, jurors rely heavily on a summary of the trial evidence in the form of a narrative story. The Story Model seems intuitively correct to professionals who try legal cases for a living (e.g., Amsterdam and Bruner 2000; Moore 1989). In addition, competitive scientific tests favor the descriptive validity of the Story Model over competing hypotheses (Hastie 1993; Pennington and Hastie 1992; cf. Schum and Martin 1982). Furthermore, the small stock of behavioral research on the trial judge's decision process also points toward the centrality of narrative, story evidence summaries in the trial judge's cognitive processes (e.g., Wagenaar et al. 1993).

The Story Model for Juror Decision Making

Most juror and judge decisions in criminal and civil trials can be described in terms of a general model of *explanation-based judgment* (Hastie 1999, 2001; Hastie and Pennington 1994, 1996; Pennington and Hastie 1981, 1986, 1988, 1991, 1992, 1993; for similar views, see also Bennett and Feldman 1981; Wagenaar et al. 1993). Legal decision makers reason about evidence to construct a summary in the form of a mental model of important, decision-relevant events and the causal relations between them. Then, this intermediate representation, rather than the original "raw" evidence, is the basis of the final decision. Interposition of this causal representation facilitates evidence comprehension, directs additional inferences, and is the primary determinant of the confidence assigned to the decision. Researchers have proposed comprehension-based interpretations of other simpler decisions (e.g., Simon and Holyoak 2002; Kintsch 1998; Trabasso and Bartolone 2003) and some have shown how simple causal models underlie well-known judgment errors (e.g., base rate neglect: Sloman et al. 2003; framing effects: Jou et al. 1996; the conjunction fallacy: Kintsch 1998; the planning fallacy: Buehler and Griffen 2003). The explanation-based approach to judgment parallels studies of the role of explanations in categorization behavior (Ahn et al. 1995; Keil and Wilson 2000; Murphy and Medin 1985; Rehder and Hastie 2001), category learning (e.g., Schank et al. 1986), planning (Wilensky 1983), and learning by generalization from examples (e.g., Lewis 1988).

The American lay juror's decision task is a prototype of the tasks to which explanation-based models apply: First, a massive "database" of evidence is encountered at trial, frequently requiring several days to present. Second, the evidence comes in a scrambled order in which several witnesses and exhibits convey pieces of a historical puzzle in a jumbled temporal sequence. Third, the evidence is piecemeal, and there are many gaps in its depiction of the historical events that are the focus of reconstruction: event descriptions are incomplete, usually some critical events were not observed by the available witnesses, and information about personal reactions and motivations is not presented (usually because of the rules of evidence in American courts). Finally, subparts of the evidence (e.g., individual propositions or episodes) are interdependent in their probative implications for the verdict (Anderson and Twining 1991; Schum 1994; Wigmore 1937). The meaning of one statement cannot be assessed in isolation because it depends on the meanings of related statements.

The juror's decision process in a criminal trial can be broken down into three component processes (see Figure 17.1). First, an explanation is constructed, in the form of a narrative story, to account for the evidence; second, the choice set of decision alternatives is learned by comprehending the verdict categories presented in the instructions on the law; and, third, a decision is reached by classifying the story into the best-fitting verdict category. The major variations on this model in American trials apply to the verdict categories. In civil trials, the instructions often convey information about how to infer causality, responsibility, and motivations from the evidence (in practice, from the evidence-based story), and thus the choice set is often not structured as a set of categorical attributes, as it is in criminal cases. In contrast to jurors, usually judges know the relevant verdict categories before they hear the evidence (from which they also construct narrative summaries), and they appear to infer the verdict from analogies to prior cases, rather than from black letter law. In addition to descriptions of processing stages, the central claim of the model is that the story the juror constructs *causes* the decision. The explanation-based theory includes also four certainty principles—coverage, coherence, uniqueness, and goodness-of-fit—that govern which story will be accepted, which decision will be selected, and the confidence with which the selected decision will be made.

More generally, according to the explanation-based framework, the type of causal model constructed to explain the evidence will depend on the decision domain. Different domain-specific causal rules and knowledge structures will underlie an internist's causal model of a patient's medical condition (Patel and Groen 1991; Pople 1982), an engineer's mental model of an electrical circuit (DeKleer and Brown 1983), an epidemiologist's model of the effect of radon contamination on health (Bostrom et al. 1992), a manager's image of factors affecting his profits (Hogarth et al. 1980), an economist's cognitive maps of economic events (Sevón 1984), or a diplomat's causal map of the political forces in the Middle East (Axelrod 1976; for additional examples, see Klein et al. 1993). In short, there is a plethora of empirical, behavioral evidence that explanation-based reasoning plays a role in many fundamental judgments and decisions (Hastie and Pennington 1995, 2000).

The Juror's Decision Task

To illustrate the explanation-based decision process, I will refer to illustrations from one of the simulated trials used in our research: *Commonwealth of Massachusetts v. Johnson*. In this trial, the defendant, Frank Johnson, was charged with first-degree murder. The undisputed background events include the following: the defendant Johnson, and the victim, Alan Caldwell, had a quarrel early on the day of Caldwell's death. On that morning, Caldwell threatened Johnson with a razor. Later in the evening, they were present at the same bar.

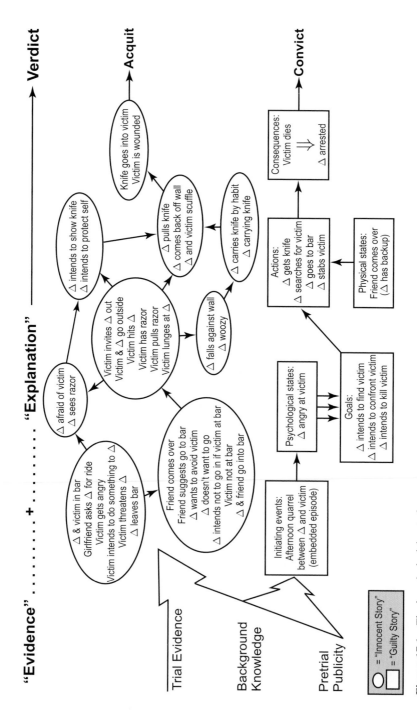

Figure 17.1 The juror's decision task.

They went outside together, got into a fight, and Johnson stabbed Caldwell, and this resulted in Caldwell's death. The events under dispute include whether or not Caldwell pulled out a razor at the evening fight, whether Johnson actively stabbed Caldwell or merely held his knife out to protect himself, how they got outside together, whether or not Johnson intentionally went home to get his knife after the morning altercation, and whether Johnson went to the bar to find Caldwell or whether he went to the bar because it was his habit.

Constructing an Explanation

Our empirical research has focused on the claim that the juror's explanation of legal evidence takes the form of a "story" in which causal and intentional relations among events are prominent. My colleagues and I have shown that, under the conditions that hold in a typical criminal jury trial, jurors spontaneously construct story structures (and not other plausible structures); jurors who choose different verdicts construct different stories; and the story summary constructed by an individual juror is the *cause* of that juror's decision. According to the theory, the story is constructed from three types of knowledge: (a) case-specific information acquired during the trial (e.g., statements made by witnesses about past events relevant to the decision); (b) knowledge about events similar in content to those that are the topic of dispute (e.g., knowledge about a similar crime in the juror's community); and (c) generic expectations about what makes a complete story (e.g., knowledge that human actions are usually motivated by goals). This constructive mental activity results in one or more *interpretations* of the evidence in the form of narrative stories. One of these interpretations (stories) will be accepted by the juror as the best explanation of the evidence. The story that is accepted is the one that provides the greatest coverage of the evidence and is the most coherent, as determined by the individual juror.

Stories involve human action sequences connected by relationships of physical causality and intentional causality between events. In its loosest form, a story could be described as a "causal chain" of events in which events are connected by causal relationships of necessity and sufficiency (Charniak 1991; Trabasso and van den Broek 1985). However, psychological research on discourse comprehension suggests that story causal chains have schematic structure, both when considering the discourse itself and when considering the reader's "mental models" of the discourse. Stories appear to be organized into units called *episodes* (Mandler 1984; Rumelhart 1977; Schank 1975; Stein and Glenn 1979). Episodes fulfill particular roles and are connected by certain types of causal relationships to form stories. In addition, within-episode *initiating events* cause characters to have psychological *responses* and to form *goals* that motivate subsequent *actions*, which cause certain *consequences* and accompanying *states*. An example of an episode in the Johnson case is the following sequence: Johnson and Caldwell are in Gleason's bar. Caldwell's girlfriend,

Sandra Lee, walks up to Johnson and asks him for a ride to the dog track the next day (initiating events). Caldwell becomes angry (internal response), pulls his razor, and threatens Johnson (actions; note that a goal is missing and must be inferred by the observer), and Johnson backs off (consequence).

In addition, stories have a schematic structure that reflects within-episode structure. In their analysis of legal decisions, Amsterdam and Bruner (2000, pp. 113–114) provide an austere definition of a narrative that resembles closely the interpretation just provided:

> A narrative can purport to be either a fiction or a real account of events; it does not have to specify which. It needs a cast of human-like characters, beings capable of willing their own actions, forming intentions, holding beliefs, having feelings. It also needs a plot with a beginning, a middle, and an end, in which particular characters are involved in particular events. The unfolding of the plot requires (implicitly or explicitly):
>
> 1. an initial steady state grounded in the legitimate ordinariness of things,
> 2. that gets disrupted by Trouble consisting of circumstances attributable to human agency or susceptible to change by human intervention,
> 3. in turn evoking efforts at redress or transformation, which succeed or fail,
> 4. so that the old steady state is restored or a new (transformed) steady state is created,
> 5. and the story concludes by drawing the then-and-there of the tale that has been told into the here-and-now of the telling through some coda—say, for example, Aesop's characteristic moral of the story.

Stories may have further structure by virtue of the fact that each component of an episode may be an episode itself. For example, the entire episode above (characterized as Caldwell threatens Johnson) is the *initiating event* in one version of the Johnson story. In this version, the morning "threat" episode causes Johnson to be angry enough to want to pay Caldwell back. Thus, a story is a hierarchy of embedded episodes. The highest-level episode characterizes the most important features of "what happened." Components of the highest-level episode are elaborated in terms of more detailed event sequences in which causal and intentional relations among subordinate story events are represented.

The structure of stories, according to our theory, plays an important role in the juror's comprehension and decision-making processes. The story constructed by the juror will consist of some subset of the events and causal relationships referred to in the presentation of evidence, *as well as* additional events and causal relationships inferred by the juror. Some of these inferences may be suggested by the attorneys while others may be constructed solely by the juror. Whatever their source, the inferences serve to fill out the episode structure of the story. Furthermore, expectations about the kinds of information necessary to make a story reveal to the juror when important pieces of the explanation structure are missing and when inferences must be made.

Knowledge about the structure of stories allows the juror to form an opinion concerning the completeness of the evidence—the extent to which a story has all its parts. The structure of episodes in a story corresponds to the structure of our knowledge about human action sequences in the world. That is, story construction is a general comprehension strategy for understanding human action (Schank and Abelson 1977, 1995). Thus, the juror can easily compare the structure that is being imposed on the evidence to already encoded prior knowledge. Finally, the hierarchical episode and causal structure of the story provides an "automatic" index of the importance of different pieces of evidence (Trabasso and Sperry 1985). In the example above, the details of the embedded "threat" episode are subordinate in importance to the details of the top-level episode, which reveal what Johnson did in order to pay Caldwell back. This indexing of importance is something that emerges from the *structure* of the story.

Learning the Choice Set (Verdicts)

The decision maker's second major task is to learn or to create a set of potential solutions or action alternatives that constitute the choice set. In criminal trials, the legal information for this processing stage is given to jurors at the end of the trial in the judge's instructions about the verdict alternatives available to the juror. These instructions provide only a sketchy outline of the decision categories, and jurors may also have prior ideas concerning the meaning of the verdict alternatives. The information contained in the judge's instructions on verdict definition is usually abstract and often couched in unfamiliar language: a crime is named and then abstract features are presented that define the crime. Features typically describe requirements of identity, mental state, circumstances, and actions that constitute the crime (Kaplan 1978).

Again, constructive inference processes are rampant, and it is common for prior conceptions of the verdicts (e.g., from news media and fictional accounts of trials) to intrude into the verdict representations (for additional empirical results on verdict representation, see Smith 1991). However, many gaps and errors remain in the jurors' operative conceptualizations of the law (cf. Elwork et al. 1977, 1987; Hastie et al. 1983).

Matching the Story to the Verdicts

The final stage in the global decision process involves matching the summary evidence representation to the decision alternatives to find the best match. It is even possible that many definitions of legally significant actions are organized in a format that matches narrative structures (i.e., the definitions of many crimes in terms of identity, mental state, circumstances, and actions may anticipate the most common organization imposed on the evidence). Because verdict categories are unfamiliar concepts, the classification of a story into an appropriate verdict category is likely to be a deliberate inferential process.

For example, a juror may have to decide whether a circumstance in the story, such as "pinned against a wall," constitutes a good match to a required circumstance, "unable to escape," for a verdict of not guilty by reason of self-defense. In this example, these inferences would depend on knowledge from the trial evidence, from the judge's instructions, and from the juror's background knowledge about human motivations (Was the defendant "trying" to escape?), mental processes (Was the person incapacitated?), and the physical world (Was it physically possible for the person to escape?).

The story classification stage also involves the application of the judge's procedural instructions on the presumption of innocence and the standard of proof. That is, if not all verdict attributes for a given verdict category are satisfied "beyond a reasonable doubt" by events in the accepted story, then the juror should presume innocence and return a default verdict of not guilty.

Confidence in Decisions

More than one story may be constructed by a juror. However, one story will usually be accepted as the "best" story, with a level of confidence ranging from high to low. We call the principles that determine acceptability of a story, and the resulting level of confidence, *certainty principles*. According to our explanation-based theory, two certainty principles govern acceptance: *coverage* and *coherence*. An additional certainty principle, uniqueness, contributes to confidence.

A story's *coverage* of the evidence refers to the extent to which the story incorporates and accounts for evidence presented at trial. The greater the story's coverage, the more acceptable the story will stand as an explanation of the evidence and the greater confidence the juror will have in the story as an explanation, if accepted. An explanation that does not account for a lot of evidence will have a lower level of acceptability as the correct explanation. Poor coverage should lower the confidence in a story and consequently lower confidence in the ultimate decision.

In addition, a story's *coherence* enters into its acceptability and level of confidence in a decision based on that story. Coherence itself can be decomposed into three components: *consistency*, *plausibility*, and *completeness*. A story is *consistent* to the extent that it does not contain internal contradictions, either with evidence believed to be true or with other parts of the explanation. A story is *plausible* to the extent that it corresponds to the decision maker's knowledge about what typically happens in the world and does not contradict that knowledge. A story is complete when the expected structure of the story "has all of its parts" (according to the rules of the episodic structure and discussion above). Missing information or lack of plausible inferences about one or more major components of the story will decrease confidence in the explanation. Thus, the coherence of the explanation reflects the consistency of the explanation with itself and with world knowledge, and the extent to which parts of the explanation can be inferred or assembled. These three ingredients of coherence (consistency, plausibility, and completeness) may be fulfilled to a greater or lesser degree, and the values of the three components will combine to yield the overall level of coherence of a story. Combination of these ingredients, however, is not strictly additive. For example, completeness interacts with plausibility. If a story is plausible, then completeness increases confidence. However, if a story is implausible, completeness does not increase confidence. (It might be thought that completeness of an implausible story would actually decrease confidence, but this is not the case.)

Finally, if more than one story is judged to be coherent, then the stories will lack *uniqueness*, which contributes to confidence in a story and in a decision. If there are multiple coherent explanations for the evidence, belief in any one of them over the others will be lessened (Einhorn and Hogarth 1986; Van Wallendael 1989). If there is one coherent story, this story will be accepted as the explanation of the evidence and will be instrumental in reaching a decision. (McKenzie et al. [2002] have demonstrated the comparative nature of juror decisions by showing that a weak affirmative case can actually reduce belief more than no case at all, when confronted by a strong opposing case.)

Inferences in the Service of Explanation-based Decisions

The juror's global decision process is best described as an active, constructive comprehension process in which evidence is organized, elaborated, and interpreted during the course of the trial to create a summary mental model of what happened during the events under dispute. Some story elements are accepted as true directly on the basis of their appearance as evidence from one or more credible sources (or occasionally because they are asserted by a persuasive attorney); that is, they are reasonably well established as fact. For example, an evidence item, "Caldwell was in Gleason's Bar," is direct testimony, is not a matter of dispute, and it appears in all jurors' individual stories. Where in the story an event will appear, depends on its causal relationships to other events.

Many pieces of the story are, however, produced as a result of inferences and judgments. This is the role Pennington and Hastie assign to heuristics and other reasoning processes, and this is the view of the comprehension process held by many cognitive psychologists today. To illustrate, take the following simple narrative:

> Billy went to Johnny's birthday party. When all the children were there, Johnny opened his presents. Later, they sang *Happy Birthday* and Johnny blew out the candles.

Many would infer spontaneously, and most would agree when asked, that there was a cake at the birthday party. Yet, no cake is mentioned in the sentences above. The cake is inferred because we share knowledge about birthday party traditions and the physical world (the candles had to be on something). Another illustration comes with the comprehension of the sentence, "The policeman held up his hand and stopped the car." Most of us understand this sentence in the cultural context of the policeman's authority, shared signals, a driver watching the policeman while controlling the car, etc. Indeed, this is a sentence that would be puzzling to a person from a different culture.

Probably the most common inferences are best described as *modus ponens* or condition–action rule applications (Smith et al. 1992). Pennington and Hastie (1993) documented many of these logic-like inferences that jurors mention when they report on their decision processes. For example, a typical deduction from world knowledge in the "Johnson case" consists of the following premise (P1–P2) and conclusion (C) structure:

> P1. A person who is violent causes other people to be afraid. (world knowledge)
> P2. *Caldwell was violent.* (evidence)
> C. Johnson was afraid of Caldwell. (inferential conclusion)

In this example, the juror matches features of Caldwell from undisputed evidence (P2) and a previous inferential conclusion (P3) to world knowledge about the consequences of being confronted with such a person (P1) to infer that Johnson was afraid (C). More impressive are the many inference forms that illustrate more complex logical inference rules, such as *modus tollens* (which are rarely observed in laboratory studies of deductive reasoning).

> P1. If Johnson was afraid of Caldwell, he would never go back to the scene of the fight. (world knowledge)
> P2. *Johnson did go back to the scene of the fight.* (evidence)
> C. Johnson was not afraid. (inferential conclusion)

Pennington and Hastie (1993) used a taxonomy to describe inference procedures based on a system proposed by Allan Collins and his colleagues (Burstein et al. 1991; Collins and Michalski 1989). The Collins' system is an elaboration of traditional logical inference rule systems (for a comprehensive theory of inference processes, see Rips 1983, 1994). Pennington and Hastie proposed that inference rules are the primary tools for the construction, interpretation, and application of an explanatory mental model to perform an overarching decision task; this proposal may be a partial resolution of the dispute between Johnson-Laird and Byrne (1991) and Rips (1986, 1989).

Conscious and Nonconscious Cognitive and Emotional Processes within the Explanation-based Framework

Most of the computations carried out by the brain and labeled cognitive and emotional processes occur outside of awareness and can be called "nonconscious."

Traditionally, "awareness" has been defined as verbally reportable. Almost all cognitive researchers would acknowledge that the verbal report criterion is a little fuzzy and that more percepts and concepts are conscious than can be reported (cf. Anderson 1993). Furthermore, within typical information-processing models, theorists propose that it is the contents of working memory or of active declarative memory that are potentially reportable (Ericsson and Simon 1984; for a thoughtful argument that consciousness extends a bit further into the cognitive system, see Block 2007). What is notable is how much of cognitive–emotional processing is nonconscious according to these operational and conceptual criteria. In fact, as many theorists have noted, the true fundamental puzzle is why any cognitive material is consciously reportable. The best functional conjecture, at the moment, is doubtless biased by the "reportability criterion" itself: Perhaps consciousness has a primary function of serving (or signaling) communication of important private information to others.

Two Systems or a Continuum?

Several influential theorists have proposed that there are two fundamental and partly independent cognitive–emotional processing systems: system 1 (intuition) is associative, mostly nonconscious, emotion-laden, fast, parallel, automatic, and phylogenetically primitive; system 2 (reasoning) is rule-based, partly conscious, slow, serial, more controllable, and more recent in evolution (Sloman 1996; Stanovich and West 2000; Kahneman 2003; Cohen 2005). Some theorists assert that the two systems can operate completely independently, so that system 1 and system 2 can reach contradictory conclusions to a judgment problem (Sloman 1996). Other theorists imply that system 1 can reach a conclusion by itself, but that system 2 always operates in concert with system 1 (Kahneman 2003). A popular interpretation is that system 1, the fast intuitive one, starts prompting responses very quickly and system 2, the slow deliberate one, kicks in later to correct biases in system 1. (There are suggestions, however, that in some tasks, system 2 may add error to more accurate system 1 responses; see following discussion on intuitive choice.)

I believe there are many component processes that are assembled to create cognitive strategies to perform various explicit judgment and decision tasks such as those induced by the juror or judge's decision task (this multi-strategy interpretation is closest to the general approach illustrated by the "Adaptive Decision Maker" research program; Payne et al. 1993). Different people performing identical tasks may rely on different strategies and processes; the same person performing the same task on different occasions may even rely on different strategies. *All* strategies involve both conscious and nonconscious components. Some strategies produce more reportable traces than others; some components are more resource demanding than others; different components are susceptible to interference from different secondary tasks; and different components involve more emotional responses than others. Thus, it is a basic problem in all cognitive research to design tasks and provide collateral measures to constrain participants' use of strategies to one or a few, or to identify the specific strategy adopted by individual participants. Solving the "strategic variety" problem is always one of the highest priority methodological tasks in all cognitive research.

The best behavioral research methods analyze a judgment strategy of interest into its components and then summarize the strategy as an information-processing flowchart (or some other explicit process model). When this is done, the most opaque strategies are likely to be identified as case-based reasoning (also termed recognition-primed decision making; Klein et al. 1993), category-based judgment (sometimes called "prejudice" or representativeness; Hastie and Wittenbrink 2006), and affect-based judgment (sometimes called the somatic-marker process; Slovic et al. 2002). The most transparent, cognitively accessible strategies are likely to be the more inference-rich, reason-seeking strategies or choice strategies like those identified in many studies of multi-attribute choice (elimination by aspects, satisficing, etc.). Strategies like the ubiquitous anchor-and-adjust family of many substrategies probably lie in the middle of this continuum, with substantial unconscious (anchoring) and conscious (adjustment) components.

It is useful to order strategies on a continuum, from highly transparent (with many verbally reportable byproducts, system 2) to opaque (mostly nonconscious, system 1). Hammond (1996) provides the clearest statement of such a "cognitive continuum theory" (summarized in Cooksey 1996). An important assumption of the cognitive continuum theory framework is that judges and decision makers can deliberately (or inadvertently) shift up and down along the continuum, adapting more and less intuitive strategies as a function of motivation, accountability, judgment task demands, and so forth. Hammond has identified some conditions that are known to push the strategy toward the more deliberate (or intuitive) ends of the continuum; for evidence that motivation (consequentiality) can shift people from quick, intuitive choice strategies to slower, deliberate strategies, see Payne et al. (1993).

Which System Makes the Best Decisions?

An interesting question concerns the conditions under which more intuitive, automatic judgments and choices are superior to judgments that involve more deliberate, conscious, controlled processes. Wilson and his colleagues (Wilson et al. 1993; Wilson and Schooler 1991) have presented suggestive evidence that simple aesthetic and gustatory choices yield more long-term consumption satisfaction when made via an intuitive, unanalyzed strategy, as compared with a strategy in which the experimenter required the chooser to provide written reasons to justify the outcome; Dijksterhuis and van Olden (2006) provide a systematic replication of the Wilson et al. (1993) findings. Wilson and colleagues' interpretation makes good sense: When people evaluate habitually according to an intuitive strategy, requiring them to perform a novel, distracting verbal task will most likely interfere with the execution of the habitual strategy and degrade the quality of choices based on the strategy.

A more puzzling set of experiments has been reported by Dijksterhuis et al. (2006) in which experimental participants made memory-based choices between four hypothetical cars (or apartments to rent; Dijksterhuis 2004). In one experimental "unconscious thought" condition, participants were presented information about the attributes of the cars and then distracted for four minutes by an anagram problem-solving task before making their choices. In the "conscious thought" condition, participants were instructed to concentrate on their memories of the cars and to think about their choice for four minutes. Participants were likelier to choose the objectively best alternative within the choice set when distracted before making their choices. Dijksterhuis assumes that the distraction treatment induces participants to make the choice using nonconscious intuitive evaluation processes and concludes that "deliberation-without-attention" is a superior choice strategy when choice sets are composed of complex, multi-attribute options. This result is puzzling because this does not seem to be the type of choice that people usually make by relying on quick intuitive hunches; when choosing a car or an apartment, people usually scrutinize the attributes systematically and seek explicit "reasons for" their final choices (cf. Payne et al. 1993; Shafir et al. 1993). It may be important that none of Dijksterhuis's choice conditions included a natural, "just make the choice as you would normally" condition; that is, in the "conscious thought" choice condition, participants were required to spend four minutes "thinking very carefully about each option." Furthermore, these choices are not usually made in a memory-based manner with a large "load" of disorganized choice attributes in memory (Dijksterhuis presented the 48+ attributes of each car or apartment in a scrambled list and required participants to rely on their memories for all information while deliberating on their choices.) This means that Wilson and colleagues' plausible interpretation, in terms of a mismatch between customary choice strategies and the strategy induced by instructions to "deliberate," would *not* apply to these findings. Dijksterhuis provides a provocative interpretation of his findings in terms of hypothesized differences in conscious versus nonconscious systems' processing capacity; he asserts that the nonconscious processing system (system 1) has a much higher capacity than the conscious system. (It should be noted that Dijksterhuis' assumption that system 1 has virtually unlimited processing capacity has no independent scientific support and has a low prior probability of validity.)

For the present, it seems that simple aesthetic ("Which poster do I want on my apartment wall?") or gustatory ("Which jam do I want on my toast this morning?") choices are best made via a quick, mostly nonconscious strategy. It makes sense that such choices are usually based on quick, intuitive evaluations (simulation of consumption, retrieval of similar cases); hence more deliberative, consciously accessible strategies will be maladaptive and produce less satisfying outcomes. Furthermore, Wilson and colleagues have provided behavioral evidence to support this claim in some typical everyday choice tasks. The more challenging claim that complex multi-attribute choices are best made in a quick, intuitive fashion seems less likely to generalize to everyday choice situations. We must, however, acknowledge Dijksterhuis' empirical evidence for this claim. As for jurors' legal judgments, nonconscious decision processes do not primarily seem to be the mode in naturalistic decision tasks, and it seems unlikely that a shift toward less conscious, more intuitive strategies would improve performance. However, this is a speculative claim.

Back to Legal Decisions

The complex judgment strategy summarized by the explanation-based Story Model for juror decisions is a multistage conglomeration of strategies. Some of the substrategies are relatively opaque (e.g., jurors' category-classification judgments to "stereotype" actors involved in the trial, cased-based memory retrieval), while others are relatively available to consciousness (e.g., the jurors' inference processes that produce the verbal reports described above; for a discussion of the role of social category-based biases in legal judgments, see Hastie and Wittenbrink 2006). Every stage of processing in the explanation-based framework involves, however, a mixture of conscious and nonconscious processes.

Legal institutions such as rules of evidence, instructions on the decision process, and trial procedures are designed primarily to push the decision processes toward the deliberate end of Hammond's "cognitive continuum." Some conventions in American jury trials are motivated partly by the goal of keeping jurors' reasoning on the analytic, deliberate end of the continuum by shielding the juror from events and materials during the trial, which might induce intuitive decision making. For example, evidence or arguments that are likely to evoke strong emotional reactions are sometimes excluded from jurors' review on the assumption that they will move the decision process toward the intuitive end of the cognitive continuum. Indeed, the requirement for a vigorous verbal discussion in the "crucible of jury deliberation" is partly aimed at making the decision process explicit and conscious. The extensive procedural instructions given to American jurors are an example of more direct efforts to keep the process deliberate and rational: presume innocence, the burden is on the prosecution, beyond reasonable doubt, in order to find, you must conclude.... At the end of the decision process, special verdict forms and hybrid interrogatory verdict forms are designed to get jurors to think deliberately, to focus on fact-finding, and to consider consciously each element of the legal requirements for a verdict. The many requirements to justify judicial decisions at trial and during the appellate review process, in courts around the world, make judges' decision processes deliberate and consciously thoughtful. There are many essays written by experienced judges prescribing system 2 modes of thinking for both jurors and judges (Levi 1949; Wasserstrom 1961; Weinreb 2005).

Concluding Remarks

All complex decisions, including all legal decisions, involve a mixture of conscious and nonconscious cognitive processes. The explanation-based, Story Model for the juror's decision process provides a framework to understand the many components of the larger cognitive achievement involved in comprehending evidence and making decisions in a typical American trial. There is considerable behavioral evidence that the framework provides a valid overview of the juror's decision and many components of the trial judge's decision process as well (comprehension of the facts to construct a story that explains those facts is central and common to both decision tasks). To date, no systematic behavioral studies have been conducted to separate conscious from nonconscious processes in jurors' and judges' decisions, but it seems indisputable that the larger process is a thorough mix of both reportable and unconscious processes.

What are the most controversial implications of the present review and analysis? At this point in time, the general validity of the Story Model framework does not seem to be in dispute. Still, the framework needs further development and specification to be able to apply the general approach to variations on the basic legal decision task (e.g., more research on trial judges' decision processes or on decisions in a "code law" inspired judiciary vs. a case law judiciary). The centrality of the evidence comprehension subtask is, however, obvious and irresistible, and the semantic network approach to modeling the cognitive products of comprehension is virtually universal in psychology and linguistics today (e.g., Kintsch 1998; Goldman and Graesser 1999). What is more controversial is the claim that the two-systems, dual-process framework can be used to describe cognitive processes; this is an over-simplification and may not be useful to describe complex decision processes. Although it is impossible to prove such a general claim, I believe that decision processes are almost always a mixture of substantial amounts of conscious, reportable processing plus nonconscious processing. I believe (without strong evidence, nor is there evidence to the contrary) that the most effective legal decisions will involve a mixture of both modes of processing. In addition, legal institutions that prompt decision makers to increase deliberate systematic review of evidence, procedural requirements, and decision criteria, *without banishing the essential associated nonconscious processing substrate*, make a positive contribution to the quality of the overall decision (i.e., I reject the implications of the Dijksterhuis et al. [2006] interpretation for the practice of legal decision making). Somewhat paradoxically, I believe that the deliberate control of the most basic attentional processes, institutional procedures that force decision makers to attend systematically to all of the relevant inputs to the decision process, will increase the effectiveness and accuracy of decisions based on a wide range of cognitive strategies.

References

Ahn, W.-K., C. W. Kalish, D. L. Medin, and S. A. Gelman. 1995. The role of covariation versus mechanism information in causal attribution. *Cognition* **54**:299–352.

Allen, W. 1967. Literary Cavalcade 2005. **57(8)**:20; reprinted in *Seriously Funny*, May 2005.

Amsterdam, A. G., and J. S. Bruner. 2000. Minding the Law. Cambridge: Harvard Univ. Press.

Anderson, J. R. 1993. Implicit memory and metacognition: Why is the glass half full? In: Implicit Memory and Metacognition, ed. L. M. Reder, pp. 123–135. Mahwah, NJ: Lawrence Erlbaum.

Anderson, T. J., and W. Twining. 1991. Analysis of Evidence. Boston, MA: Little, Brown.

Axelrod, R., ed. 1976. Structure of Decision: The Cognitive Maps of Political Elites. Princeton: Princeton Univ. Press.

Bennett, W. L., and M. S. Feldman. 1981. Reconstructing reality in the courtroom: Justice and Judgment in American Culture. New Brunswick, NJ: Rutgers Univ. Press.

Block, N. 2007. Consciousness, accessibility, and the mesh between psychology and neuroscience. *Behav. Brain Sci.* **30**, in press.

Bostrom, A., B. Fischhoff, and G. Morgan. 1992. Characterizing mental models of hazardous processes: A methodology and an application to radon. *J. Soc. Issues* **48**:85–100.

Buehler, R., and D. Griffin. 2003. Planning, personality, and prediction: The role of future focus in optimistic time predictions. *Org. Behav. Hum. Dec. Proc.* **92**:80–90.

Burstein, M. H., A. Collins, and M. Baker. 1991. Plausible generalization: Extending a model of human plausible reasoning. *J. Learn. Sci.* **1**:319–359.

Charniak, E. 1991. Bayesian networks without tears. *AI Magazine* **12(4)**:50–63.

Cohen, J. D. 2005. The vulcanization of the human brain: A neural perspective on interactions between cognition and emotion. *J. Econ. Persp.* **19(4)**:3–24.

Collins, A., and R. Michalski. 1989. The logic of plausible reasoning: A core theory. *Cogn. Sci.* **13**:1–49.

Cooksey, R. W. 1996. Judgment Analysis: Theory, Methods, and Applications. San Diego: Academic Press.

DeKleer, J., and J. S. Brown. 1983. Assumptions and ambiguities in mechanistic mental models. In: Mental Models, ed. D. Gentner and A.L. Stevens. Hillsdale, NJ: Lawrence Erlbaum.

Dijksterhuis, A. 2004. Think different: The merits of unconscious thought in preference development and decision making. *J. Per. Soc. Psychol.* **87**:586–598.

Dijksterhuis, A., M. W. Bos, L. F. Nordgren, and R. B. van Baaren. 2006. On making the right choice: The deliberation-without-attention effect. *Science* **311**:1005–1008.

Dijksterhuis, A., and Z. van Olden. 2006. On the benefits of thinking unconsciously: Unconscious thought can increase post-choice satisfaction. *J. Exp. Psychol.* **42**:627–631.

Einhorn, H. J., and R. M. Hogarth. 1986. Judging probable cause. *Psychol. Bull.* **99**:3–19.

Elwork, A., B. D. Sales, and J. J. Alfini. 1977. Juridic decisions: In ignorance of the law or in light of it? *Law Hum. Behav. 1:*163–189.

Elwork, A., J. J. Alfini, and B. D. Sales. 1987. Toward understandable jury instructions. In: In the Jury Box: Controversies in the Courtroom, ed. L. S. Wrightsman and S. M. Kassin, pp. 161–179. Thousand Oaks, CA: Sage Publications.

Ericsson, K. A., and H. A. Simon. 1984. Protocol Analysis: Verbal Reports as Data. Cambridge: MIT Press.

Goldman, S. R., and A. C. Graesser. 1999. Narrative Comprehension, Causality, and Coherence: Essays in Honor of Tom Trabasso. Mahwah, NJ: Lawrence Erlbaum.

Hammond, K. R. 1996. Human Judgment and Social Policy: Irreducible Uncertainty, Inevitable Error, Unavoidable Injustice. New York: Oxford Univ. Press.

Hastie, R., ed. 1993. Inside the Juror. New York: Cambridge Univ. Press. [See, in particular, chapters by Hastie: "Introduction to Models of Juror Decision Making," "Algebraic Models of Juror Decision Processes," as well as "The Story Model of Juror Decision Making," with N. Pennington].

Hastie, R. 1999. The role of "stories" in civil jury judgments. *Michigan J. Law Ref.* **32(2)**:1–13.

Hastie, R. 2001. Emotions in jurors' decisions. *Brooklyn Law Rev.* **66**:991–1009.

Hastie, R., and N. Pennington. 1994. Review of Anchored Narratives: The Psychology of Criminal Evidence, by Wagenaar, W. A., P. J. J. van Koppen, and H. F. M. Crombag. 1993. *J. Behav. Dec. Mak.* **7**:293–296.

Hastie, R., and N. Pennington. 1995. The big picture: Is it a story? In: Knowledge and Memory: The Real Story, ed. R. S. Wyer Jr., and J. K. Srull, pp. 133–138. Hillsdale, NJ: Lawrence Erlbaum.

Hastie, R., and N. Pennington. 1996. The O. J. Simpson stories: Behavioral scientists look at The People v. O. J. Simpson trial. *Univ. of Colorado Law Rev.* **67**:957–976.

Hastie, R., and N. Pennington. 2000. Explanation-based decision making. In: Judgment and Decision Making: An Interdisciplinary Reader, 2d ed., ed. T. Connolly, H. R. Arkes, and K. R. Hammond, pp. 212–228. New York: Cambridge Univ. Press.

Hastie, R., S. D. Penrod, and N. Pennington. 1983. Inside the Jury. Cambridge, MA: Harvard Univ. Press.

Hastie, R., and B. Wittenbrink. 2006. Heuristics for applying laws to facts. In: Heuristics and the Law, ed. G. Gigerenzer and C. Engel, pp. 259–280. Cambridge: MIT Press.

Hogarth, R. M., C. Michaud, and J. L. Mery. 1980. Decision behavior in an urban development: A methodological approach and substantive considerations. *Acta Psychologica* **45**:95–117.

Johnson-Laird, P. N., and R. M. J. Byrne. 1991. Deduction. Hillsdale, NJ: Lawrence Erlbaum.

Jou, J., J. Shanteau, and R. J. Harris. 1996. An information processing view of framing effects: The role of causal schemas in decision making. *Mem. Cogn.* **24**:1–15.

Kahneman, D. 2003. A perspective on judgment and choice: Mapping bounded rationality. *Am.Psychol.* **58**:697–720.

Kaplan, J. 1978. Criminal Justice: Introductory Cases and Materials. 2d ed. Mineola, NY: Foundation Press.

Keil, F. C., and R. A. Wilson. 2000. Explanation and Cognition. Cambridge: MIT Press.

Kintsch, W. 1998. Comprehension: A Paradigm for Cognition. New York: Cambridge Univ. Press.

Klein, G. A., J. Orasanu, R. Calderwood, and C. E. Zsambok, eds. 1993. Decision Making in Action: Models and Methods. Norwood, NJ: Ablex.

Lewis, C. H. 1988. Why and how to learn why: Analysis-based generalization of procedures. *Cogn. Sci.* **12**:211–256.

Levi, E. 1949. Introduction to Legal Reasoning. Chicago: Univ. of Chicago Press.

Mandler, J. M. 1984. Stories, Scripts and Scenes: Aspects of Schema Theory. Hillsdale, NJ: Lawrence Erlbaum.

McKenzie, C. R. M., S. M. Lee, and K. K. Chen. 2002. When negative evidence increases confidence: Change in belief after hearing two sides of a dispute. *J. Behav. Dec. Mak.* **15**:1–18.

Moore, A. J. 1989. Trial by schema: Cognitive filters in the courtroom. *UCLA Law Rev.* **37**:273–341.

Murphy, G. L., and D. L. Medin. 1985. The role of theories in conceptual coherence. *Psychol. Rev.* **92**:289–316.

Patel, V. L., and G. J. Groen. 1991. The general and specific nature of medical expertise: A critical look. In: Toward a General Theory of Expertise: Prospects and Limits, ed. K. A. Ericsson and J. Smith, pp. 93–125. New York: Cambridge Univ. Press.

Payne, J. W., J. R. Bettman, and E. J. Johnson. 1993. The Adaptive Decision Maker. New York: Cambridge Univ. Press.

Pennington, N., and R. Hastie. 1981. Juror decision-making models: The generalization gap. *Psychol. Bull.* **89**:246–287.

Pennington, N., and R. Hastie. 1986. Evidence evaluation in complex decision making. *J. Pers. Soc. Psychol.* **51**:242–258.

Pennington, N., and R. Hastie. 1988. Explanation-based decision making: Effects of memory structure on judgment. *J. Exp. Psychol.: Learn. Mem. Cogn.* **14**:521–533.

Pennington, N., and R. Hastie. 1990. Practical implications of psychological research on juror and jury decision making. *Pers. Soc. Psychol. Bull.* **16**:90–105.

Pennington, N., and R. Hastie. 1991. A cognitive theory of juror decision making: The story model. *Cardozo Law Rev.* **13**:519–557.

Pennington, N., and R. Hastie. 1992. Explaining the evidence: Tests of the story model for juror decision making. *J. Per.Soc. Psychol.* **62**:189–206.

Pennington, N., and R. Hastie. 1993. Reasoning in explanation-based decision making. *Cognition* **49**:123–163.

Pople, H. E., Jr. 1982. Heuristic methods for imposing structure on ill-structured problems: The structuring of medical diagnostics. In: Artificial Intelligence in Medicine, ed. P. Szolovits. Boulder: Westview Press.

Rehder, B., and R. Hastie. 2001. Causal knowledge and categories: The effects of underlying causal beliefs on categorization, induction, and similarity. *J. Exp. Psychol.: Gen.* **130**:323–360.

Rips, L. J. 1983. Cognitive processes in propositional reasoning. *Psychol. Rev.* **90**: 38–71.

Rips, L. J. 1986. Mental muddles. In: The Representation of Knowledge and Belief, ed. M. Brand and R.M. Harnish, pp. 128–141. Tucson: Univ. Arizona Press.

Rips, L. J. 1989. The psychology of knights and knaves. *Cognition* **31**:85–116.

Rips, L. J. 1994. The Psychology of Proof: Deductive Reasoning in Human Thinking. Cambridge: MIT Press.

Rumelhart, D. E. 1977. Understanding and summarizing brief stories. In: Basic Processes in Reading: Perception and Comprehension, ed. D. LaBerge and S. J. Samuels. Hillsdale, NJ: Lawrence Erlbaum.

Schank, R. C. 1975. The structure of episodes in memory. In: Representation and Understanding: Studies in Cognitive Science, ed. D. G. Bobrow and A. Collins, pp. 237–272. New York: Academic Press.

Schank, R. C., and R. P. Abelson. 1977. Scripts, Plans, Goals, and Understanding. Hillsdale, NJ: Lawrence Erlbaum.

Schank, R. C., and R. P. Abelson. 1995. Knowledge and memory: The real story. In: Knowledge and Memory: The Real Story, ed. R. S. Wyer., Jr., pp. 1–86. Hillsdale, NJ: Lawrence Erlbaum.

Schank, R. C., G. C. Collins, and L. E. Hunter. 1986. Transcending inductive category formation in learning. *Behav. Brain Sci.* **9**:639–686.

Schum, D. A. 1994. The Evidential Foundations of Probabilistic Reasoning. New York: Wiley.

Schum, D. A., and A. W. Martin. 1982. Formal and empirical research on cascaded inference in jurisprudence. *Law Soc. Rev.* **17**:105–151.

Sevón, G. 1984. Cognitive maps of past and future economic events. In: Research Perspectives on Decision Making under Uncertainty, ed. K. Borcherding, B. Brehmer, C. A. J. Vlek and W. A. Wagenaar, pp. 71–78. Amsterdam: North Holland.

Shafir, E., I. Simonson, and A. Tversky. 1993. Reason-based choice. *Cognition* **49**:11–36.

Simon, D., and K. J. Holyoak. 2002. Structural dynamics of cognition: From consistency theories to constraint satisfaction. *Pers. Soc. Psychol. Rev.* **6**:283–294.

Sloman, S. A. 1996. The empirical case for two systems of reasoning. *Psychol. Bull.* **119**:3–22.

Sloman, S. A., D. Over, L. Slovak, and J. M. Stibel. 2003. Frequency illusions and other fallacies. *Org. Behav Hum. Dec. Proc.* **91**:296–309.

Slovic, P., M. Finucane, E. Peters, and D. G. MacGregor. 2002. The affect heuristic. In: Heuristics and Biases: The Psychology of Intuitive Judgment, ed. T. Gilovich, D. Griffin, and D. Kahneman, pp. 397–420. New York: Cambridge Univ. Press.

Smith, V. L. 1991. Prototypes in the courtroom: Lay representations of legal concepts. *J. Pers. Soc. Psychol.* **61**:857–872.

Smith, E. E., C. Langston, and R. E. Nisbett. 1992. The case for rules in reasoning. *Cogn. Sci.* **16**:99–112.

Stanovich, K. E., and R. F. West. 2000. Individual differences in reasoning: Implications for the rationality debate. *Behav. Brain Sci.* **23**:645–665.

Stein, N. L., and C. G. Glenn. 1979. An analysis of story comprehension in elementary school children. In: New Directions in Discourse Processing, vol. 2, ed. R. O. Freedle, pp. 83–107. Norwood, NJ: Ablex.

Trabasso, T., and J. Bartolone. 2003. Story understanding and counterfactual reasoning. *J. Exp. Psychol.: Learn. Mem. Cogn.* **29**:904–923.

Trabasso, T., and L. L. Sperry. 1985. Causal relatedness and importance of story events. *J. Mem. Lang.* **24**:595–611.

Trabasso, T., and P. van den Broek. 1985. Causal thinking and the representation of narrative events. *J. Mem. Lang.* **24**:612–630.

Van Wallendael, L. R. 1989. The quest for limits on noncomplementarity in opinion revision. *Org. Behav. Hum. Dec. Proc.* **43**:385–405.

Wagenaar, W. A., P. J. J. van Koppen, and H. F. M. Crombag. 1993. Anchored Narratives: The Psychology of Criminal Evidence. Hertfordshire, UK: Harvester Wheatsheaf.

Wasserstrom, R. 1961. The Judicial Decision: Toward a Theory of Legal Justification. Stanford: Stanford Univ. Press.

Weinreb, L. L. 2005. Legal Reason: The Use of Analogy in Legal Argument. New York: Cambridge Univ. Press.

Wigmore, J. H. 1937. The Science of Judicial Proof, as Given by Logic, Psychology, and General Experience, and Illustrated in Judicial Trials, 3d ed. Boston: Little, Brown.

Wilensky, R. 1983. Planning and Understanding: A Computational Approach to Human Reasoning. Reading, MA: Addison-Wesley.

Wilson, T. D., D. J. Lisle, J. W. Schooler, S. D. Hodges, K. J. Klaaren et al. 1993. Introspecting about reasons can reduce post-choice satisfaction. *Pers. Soc. Psychol. Bull.* **19***:*331–339.

Wilson, T. D., and J. W. Schooler. 1991. Thinking too much: Introspection can reduce the quality of preferences and decisions. *J. Pers. Soc. Psychol.* **60***:*181–192.

18

Institutions for Intuitive Man

Christoph Engel

Max Planck Institute for Research on Collective Goods, 53113 Bonn, Germany

Abstract

By its critics, the rational choice model is routinely accused of being unrealistic. For all nontrivial problems, calculating the best response is cognitively way too taxing. This, however, is true only for the consciously controlled handling of information. The automatic system handles huge amounts of information in almost no time. Only the end result is propelled back to consciousness as an intuition. Consequently, in appropriate contexts, institutions should in principle see to it that decision makers trust their intuitions. However, accountability, predictability, and regulability are hard to guarantee for intuitive decision making. Intuitive decision making is even more desirable if the underlying social problem is excessively complex or ill-defined. For instance, in simple social dilemmas, a combination of cheater detection and punishing sentiments does the trick. However, intuition can be misled. For instance, punishing sentiments are triggered by a hurt sense of fairness. Now in more complex social dilemmas, there are competing fairness norms, and people intuitively choose with a self-serving bias. In such contexts, institutions must step in so that clashing intuitions do not lead to social unrest.

Institutions and Behavior

People want to be in control. This at least is a cultural trait of modern Western civilizations. By definition, the nonconscious mental apparatus is not under (direct) conscious control. In the past this has led, for example, to exorcisms aimed at liberating the victim from the foreign being by which it is possessed. Freudian psychoanalysis views the subconscious as the source of serious mental disorder. In this chapter I adopt a more pragmatic perspective. Like any human ability, the nonconscious mental apparatus is assumed to serve a function that, at least in the past when the neuronal structure underlying it developed, gave human genes an evolutionary advantage. As I will try to demonstrate, this advantage is large and it still persists. However, what is beneficial in most contexts can be dysfunctional in others. It can be in the best interest of the individual, and of society for that matter, to exploit the power of intuition, or to prevent intuitive decision making from doing harm, depending on the specific context. To that end, an individual can design its own decision aids or it can voluntarily seek the support of a coach or of technology. Yet modern societies do not always wait for that. Formal and informal institutions impose themselves. The intention can be paternalistic. They can aim at curing a perceived social ill, or they can merely exert power to exploit those who are under their spell.

There are many reasons why institutional designers ought to be cautious. Many institutions are informal, and frequently they emerge, rather than being purposefully designed (Hodgson 1988). Likewise, the target of institutional intervention, human behavior, is usually socially embedded (Granovetter 1985). To be effective, institutional intervention must therefore set in motion a learning process (Engel 2008). Usually, those deciding on the introduction of new institutions are not disinterested (Buchanan and Tullock 1962). This does not imply necessarily that existing formal institutions miss their stated purpose of social betterment. They are, however, likely to pick those solutions that give well-organized political forces a distributional advantage (J. Knight 1992). Once the legislator has promulgated a new rule, it is turned over to the legal system. Like any subsystem of society, the legal system will apply its own internal logic, which may well be at variance with the original political intention (Teubner 1989). Conversely, institutional addressees have the ability to mute the institution creatively (Wegner 1997).

Despite all these caveats, in modern industrialized countries, a legislator produces thousands of new rules in a year. If there is a written constitution, and a Supreme Court to enforce it, the legislator must be able to defend any new intervention into freedom or property. A consistent story must relay why there is a social problem, and how it is solved by the intervention; it will also help in generating political support. Moreover, seeing a new bill through to adoption requires a lot of zeal and may well be costly, for example, in terms of log-rolling. One must assume a high degree of illusionary thinking to claim that all or at least most of this activity misses the point. If institutions are, at least in principle, effective, institutional designers want to reconstruct them as governance tools to cure a (perceived) social ill.

Traditionally, social problems are reconstructed as incentive problems. Individually, institutional addressees are better off if they behave in a socially detrimental way. Institutional intervention realigns individual with social well-being. This reconstruction relies on rational choice theory. Rational choice theory has been exposed to two lines of criticism. The first line focuses on behavioral assumptions (Kahneman and Tversky 2000). It accepts rational choice theory to be the norm and is interested in knowing whether human decision makers live up to this norm. It thus explores a potential gap between the norm and the neuronal and psychological algorithms by which human decision makers try to implement the norm. Actually, it is only in this outside perspective that rational choice theory advances to a behavioral norm. In positive economic theory it is only a conceptual tool. Neoclassical economists do not claim that people truly take decisions in accordance with the axioms of rational choice theory. They only make this assumption to understand how behavior responds to changes in the opportunity structure (Friedman 1953).

The second line of criticism focuses on the norm. It is an established piece of wisdom from normative philosophical theory that all norms for good behavior ultimately rest on a specific construction of reality (Kersting 1994). The critics of rational choice theory claim that this theory assumes an inappropriately certain world (Gigerenzer et al. 1999). Rational choice theory only works if individuals interact in a relatively certain world. At the minimum, all who interact must hold the same beliefs about how their interaction partners reconstruct the situation (Savage 1954). Usually, rational choice models assume a well-defined problem. They exclude situations of ignorance (Kirzner 1994), and usually situations of uncertainty. In rational choice theory, a situation is called uncertain if the problem space is well-defined, but there is uncertainty about the probabilities attached to each potential state of nature. If probabilities are known, this is called risk (F. H. Knight 1921). In situations of risk, expected values may be calculated.

If one properly accounts for the nonconscious mental abilities, the first line of criticism is considerably weakened. Specifically, at the nonconscious level, human decision makers have many more cognitive resources at their disposition. However, the second line of criticism gets additional support: Not only is rational choice theory an inadequate reconstruction of decisions in a fundamentally uncertain world. Many features of the nonconscious mental apparatus are highly functional precisely if the individual has to decide routinely on an incomplete factual basis. In the following, both stories will be presented.

The Incentive Story

Social Problems Are Dilemma Situations

The incentive story is epitomized by the Prisoner's Dilemma (Figure 18.1): an individual is best off if others contribute to the public good, while she gets a free ride. Writing C for contribution and D for defection, and using the first letter for one's own action and the second for the action of others, in a Prisoner's Dilemma each individual holds the following preferences:

$$DC > CC > DD > CD. \tag{1}$$

An equilibrium (in pure strategies) presupposes that two best responses come together in one cell. The only cell for which this is true is the defection/defection cell. This is a dilemma since both players would be better off contributing. This would give both of them their second best outcome, rather than only the third best. However, if they only interact once, and if binding and enforceable agreements are not available, the parties miss this outcome. A combination of

	Contribution	Defection
Contribution	2, 2	0, <u>3</u>
Defection	<u>3</u>, 0	<u>1</u>, <u>1</u>

Figure 18.1 Prisoner's Dilemma. The numbers in the cells are the players' payoffs, where the first number is the payoff of the row player, and the second number the payoff of the column player. Payoffs are represented by the rank in the respective player's preference order, and best responses are underlined.

greed and fear leads to the socially detrimental result (Macy and Flache 2002). Greedy individuals try to get at their individually best outcome (i.e., the free ride). Fearful individuals anticipate this and defect because they do not want to be the sucker.

Although game theorists rightly caution against the abuse of this model, it captures nonetheless the essence of problems as diverse as climate change, arms races, or incentives for innovation in the absence of intellectual property (Hardin 1968). Relying on the sovereign forces of the state, institutional intervention is able to change a Prisoner's Dilemma so that the socially desirable result is achieved. There are several options for this: A tax may reduce the benefit from unilateral defection. A subsidy may increase the benefit from unilateral contribution. Those who have contributed may be given the enforceable right to exclude those who have not from the benefit. At a first stage, the players may be allowed to conclude a binding and enforceable contract (Baird et al. 1994).

Behavioral Critique

A Prisoner's Dilemma is a dilemma, because both players consider exclusively their own utility. In so doing, a player is smart: Not only does she assess correctly which outcome she expects in every possible state of the world. She also assumes that all others with whom she is interacting do the same. Given this assumption, she calculates a best response function and finds her action by maximizing over this function (Fudenberg and Tirole 1991). In all but extremely simple games, this is a daunting intellectual task. For a long time, critics have objected that only demons, not humans, are able to perform the necessary intellectual operations (H. A. Simon 1957; Gigerenzer et al. 1999). Indeed, experimental evidence shows that untrained subjects violate all kinds of mathematical and statistical norms (Conlisk 1996).

The critics have concluded that rational choice models are inappropriate to capture behavior in real-life situations. They have suggested that individuals use instead radically simple decision rules, which they call heuristics. Heuristics deliberately ignore information. They often are lexicographic. Decision makers go through predefined decision trees. They only go to lower branches if the criteria for taking a decision at a higher branch have been inconclusive.

Normally, the criterion at each branch is just one cue. Similar rules tell the decision maker how much effort should be invested when searching for evidence. To keep this effort low, search is usually stopped early in the process (Gigerenzer 2004).

Critique of the Critique

If the heuristics approach is an accurate model of human decision making, the implications for institutional design are profound (Gigerenzer and Engel 2006). However, does the approach rest on an incorrect factual basis? Is the idea that human cognitive abilities are severely limited flawed? Specifically, are the apparent limitations confined to conscious reasoning, whereas the nonconscious mental apparatus offers so many resources that the quest for radically simple decision rules is no longer warranted? Does the heuristics approach suffer from aiming too high? Is the heuristics program only justified if the decision rule remains the same when performed consciously? Is rational choice reinstalled, once one properly accounts for nonconscious abilities? Specifically, does rational choice theory turn out to have not only paramorphic, but even isomorphic quality (cf. Fischhoff et al. 1981)?

There is evidence that points in this direction. Psychologists have demonstrated that individuals take a large amount of evidence into account when deciding on a problem with multiple attributes (Glöckner 2007). Neuroscientists have shown that even monkeys carefully record information on cue validities, and that they use the information in a way that can be modeled by one of the most demanding concepts of rational choice theory, Bayesian updating (Glimcher 2003). The human brain is much larger than the brain of monkeys. It is therefore highly plausible that human decision makers do not only possess the same ability, but that they are even better at it. Anecdotal evidence supports this: If people did not possess a powerful nonconscious mental apparatus, speed reading would not be a possibility. In experts, a lack of conscious awareness is often taken to be a sign of professionalization (Coward 2005, p. 323).

Before institutional intervention can be targeted to nonconscious mental abilities, one should, of course, understand them better. Consciousness only speaks to mental awareness, which is a precondition for deliberate online control. It does not explain how the information is processed nonconsciously. It seems that several inputs are processed in parallel. Parallel constraint satisfaction models explain decision making the following way: an option is chosen that receives the highest activation, provided the system has reached a predefined level of stability, due to attempts at reducing local conflicts between positive and negative activation (Glöckner 2007). For consciousness, only the result of this process is returned. It is perceived as an intuition. Here, much more knowledge is obviously needed.

C. Engel

Implications for Institutional Design

Even at this early stage, first implications for institutional design can be discerned[1]. They point in two opposing directions. First, if the nonconscious mental apparatus is indeed so much more powerful than the conscious apparatus, institutions should see to it that, in appropriate circumstances, decision makers are free to use the better mental machinery. For that purpose, sometimes it will be enough to just point them into the right direction. It is said that a picture speaks a thousand words. Arguably this is due to the fact that pictures convey a lot of information simultaneously that the nonconscious apparatus is able to handle properly. Specifically, pictures are able to inform about a complex relational graph, without giving an explicit definition of the individual relations. Normally, there is not much opposition to using pictures. It may suffice to encourage decision makers to rely on their visualizing skills.

If information is processed nonconsciously, however, those relying on this information yield control. At most they can use their guts to decide whether they feel comfortable with the resulting intuition. It may be necessary to train people that they should indeed trust their intuitions; however, this will not likely be appropriate in all circumstances. Institutions could therefore ensure that addressees gain expertise at the meta-level, learning about situations where intuitive decision making is indeed best policy. The institutional arrangements for professional training may be interpreted as doing exactly this. Moreover, accountability research shows that when the stakes are raised, people work harder but are not necessarily smarter (Wilson and Schooler 1991). They focus attention on what they are good at doing and seek out justifications, should ambient risks materialize (Tetlock 1985). Where intuitive decision making is socially desirable, institutions should therefore not hold decision makers ostensibly liable (as illustrated by rules that strictly limit the personal liability of public officials, or the business judgment rule that shields managers from personal liability; Hansen 1993).

Conversely, although relying on intuition would be good for decision quality, institutional designers may want to impose conscious decision making for competing normative reasons. If they do, they face a dilemma. Furthering the competing goal may very well deteriorate the quality of decisions. Good institutional design ought to get this balance right. Nonetheless, intuitive decision making may not be desired. Institutional intervention may seek to change the way in which addressees take a decision, rather than (only) behavioral output (Engel and Weber 2007). The three main reasons for this are related to each other. In principle, they affect private and public decision makers alike. Yet

---

[1] Of course, the choice set of institutional designers is broader than just impacting on the behavior of individuals who have to live up to their cognitive limitations. Institutions can bring in technological aids (like powerful computers), can impose expert advice, or address a complex social problem by a rule simple enough that everyone can grasp it. However, frequently, legislators are not able to use one of these routes to bypass the limits of human cognition.

since public officials exercise sovereign powers, frequently these secondary concerns will matter more for their decisions.

By definition, nonconscious decision making is not under conscious control. Consequently, the person who has had the intuition is unable to convey to outsiders anything but the final outcome. At most, learning that one person has had a particular intuition may trigger the nonconscious formation of the same intuition in others; otherwise they must trust the foreign intuition. In many contexts, this is deemed insufficient. For instance, most legal orders oblige judges to give explicit, written reasons for the decisions they are taking on behalf of the People (Engel 2007). This is not only a measure of social hygiene. If their intuitions go unchecked, judges might have been influenced nonconsciously by stereotypes and prejudices, rather than unbiased judgment. The same holds for legislators and regulatory agencies. Likewise tort law effectively forces doctors to be able to give explicit reasons for the treatments they order. In the light of the scandals that led to the Sarbanes-Oxley Act, shareholders increasingly force Chief Executive Officers to give reasons for their business decisions as well.

The second and third reasons become even stronger once one drops the assumption of a well-defined problem space. However, even under the more restrictive assumption, predictability and regulability are an issue. Then the power of intuition results from the fact that large amounts of information may be processed nonconsciously in very little time (Kahneman and Frederick 2002). This information need not be taken online from the environment. It may be retrieved from memory. This makes it difficult for interaction partners to predict foreign intuition. They may have overlooked many facets of the situation that have induced the decision maker to form a certain intuition. Even with perfect attention to the situation, it is impossible to second guess the elements of declarative memory that the decision maker's brain adds to the material from which it forms the intuition. One would have had to accompany the decision maker throughout her entire previous life. With imperfect prediction, social interaction becomes at least risky, if not impossible to bring about (Engel 2005). Of course, intuitive decision making is not always and necessarily less predictable. An example to the contrary is behavior guided by strong and persistent emotions, such as vengeance.

Predictability is also of utmost importance for regulation. Most social problems originate in human behavior. Admittedly, there are exceptions. If a volcano bursts, one cannot hold a person liable. Instead, one can implement an early warning system and evacuate neighboring regions once the alert system is triggered. However, an ever smaller part of institutions is meant to contain pure natural risk. Even risks as apparently natural as global warming are very likely to result from human behavior. Most problems addressed by institutions result from strategic interaction. They are thus purely human in origin.

Whenever human behavior is at least part of the explanation for the problem, regulators must interpret this behavior correctly. They are in the business of prediction. Prediction is inevitable for the second component of institutional design: defining the precise shape of the institution itself. This presupposes anticipating how addressees will react to the intervention. If addressees use their intuition for this purpose, the intervention is bound to be only one out of many elements being processed. It is next to impossible for institutions to get addressees' intuition under control. Understanding the nonconscious mental apparatus, therefore, radicalizes an observation from the evolutionary theory of institutions. The effect of institutional intervention is not only unpredictable if addressees, on purpose, try to mute the impulse creatively (Wegner 1997). The predictability problem already exists whenever addressees use their nonconscious mental apparatus.

In appropriate contexts, institutional designers may respond by shifting to two-level governance. Through a first intervention, they induce addressees to keep their decision under full conscious control. The second intervention exploits the much better predictability for doing something about the underlying social problem. Visibly raising stakes is the most popular way to achieve this. The most drastic intervention to that end is holding managers liable under criminal law, as in the environmental legislation of many countries (for an overview, see O'Hear 2004). A justification requirement has a similar effect (Tetlock et al. 1989). However, this strategy comes at a high price. Precisely since the nonconscious mental apparatus is so much more powerful, institutional designers face a hard choice between higher predictability and better decision quality.

Although predictability is the most visible, it is not the only challenge to regulability resulting from intuition. By definition, only the final outcome becomes conscious. The mental process of forming an intuition is beyond conscious control. It is therefore not a matter of willpower whether a person has an intuition, and which are its contents. The standard suggestion from rational choice theory for the design of institutions is mute. Raising the stakes, be it via imposing sanctions or handing out subsidies, is pointless if the addressee is unable to control the target activity. Specifically, institutional designers would have to be sure that higher stakes do not only influence conscious decision making, but find a way to impact the nonconscious formation of an intuition. Preparing for future intuitive decision making may be easier to influence.

This casts new light on the legal concept of negligence. Negligence is stricter than intent. A tort feasor, or a person bound by a contract, is not only sanctioned if she has violated her duty on purpose. She is also held liable if she could have been expected to prevent the violation from happening. It would make sense to at least partly reconstruct this as liability for not having properly trained one's intuitions. If this holds true, it has an important implication for institutional design. Since training intuitions takes time, effective institutional intervention must start very early. Institutional designers, and the political and legal constituencies that control them, must be sufficiently patient. It is possible that additional institutions must see to it that the respective task is only performed by those who have undergone training. The institutional arrangements around the liberal professions may serve as an illustration. For instance, the training of future doctors is not confined to transmitting explicit knowledge. They are also sent to hospitals to practice under supervision. This is meant to imbue them with the implicit knowledge of the discipline (cf. the distinction between explicit and implicit knowledge in Cowan et al. 2000).

Although the nonconscious mental apparatus is able to handle a huge amount of information in very little time, it might well not be perfect. Even the many more resources must have their limits. Take the following, deceptively simple, problem: Two players interact. Each of them has three options. At every instance of interaction, the options of either player may therefore be combined in nine different ways. Each player may rank each of these nine outcomes differently. This apparently simple structure already makes for $9! = 362,880$ possible different games. The human mind may be able to solve problems as complex as this. The fact that people solve the traveling salesman problem so easily points in this direction. Doing so involves mental operations in this order of complexity. Ultimately, however, there must be a limit. If each player has four options, this already makes for $16! = 20,922,798,888,000$ combinations, and interacting with just one other person that may order four items in her utility function in every possible way is not an outlandish situation. Therefore, it is highly likely that there are situations for which even the limitations of the nonconscious mental apparatus matter.

It still seems to be largely unclear whether the nonconscious mental apparatus has not only quantitative, but also qualitative limitations. A hint is provided by work that shows how expert intuition is, in appropriate contexts, beaten by statistical evidence (Meadow and Sunstein 2001). This issue is related to a second one: Why does the human species have an evolutionary advantage to develop the ability to override the nonconscious apparatus consciously? Does the nonconscious apparatus have too many degrees of freedom? A clue comes from twin studies: when twins grow up together, they tend to create more divergence than if they grow up in different places. Does the human mind thus suffer from an embarrassment of riches? Does the nonconscious apparatus lack the ability to self-program or to direct an active search for information? Is it too easily trapped by the surface structure of a problem, and risks neglecting what is already known about the underlying basic structure? Related to this, one might ask: Is it difficult for intuitive decision making to ignore history and to decontextualize? Is intuition too good at finding an acceptable solution for the problem at hand, and does it run the risk of neglecting the consequences for future similar situations? Are institutions needed where the socially desirable outcome is counterintuitive?

It probably is too early to build institutional interventions on any of these speculations. Until our knowledge about the limitations of the nonconscious mental apparatus has further advanced, these ideas may, however, at least serve as an additional explanation for interventions that are already found in institutional practice. The last point provides a good illustration for this. In principle, the law of torts is an elegant institution. All the legislator has to do is to promulgate that tort feasors are held liable, maybe with the restriction that they can be found negligent. What this general rule means in practice is, step-by-step, developed by the courts, in the light of concrete conflicts. Through this decentralized mechanism, much more local knowledge goes into the actual shaping of the rule. However, since the general rule, at least originally, is underspecified, the courts are likely to rely on their intuition when making it more concrete. Many have complained that this often creates a bias. In the interest of being fair with the victim, the courts generate rules that, for the general public, are overly stringent (Rachlinski 2000). It has been one of the hallmarks of law and economics to teach the courts to see the long-term implications of negligence standards (Posner 2003). Thus far, this discussion has used different language. One might, however, reconstruct the law and economics of torts as a tool for correcting intuitive decision making where it leads to socially undesirable results.

Along the same lines, one may wonder whether institutions play a role in shaping the interaction between the intuitive and the deliberate mental apparatus. It has been claimed that the nonconscious and the conscious, the intuitive and the deliberate, the parallel and serial are not tightly separated from each other, but may interact (Strack and Deutsch 2004). Again it probably is too early to suggest new institutions for the socially more desirable fine tuning of this interaction. Suffice it to point to one existing institutional arrangement that may be reconstructed as doing exactly this. It goes to the core of the legal profession. Decision making in the courts has been demonstrated to rely heavily on "coherence-based reasoning" (D. Simon 2004). Given the institutional framework, and the need to give explicit reasons for the decision taken in particular, one could not possibly claim that judges rely exclusively on their intuition. It is also beyond doubt that legal decision making is not just a matter of calculus. The legal method is hermeneutical. It asks the lawyer to match an overly rich reality to an abstract rule. Judges get at this syllogism by deliberating, permanently checking inputs and potential outputs against their intuition. In light of this, one may interpret the compulsory training of future lawyers and the organization of the court system as tools for bringing about the socially desired interaction between intuition and deliberation.

Finally, clever institutional design might be able to get at the best of both worlds. There might be interventions that leave enough room for the power of intuition, and nonetheless provide society with accountability, predictability and regulability. Again, judicial procedure might provide an illustration. Judges are obliged to give explicit reasons for their decisions. They are not obliged, however, to report the mental process by which they have found the solution to the case. The separation between the context of discovery and the context of representation might do the trick (Engel 2007). It has been claimed that this is also how morality serves as a post hoc control of individual behavior

(Haidt 2001). If mere predictability is enough, standardizing context might suffice, if certain intuitions predictably go with this context (Engel 2005). This might be due to the fact that the mental representation of the standardized setting is reliable. Obviously, more experimental work is needed.

Navigating a Fundamentally Uncertain World

Defining Uncertainty

As long as individuals have to make choices from a well-defined problem space, the (evolutionary) advantage of intuition boils down to a question of quantity. If individuals rely on their intuition, they can muster many more resources for decision making. The fact that the problem or the socially desired solution is complicated does not mean necessarily that the individual is unable to solve it. The full power of intuition is seen only if one drops the assumption that the problem space is well-defined. Many problems that individuals and societies have to solve are indeed ill-defined. Frequently, social problems are a moving target. At most, the institutional designer is able to show that today's state of the world is at variance with some accepted normative standard. Whether the problem persists in the future depends on a plurality of contextual factors to which the institutional designer can at best express beliefs. By definition, the future is uncertain. In addition, the reconstruction of the present state of affairs is often based on shaky grounds. If time series information is needed to prove the existence of a problem or show something meaningful about causality (Leamer 1983), the necessary data will often not be available. Things become worse if individual events must be reconstructed. As court procedure demonstrates, true certainty is almost never achieved. Eyewitnesses are particularly unreliable. Memory decays over time and is reconstructive rather than photographic in the first place (Sporer et al. 1996).

Even if, in a categorical sense, the problem is well-defined, it may not be rigorously tractable. This statement holds even if one expects the nonconscious mental apparatus to be more powerful than it probably is. Let us recall, from the previous section, the instance of strategic interaction as simple as one having only two players, each with three options; this already constitutes a set of $9! = 362,880$ different games. Calculating this degree of complexity, however, would not be difficult for a personal computer nowadays. But a game on par with chess is no longer open to canonical analysis and decision making, although a chessboard does not have more than 64 fields. Of course, Deep Blue was able to beat the world champion at chess ten years ago. In so doing, however, it did not use brute force; it worked with approximations, not with simple calculus. A limit of principle is reached once a problem is "NP-hard"; that is if, by calculus, the problem cannot be solved in defined time, whatever the amount of resources used for calculation (Garey and Johnson 1979). This is already the case if the dependent variable is in the exponent, as in the following, deceptively simple, equation, $y = a^x$, where a is a constant and $y = f(x)$.

Finally, for pragmatic reasons, decision makers may prefer to reduce mental effort and to solve problems in a noncanonical way, although this would, in principle, be possible. Indeed Oaksford and Chater (2001) have shown experimentally that this is what many people do. It seems that many people use trust, rather than any version of game theory, to decide upon action in situations of strategic interaction, even if they are experienced (Selten et al. 1997). This may be a strategy to save mental resources for competing tasks. The strategy may also be triggered by time pressure. Still, it seems that, even beyond such cost-benefit analysis, most people are "cognitive misers" (Tetlock et al. 1989, p. 633).

Decision Making Adapted to a Fundamentally Uncertain World

The remarkable power of the nonconscious mental apparatus casts some doubt on the first argument brought forward in support of the heuristics program: cognitive limitations. Yet the main argument has always been that most real-life problems are either ill-defined or NP-hard (Gigerenzer 2004). This second argument is not affected by the criticism. However, the heuristics program suffers from a lacuna. By now, there is ample evidence that fast and frugal heuristics can perform surprisingly well, although the decision rule asks decision makers to ignore deliberately most of the available information. This statement, however, holds only if the appropriate heuristic is applied. Thus far, the heuristics program is not able to say much about appropriateness, and even less about the way in which people learn about it (cf. Rieskamp and Otto 2006). Heuristics are good if and when they are "ecological." They perform poorly if they are used out of their respective domain (Engel 2006). Intuition provides the missing link. Defining the proper domain of a heuristic, and assessing whether the case at hand fits the definition, is bound to be an information-rich activity. Precisely because intuition is able to handle large amounts of information rapidly, it is possible that decision makers apply a certain heuristic where it is indeed likely to lead to a good decision.

Actually, the power of intuition goes even beyond this. Decision makers can use their intuition to match features from the environment to schemas (Bartlett 1932, p. 199–204) and exemplars (Anderson 2000, p. 350–352). In either concept, not each and every element from the description of the schema or the exemplar must be met by observation. Some may miss. It depends on the relevance of the missing element whether the case at hand is assimilated nonetheless to the domain of the heuristic. Intuition has a further advantage for the concept of heuristics. The result of the nonconscious processing can be made consciously available. This opens up the possibility that decision makers check nonconsciously whether they dispose of an appropriate heuristic, and then apply it consciously. This fits the heuristics program, since this research has normally not specified whether the heuristic is applied consciously or not, and it is certainly open to the idea that the decision tree itself is processed consciously.

There is an alternative possibility: decision making can rest entirely on intuition. If this is the case, the decision maker uses not only a lot of information to assess whether a certain heuristic is applicable, she also takes many elements into account when making the actual decision. Specifically, she may consider not only multiple cues, but also attach different weights to each of them and allow for cue weights to be changed via the interaction with competing cues (Glöckner 2007). Ultimately, this is an empirical question. The existing evidence makes it probable that the meta-decision on how to decide is influenced by the perceived situation and by personality. The stronger the time pressure, and the higher the load of competing tasks, the more parsimonious the decision rule. Some people, most of the time, prefer relatively simple rules whereas others tend to spend more (nonconscious!) effort on the processing of information (Glöckner 2007).

In functional terms, nonconscious parallel processing of information enables decision makers to use Bayesian statistics (Bolstad 2004). They are thus not confined to using the information to which they have access at the moment of decision making. Rather they can use the new information to update their provisional knowledge about the environment (Oaksford and Chater 1994). In addition, they are able to engage in mental simulation (Stone and Davies 1995).

All of this is extremely helpful in navigating an (fundamentally) uncertain environment. The individual may find critical situations by looking for outliers: "something is fishy here." The early alert system becomes even more powerful if the individual can quickly check whether single features of an otherwise familiar situation are novel, or even similar to the characteristics of a dangerous event. Individuals are able to engage in sense making (Weick 1995), in constructing mental models (Johnson-Laird 1983), and in observational learning (Bandura 1986). They can transpose solutions that have been successful in the past to new situations, once the current problem has been identified as sufficiently similar to the earlier one (Gilboa and Schmeidler 1995). Thus, they can exploit the power of associations (Coward 2005, p. 305).

Intuition as a Solution to Social Problems

Occasionally, once one accounts for the power of intuition properly, there is no longer any need for institutional intervention. In appropriate circumstances, this even holds for the classic rational choice justification for institutional intervention: the Prisoner's Dilemma. In principle, the dilemma persists if the two players are allowed to communicate. It is in the best interest of both of them to agree on the cooperative solution. However, this only shifts the original conflict to the implementation stage. Once they have agreed, either player is best off if the other is loyal to the agreement while she defects. This even holds if the agreement allows the victim, or any member of a larger group, to impose a sanction on those who violate the agreement, for punishment is costly. Again those individuals are best off who have others do the costly punishing. The original dilemma repeats itself (Heckathorn 1989).

Lawyers tend to be unconvinced by this story. It clashes with their experience that the conclusion of a contract matters, even if the contract cannot be enforced. The experience is particularly pronounced in public international law. Since there is no world government, the enforcement of international treaties may not often be taken for granted. Nonetheless states are reluctant to accept treaty provisions if they know that they will not want to implement them at a later date. There are rational choice explanations for this: A state might be afraid of gaining a bad reputation, which could be costly in future negotiations. But legal experience seems to point to the fact that there is more to it than just repeated or nested games. One possible explanation of the add-on fits here.

It has been demonstrated that people dispose of a very sensitive cheater detection mechanism (Cosmides 1989). Further evidence shows that most people hold strong punishing sentiments if they suspect others to have cheated on an earlier promise (Fehr and Gächter 2000). The combination of both mechanisms offers a solution to the Prisoner's Dilemma: Players are allowed to communicate and to punish free riders.

Intuition helps us understand a frequent observation from political practice and legal discourse. Since contestants cannot agree on fundamentals, they content themselves with an "incompletely theorized agreement" (Sunstein 1995). They are happy to agree on an outcome, although each may hold different convictions as to why it is justified. This may be due to the fact that each of them is able to give a consistent justification, only starting from different premises. However, in legal practice, the experience is a different one. Someone suggests a solution. Everyone accepts it quickly as a good one. Conflict breaks out once one side starts giving reasons. After a long and vigorous fight, both sides agree finally to leave the reasons aside, since they still feel happy with the original suggestion for a solution. This line of events can only be explained if some contextual, but hard to formulate, element pushes the decisions of all of them into the same direction.

This explanation also holds for another frequent observation. When they learn about the latest theoretical achievements in one of the social sciences, lawyers have often responded: oh yes, we have been attentive to this for a hundred years. There have, for instance, been many legal rules taking care of the anti-commons problem before the term was even coined (Heller 1998). This statement is not meant to depreciate the advancement of the social sciences. Being able to articulate a problem precisely has value. However, the fact that the (legal) solution so often predates the precise formulation of the problem can only be explained if, intuitively and hence nonconsciously, legal decision makers have already grasped the essence of the problem.

Intuition Misled

Although intuition is a powerful tool for navigating an uncertain environment, it is not foolproof. Intuition can easily be misled. Under experimental conditions, judges have discounted pieces of evidence to generate coherence when the material presented to them did not allow for this (D. Simon et al. 2001). Legal professionals have at most only a very small advantage over laypeople when it comes to telling a credible eyewitness from one who is lying. However, the professionals feel much more comfortable with their assessment (Sporer 2007). If decision makers have been exposed to a biased sample, they build intuitions that are inappropriate for the true population (cf. Fiedler 2000). Interested outsiders can specialize in manipulating foreign intuition to their advantage. A classic example is subliminal advertising, where the target group is primed in favor of buying a product without consciously noticing (Greenwald et al. 1995).

Intuition seems to be much better at finding a locally, rather than a globally, acceptable solution. Economists, for instance, claim that non-economists are very bad at capturing multiple, interrelated effects (e.g., the co-presence of substitution and income effects (Hellwig 2007). Note that the explanation for the phenomenon would not be sheer complexity. Rather the nonconscious apparatus would be more or less well prepared to execute some (mildly) complicated mental operation. In this explanation, the problem originates in the fact that socially relevant mental operations are "counterintuitive." This might be due to the fact that individuals are genetically prepared to interpret the situation otherwise, or they might have acquired this inclination through enculturation.

Intuitive decision making becomes particularly socially disruptive if individuals must cooperate when intuitions clash. The problem is so hard precisely because the individuals do not have access to the underlying mental process. All they have is the result, the intuition, which they cannot but believe to be true. The very instance that has served to demonstrate the potential of the nonconscious for the solution of social problems illustrates as well the most profound risk in this. The Prisoner's Dilemma is overcome if players use intuition to detect cheaters and are willing to punish them. However, what if cheating is a matter of interpretation? In the standard game presented above, there is no room for ambiguity. Both players have identical endowments. The optimal solution for the community of the two players is precisely defined. The game is fully symmetrical. Both players know this. It is easy for them to calculate their own payoffs, as well as the payoffs of the other player, for each combination of actions. Real-life conflicts are hardly ever that tidy. The potential for gains and losses is distributed asymmetrically (Rapoport and Chammah 1965). The players are informed asymmetrically as well. The structure of the game and the payoffs are not beyond doubt. The players bring different endowments to the game.

The cheater detection mechanism rests on assessing fairness. Once one gets away from the tidy situation, different fairness norms can be applied. Rather than formal equality, desert, entitlement or status could be used (Hoffman and Spitzer 1985; Hoffman et al. 1998). Depending on which norm is chosen, the definition of cheating will be different. Specifically, whereas one norm would give one of the players a distributional advantage, a competing one would advantage frequently the other player. Take, for instance, an asymmetric game. Is it unfair for the player who is advantaged by the structure of the game to insist on the equilibrium solution? Unfortunately, individuals have a strong self-serving bias in defining the fairness norm. Actually, they firmly believe that fairness could only be assessed in this and in no other way (Konow 2005). Their intuition traps them in two ways: (a) in picking a fairness norm and (b) in believing that the other player has cheated since she has violated this norm. In such situations, conflict is bound to escalate, for the first player feels the urge to punish the "cheater." This player, in turn, feels treated unfairly and punishes in return (Denant-Boèment et al. 2007).

Implications for Institutional Design

In principle, in an uncertain environment, the implications for institutional design are similar to the ones delineated for a well-defined problem space. Where intuition is more powerful than conscious deliberation, institutions should build trust in intuition. Where intuition risks being misled in an individually or socially detrimental way, institutions may choose among one of two aims: (a) they may try to induce their addressees to use a less problematic mental mechanism, be that just conscious reasoning, or some combination of intuitive and deliberate elements, or (b) they may try to shape the environment such that addressees form more appropriate intuitions. The problems of control, predictability, and regulability are the same as in a well-defined problem space, as are potential solutions.

In terms of conflicting intuitions, social norms have been demonstrated to guide people in the formation of not necessarily identical, but coordinated fairness norms (Kahan 2005). Formal legal rules could have the same effect if they are properly translated into more contextualized normative expectations (Engel 2008). Coordinating intuitions becomes, of course, easier, the more homogeneous a society. Responses to perceived fundamental uncertainty have been shown to be culturally contingent (Nisbett et al. 2001; Sperber and Hirschfeld 2004). Making societies more homogeneous, however, is not usually an option for policy makers. Shaping the representation of the situation and organizing feedback could be, however, at least of some help.

Acknowledgments

Helpful comments by Matthew Adler, Paul Glimcher, Andreas Glöckner, Stefan Magen, Jeffrey Rachlinski and Wolf Singer on an earlier version are gratefully acknowledged.

References

Anderson, J. R. 2000. Learning and Memory: An Integrated Approach. New York: Wiley.

Baird, D. G., R. H. Gertner, and R. C. Picker. 1994. Game Theory and the Law. Cambridge, MA: Harvard Univ. Press.

Bandura, A. 1986. Social Foundations of Thought and Action: A Social Cognitive Theory. Englewood Cliffs, NJ: Prentice Hall.

Bartlett, F. C. 1932. Remembering: A Study in Experimental and Social Psychology. Cambridge: Cambridge Univ. Press.

Bolstad, W. M. 2004. Introduction to Bayesian Statistics. New York: Wiley.

Buchanan, J. M., and G. Tullock. 1962. The Calculus of Consent: Logical Foundations of Constitutional Democracy. Ann Arbor: Univ. of Michigan Press.

Conlisk, J. 1996. Why bounded rationality? *J. Econ. Lit.* **34**:669–700.

Cosmides, L. 1989. The logic of social exchange: Has natural selection shaped how humans reason? Studies with the Wason selection task. *Cognition* **31**:187–276.

Cowan, R., P. A. David, and D. Foray. 2000. The explicit economics of knowledge codification and tacitness. *Ind. Corp. Change* **9**:211–253.

Coward, L. A. 2005. A Systems Architecture Approach to the Brain: From Neurons to Consciousness. New York: Nova Biomedical Books.

Denant-Boèment, L., D. Masclet, and C. Noussair. 2007. Punishment, counter-punishment and sanction enforcement in a social dilemma experiment. *Econ. Theory*, in press.

Engel, C. 2005. Generating Predictability: Institutional Analysis and Design. Cambridge: Cambridge Univ. Press.

Engel, C. 2006. Social dilemmas revisited from a heuristics perspective. In: Heuristics and the Law, ed. G. Gigerenzer and C. Engel, pp. 61–85. Cambridge, MA: MIT Press.

Engel, C. 2007. The psychological case for obliging judges to write reasons. In: The Impact of Court Procedure on the Psychology of Judicial Decision Making, ed. C. Engel and F. Strack, pp. 71–109. Baden-Baden: Nomos.

Engel, C. 2008. Learning the law. *J. Inst. Econ.*, in press.

Engel, C., and E. U. Weber. 2007. The Impact of Institutions on the Decision how to Decide. *J. Inst. Econ.*, in press.

Fehr, E., and S. Gächter. 2000. Cooperation and punishment in public goods experiments. *Am. Econ. Rev.* **90**:980–994.

Fiedler, K. 2000. Beware of samples! A cognitive-ecological sampling approach to judgment bias. *Psychol. Rev.* **107**:659–676.

Fischhoff, B., B. Goitein, and Z. Shapira. 1981. Subjected expected utility: A model of decision making. *J. Am. Soc. Info. Sci.* **32**:391–399.

Friedman, M. 1953. Essays in Positive Economics. Chicago: Univ. Chicago Press.

Fudenberg, D., and J. Tirole. 1991. Game Theory. Cambridge, MA: MIT Press.

Garey, M. R., and D. S. Johnson. 1979. Computers and Intractability: A Guide to the Theory of NP-Completeness. San Francisco: W. H. Freeman.

Gigerenzer, G. 2004. Fast and frugal heuristics: The tools of bounded rationality. In: Handbook of Judgement and Decision Making, ed. D. Koehler and N. Harvey. Oxford: Blackwell.

Gigerenzer, G., and C. Engel, eds. 2006. Heuristics and the Law. Cambridge, MA: MIT Press.

Gigerenzer, G., P. M. Todd, and the ABC Research Group. 1999. Simple Heuristics That Make Us Smart. New York: Oxford Univ. Press.

Gilboa, I., and D. Schmeidler. 1995. Case-based decision theory. *Qtly. J. Econ.* **110**(3):605–639.

Glimcher, P. W. 2003. Decisions, Uncertainty, and the Brain: The Science of Neuroeconomics. Cambridge, MA: MIT Press.

Glöckner, A. 2007. Does intuition beat fast and frugal heuristics? A systematic empirical approach. In: A New Look on Intuition, ed. H. Plessner, C. Betsch, and T. Betsch. Mahwah, NJ: Lawrence Erlbaum, in press.

Granovetter, M. 1985. Economic action and social structure: The problem of embeddedness. *Am. J. Soc.* **91**:481–510.

Greenwald, A. G., M. R. Klinger, and E. S. Schuh. 1995. Activation by marginally perceptible ("subliminal") stimuli: Dissociation of unconscious from conscious cognition. *J. Exp. Psychol.: Gen.* **124**:22–42.

Haidt, J. 2001. The emotional dog and its rational tail: A social intuitionist approach to moral judgment. *Psychol. Rev.* **108**:814–834.

Hansen, C. 1993. The duty of care, the business judgment rule, and the American Law Institute corporate governance project. *Business Lawyer* **48**:1355–1376.

Hardin, G. 1968. The tragedy of the commons. *Science* **162**:1243–1248.

Heckathorn, D. D. 1989. Collective action and the second-order free-rider problem. *Ration. Soc.* **1**:78–100.

Heller, M. A. 1998. The tragedy of the anticommons: Property in the transition from Marx to markets. *Harvard Law Rev.* **111**:621–688.

Hellwig, M. 2007. Zur Kategorie der Kausalität in den Wirtschaftswissenschaften. Kausalität, pp. 47–63. Berlin: Berlin Brandenburgische Akademie der Wissenschaften.

Hodgson, G. M. 1988. Economics and Institutions: A Manifesto for a Modern Institutional Economics. Philadelphia: Univ. Pennsylvania Press.

Hoffman, E., K. McCabe, and V. L. Smith. 1998. Behavioral foundations of reciprocity: Experimental economics and evolutionary psychology. *Econ. Inq.* **36**:335–355.

Hoffman, E., and M. L. Spitzer. 1985. Entitlements, rights, and fairness: An experimental examination of subjects' concepts of distributive justice. *J. Legal Stud.* **14**:259–297.

Johnson-Laird, P. N. 1983. Mental Models: Towards a Cognitive Science of Language, Inference and Consciousness. Cambridge: Cambridge Univ. Press.

Kahan, D. 2005. The logic of reciprocity: Trust, collective action, and law. In: Moral Sentiments and Material Interests, ed. H. Gintis, S. Bowles, R. Boyd, and E. Fehr, pp. 339–378. Cambridge, MA: MIT Press.

Kahneman, D., and S. Frederick. 2002. Representativeness revisited: Attribute substitution in intuitive judgment. In: Heuristics and Biases: The Psychology of Intuitive Judgment, ed. T. Gilovich, D. W. Griffin, and D. Kahneman, pp. 49–81. New York: Cambridge Univ. Press.

Kahneman, D., and A. Tversky, eds. 2000. Choices, Values, and Frames. Cambridge: Cambridge Univ. Press.

Kersting, W. 1994. Die politische Philosophie des Gesellschaftsvertrags. Darmstadt: Wiss. Buchgesellschaft.

Kirzner, I. 1994. On the economics of time and ignorance: The market process. In: Essays in Contemporary Austrian Economics, ed. P. J. Boettke and D. L. Prychitko, pp. 38–44. Brookfield: Elgar.

Knight, F. H. 1921. Risk, Uncertainty and Profit. Boston: Houghton Mifflin.

Knight, J. 1992. Institutions and Social Conflict. Cambridge: Cambridge Univ. Press.

Konow, J. 2005. Blind spots: The effects of information and stakes on fairness bias and dispersion. *Soc. Justice Res.* **18**:349–390.

Leamer, E. E. 1983. Let's take the con out of econometrics. *Am. Econ. Rev.* **23**:31–43.

Macy, M. M., and A. Flache. 2002. Learning dynamics in social dilemmas. *Proc. Natl. Acad. Sci.* **99**:7229–7236.

Meadow, W., and C. R. Sunstein. 2001. Statistics, not Experts. *Duke Law J.* **51**:629–646.

Nisbett, R. E., K. Peng, I. Choi, and A. Norenzayan. 2001. Culture and systems of thought: Holistic versus analytic cognition. *Psychol. Rev.* **108**:291–310.

Oaksford, M., and N. Chater. 1994. A rational analysis of the selection task as optimal data selection. *Psychol. Rev.* **101**:608–631.

Oaksford, M., and N. Chater. 2001. The probabilistic approach to human reasoning. *Trends Cogn. Sci.* **5**:349–357.

O'Hear, M. M. 2004. Sentencing the green-collar offender: Punishment, culpability, and environmental crime. *J. Crim. Law Criminology.* **95**:133–275.

Posner, R. A. 2003. Economic Analysis of Law. New York: Aspen Publishers.

Rachlinski, J. J. 2000. A positive psychological theory of judging in hindsight. In: Behavioral Law and Economics, ed. C. R. Sunstein, pp. 95–115. Cambridge: Cambridge Univ. Press.

Rapoport, A., and A. M. Chammah. 1965. Prisoner's Dilemma: A Study in Conflict and Cooperation. Ann Arbor: Univ. Mich. Press.

Rieskamp, J., and P. E. Otto. 2006. SSL: A theory of how people learn to select strategies. *J. Exp. Psychol.: Gen.* **135**:207–236.

Savage, L. J. 1954. The Foundations of Statistics. New York: Wiley.

Selten, R., M. Mitzkewitz, and G. R. Uhlich. 1997. Duopoly strategies programmed by experienced players. *Econometrica* **65**:517–555.

Simon, D. 2004. A third view of the black box: Cognitive coherence in legal decision making. *Univ. Chicago Law Rev.* **71**:511–586.

Simon, D., L. B. Pham, Q. A. Le, and K. J. Holyoak. 2001. The emergence of coherence over the course of decision making. *J. Exp. Psychol.: Learn. Mem. Cogn.* **27**:1250–1260.

Simon, H. A. 1957. Models of Man: Social and Rational Mathematical Essays on Rational Human Behavior in a Society Setting. New York: Wiley.

Sperber, D., and L. A. Hirschfeld. 2004. The cognitive foundations of cultural stability and diversity. *Trends Cogn. Sci.* **8**:40–46.

Sporer, S. L. 2007. Evaluating eyewitness testimony: The fallacies of intuition. In: The Impact of Court Procedure on the Psychology of Judicial Decision Making, ed. C. Engel and F. Strack, pp. 111–150. Baden-Baden: Nomos.

Sporer, S. L., R. S. Malpass, and G. Köhnken. 1996. Psychological Issues in Eyewitness Identification. Mahwah, NJ: Lawrence Erlbaum.

Stone, T., and M. Davies, eds. 1995. Mental Simulation: Evaluations and Applications. Oxford: Blackwell.

Strack, F., and R. Deutsch. 2004. Reflective and impulsive determinants of social behavior. *Pers. Soc. Psychol. Rev.* **8**:220–247.

Sunstein, C. R. 1995. Incompletely theorized agreements. *Harvard Law Rev.* **108**:1733–1772.

Tetlock, P. E. 1985. Accountability: The neglected social context of judgment and choice. *Res. Org. Behav.* **7**:297–332.

Tetlock, P. E., L. Skitka, and R. Boettger. 1989. Social and cognitive strategies for coping with accountability: Conformity, complexity, and bolstering. *J. Pers. Soc. Psychol.* **57**:632–640.

Teubner, G. 1989. Recht als autopoietisches System. Frankfurt: Suhrkamp.

Wegner, G. 1997. Economic policy from an evolutionary perspective: A new approach. *J. Instit. Theor. Econ.* **153**:485–509.

Weick, K. E. 1995. Sensemaking in Organizations. Thousand Oaks: Sage Publications.

Wilson, T. D., and J. W. Schooler. 1991. Thinking too much. Introspection can reduce the quality of preferences and decisions. *J. Pers. Soc. Psychol.* **60**:181–192.

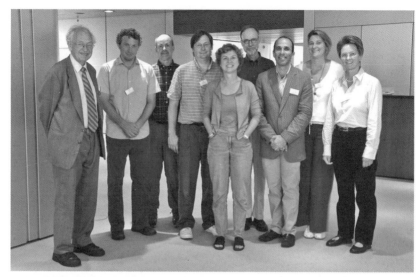

Left to right: Reinhard Selten, Mark Lubell, Reid Hastie, Jeff Rachlinski, Elke Weber, Christoph Engel, Paul Glimcher, Tania Singer, and Bettina Rockenbach

19

Institutional Design Capitalizing on the Intuitive Nature of Decision Making

Mark Lubell, Rapporteur

Christoph Engel, Paul W. Glimcher, Reid Hastie,
Jeffrey J. Rachlinski, Bettina Rockenbach, Reinhard Selten,
Tania Singer, and Elke U. Weber

Neural and Psychological Processes as the Substrate of Institutional Design

What insights about institutional design can be gained by considering that the processing of information is not always under conscious control? At first, it might seem that the very purpose of most institutional efforts to control decision making is to produce decisions that are conscious, slow, deliberative, effortful, rational, and unemotional. Institutional design would thus seem targeted to produce what psychologists sometimes refer to as "system 2" thinking (Kahneman 2003; Kahneman and Frederick 2005). From this perspective, institutional interventions should drive out cognitive processes that are unconscious, rapid, automatic, associative, holistic, and emotional; that is, to reduce to "system 1" thinking. If there is reason to believe that system 1 processes will be at work, additional institutions would aim at bringing cognition under conscious control, or at least at limiting the undesirable influence of system 1 thinking on decisions and behavior.

In this report we demonstrate that institutional efforts to improve decision making are not, and should not be, directed solely at producing system 2 thinking. No cognitive process is superior in all settings. Consequently, good institutional design ought to aim at the best match between cognitive processes and tasks. In appropriate contexts, this includes capitalizing on the power of intuition.

As other chapters in this volume reveal, the distinction between conscious and unconscious is a somewhat artificial construct (Platt et al., this volume). So, too, is the supposed "system 1" versus "system 2" distinction (Keysers et al., this volume). Human behavior is certainly the product of a combination of processes that implicate concepts of consciousness and intentionality in different ways. Since the cognitive revolution, psychologists have worked to identify and define cognitive processes, without regard to the level of awareness that they implicate. The picture becomes exponentially more complicated if one also takes the underlying neural structure into account.

Despite the artificial nature of the distinction between conscious and unconscious processing, many social institutions assume that such a distinction exists and is important. For example, the urge to impose a sanction on another person if one has been hurt "intentionally" is felt more intensely than if the same mischief has been caused by this person's negligence (Falk et al. 2000). In addition, institutional settings often provide instructions to decision makers to make careful, deliberative choices, as in the jury system (discussed below). The use of the conscious/unconscious distinction as a useful shorthand at the institutional level, however, produces methodological and practical challenges for social scientists, which we illustrate in Figure 19.1.

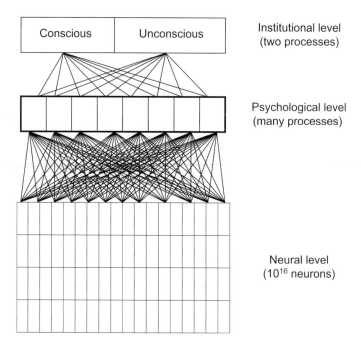

Figure 19.1   A mapping of institutional, psychological, and neurological processes.

Figure 19.1 reveals the impediment to converting an understanding of neural processes into institutional design. This might seem obvious to many; after all, understanding a tiny neuron could hardly be translated easily into understanding a complex social institution. It is tempting to think of Figure 19.1 as an inverted pachinko machine: a neural firing at the bottom level could translate into any number of different, unpredictable cognitive processes, which in turn translate into either a conscious or unconscious cognitive mechanism, thereby producing almost any conceivable behavioral output. The case studies, below, suggest that the analogy is not quite apt. We believe that, if used appropriately, psychological and even neurological knowledge can indeed help improve institutional design (although, we admit, pachinko players also harbor such beliefs, and they are certainly mistaken).

In this chapter, we identify three cases in which consciously inaccessible mental processes matter for institutional design. In principle, the distinction between the conscious and unconscious affects the analysis of all institutions. This distinction affects the constellations of formal rules and informal social norms that structure human behavior and thereby define social institutions (North 1990). It should be relevant, whether the institution has been deliberately designed or emerged through some evolutionary process, and whatever its stated or constructed goal. In our case studies, however, we rely predominantly on legal institutions: judicial decision making by judges or jurors, the interaction between legal contracts and interpersonal trust in shaping cooperative relationships, and standards of criminal responsibility. Our three case studies track the different types of interactions between the conscious/unconscious distinction and the legal system. This distinction influences the development of rules and structures that the legal system uses to advance the quality of decisions it makes; it influences how the system attempts to affect the behavior of citizens; and it guides how the system judges the conduct of its citizens. For the first case, we focus on the mental activity of the people who make decisions within the legal system; that is, judges or jurors. In the second and third cases, we investigate the efforts of the legal system to shape behavior. The first case may spur us to formulate questions that neuroscience might be able to answer in the future. For the other two cases, neuroscience data exists upon which legal institutions might build. In the case of legal contracts and trust, a better understanding of psychological and neural processes would without a doubt be helpful for institutional analysis and even design. In criminal responsibility, however, understanding the underlying mental forces may make it more difficult for the legal system to serve its historical function.

Judge and Jury Decision Making

Reid Hastie (this volume) describes a simulated trial in which the defendant Frank Johnson was charged with the first-degree murder of his drinking buddy,

Alan Caldwell. Although many of the events in the trial are undisputed (e.g., Johnson definitely stabbed Caldwell), a series of disputed facts exist such as whether or not Johnson acted in self-defense. The disputed facts all bear on legal standards that define guilt and type of offense, as well as punishment severity.

In this context, the goal of the jury system as an institution is to determine whether or not Caldwell is guilty according to the legal standards. The task of the judge or jury in such cases is "to get the story right" in order to apply the relevant standards correctly. The legal system desires to avoid both wrongful convictions and false acquittals, but it is weighted more heavily toward avoiding wrongful convictions, as most legal systems treat these as much more destructive than false acquittals.

Designing an institution to maximize correct verdicts while satisfying the criteria of weighing wrongful convictions more heavily than false acquittals would be simple enough, if the decision maker relies solely on conscious, system 2 processes. The judge or jury would observe the evidence presented by both sides, weigh the evidence appropriately in reference to the legal standards, and then integrate the available evidence into an unbiased summary judgment. The procedural rules for such a decision maker would need to be designed to ensure an efficient presentation of the evidence. Live presentation, for example, would hardly be meaningful, unless it enhanced the decision maker's memory of the relevant facts. Likewise, the order of the presentation would matter little. Oral arguments by attorneys would be unnecessary, except insomuch as they would remind the decision maker of the task or evidence. The emotional state of the witnesses would be of little worth, unless it provided a clear indication of the witnesses' mental state. Likewise, invidious influences (e.g., race, income, or gender) of the parties or witnesses would matter only to the extent of their strict Bayesian relationship to the underlying facts. Finally, any decision maker with the cognitive skills necessary to master the rules of inference and process the evidence would suffice.

Of course, this scenario depicts no process in use by any country. Trials are messy everywhere, and decision makers less predictable. The prosecution and the defense bring forth pieces of evidence in a scrambled order, based on witness availability and attorney strategy. Both sides are represented by professionals, who know they get a high premium if they successfully shift how the decision maker views the case. Legal systems adopt rules that carefully prescribe the mode, order, and content of evidence presentation as if all of these seemingly extraneous rational factors affect judgment. Research supports the influence of such factors.

How does the decision maker react to all of this? Hastie presents a "story model" of juror and judge decision making that is described in terms of general models of explanation-based judgment (Hastie 1999, 2001, this volume; Hastie and Pennington 2000). The basic intuition of this model is that legal decision makers reason about the evidence to form a mental model of events and causal relations; thereafter they compare that abstract mental model to relevant legal classifications to arrive at a decision. The legal decision makers will consider multiple possible models and choose the model with the highest level of confidence, as determined by criteria such as coverage (taking into account all the facts), consistency, plausibility, and completeness (Hastie, this volume).

Hastie's story model, however, does not fit easily into the simple distinction between conscious and unconscious. To refer back to Figure 19.1, the story model is a construct that operates at the psychological level. Nevertheless, it seems to describe the juror decision-making process accurately. Hence, institutional-level approaches that embrace a binary distinction between rational or conscious cognitive processes and the irrational or unconscious cognitive process will necessarily miss the mark in terms of their value to accurate fact-finding. The story model would generally encourage procedural rules that facilitate jurors' natural tendencies to try to construct an accurate account of the events. This might include such reforms as allowing jurors to ask questions or take notes. Judges might also provide instructions at the beginning of the case, rather than at the end, to provide jurors with a cognitive template to organize the evidence that they will receive. Furthermore, a court might attend more carefully to the order in which the evidence is presented, perhaps ensuring a chronological presentation, to facilitate the construction of a stable story.

In the United States, at least, evidentiary rules do not embrace the psychological-level concept of the story model; instead, they are attuned to concerns about the distinction between conscious and unconscious processing. The system distrusts unconscious influence, in some instances, and embraces rules to constrain the influence of unconscious processes. In other contexts, the system attempts to take advantage of the strengths of unconscious inference processes. Finally, legal systems rely sometimes on the intuition of the decision maker assessing the appropriate level of confidence in their judgment. Below, we review briefly each of these three approaches to the distinction between conscious processing.

In the U.S., the legal system has adopted numerous procedural rules to limit the influence of seemingly undesirable unconscious influences. For example, the Federal Rule of Evidence (Rule 403) precludes the introduction of evidence that presents a risk of "unfair prejudice." The Advisory Committee to the Federal Rules of Evidence explains the rule specifically as forbidding evidence that has "an undue tendency to suggest decision on an improper basis, commonly, though not necessarily, an emotional one." A common application of this rule restricts the presentation of particularly graphic evidence, such as bloodied bodies or other evidence of physical pain (Bright and Goodman-Delahunty 2006). Graphic evidence might initiate automatic processing to evoke a desire for vengeance against the defendant, regardless of whether the evidence supports a conviction. The rule assumes that a juror exposed to such evidence will attend excessively to the single piece of graphic evidence, thereby biasing jurors' assessment of the rest of the evidence. Restrictions like this on evidence are thought to be essential to restricting emotional processes that jurors cannot control, even if they are instructed to do so.

In other cases, the legal system takes full advantage of intuitive processing and does not attempt to restrict its influence. For example, judgments of culpability and liability frequently require inferences about the motives, goals, intentions, and emotions of the actors involved. It is easy to underestimate how difficult such inferences are to make. Mental states must be reliably inferred from behavior, otherwise the system will be too erratic. Furthermore, the members of the society in which the legal system operates must have a shared system of understanding intentionality. The human brain appears to be quite adept at such inferences. Social neuroscience has started to understand the neural networks underlying such inferences, for example, through cognitive (mentalizing) and emotional perspective taking (empathizing). Mentalizing refers to our ability to represent intentions and beliefs of others, whereas empathy refers to our capacity to share feelings and motivational states with others. Empathy, in particular, has been shown to occur on an implicit level of processing; that is, people seem to represent the emotional states of others quite automatically without having to engage in deliberative thinking (Singer 2006; see also McCabe and Singer, this volume). The same networks that process the sensations of touch, pain, and disgust in one person are reactivated when that person perceives others experiencing similar emotions. These automatic empathic responses can be modulated by perceived fairness, similarity, or affective link to the other (for a more detailed account, see de Vignemont and Singer 2006; Singer 2006; Singer et al. 2004, 2006).

A legal system that bases important judgments on various mental states must depend on these automatic, neural processes. Lawyers recognize clearly the existence of such processes in their strategic presentation of evidence and jury selection. Even more significantly, the system itself depends on these processes. Basically, legal systems assume that judges and juries will be able to infer mental states reliably. Jury instructions, for example, instruct jurors to assign verdicts on the basis of mental states, but provide little or no guidance as to how they are to ascertain mental states.

The case that Hastie used to illustrate the story model is typical in the instructions it provides to jurors on how they are to infer the mental states of the actors. The instructions advise the jurors to convict the defendant of murder if the defendant intended the death of the victim when he acted. They further instruct the jurors to convict of a more serious form of murder if the defendant formed this intent in advance and planned the actions in some way. They also require that the jurors acquit the defendant if they conclude that the defendant acted out of a reasonable belief that his own life was in danger. Jurors who have the cognitive mechanisms for understanding purposive action, planning, and fear can make such judgments without further elaboration. The system provides no clear rules for making such inferences, and it need not do so. The evidence from neuroscience suggests that the human brain can perform this function to a reasonable degree of reliability on its own, without invoking an elaborate set of deductive rules. Legal systems seem to depend on this ability.

In addition, legal systems appear to rely on intuitive processes in a more indirect way. Recall that most criminal justice systems are more concerned with avoiding wrongful convictions than false acquittals. Operationalizing this concern can be challenging. The English jurist, William Blackstone, asserted that he would rather let ten guilty men go free than convict one innocent man. This aphorism provides a sense of the magnitude of the weighing, but can hardly be translated into a handy rule of inference. The American system demands that a trier of fact in a criminal case (usually a jury) not convict unless they are certain of the defendant's guilt "beyond a reasonable doubt." This phrase admits of no easy definition, but it seems to convey a sense of the mental state required, as this passage from the well-known jurist Justice Lemuel Shaw (*Commonwealth* v. *Webster* 1850) illustrates:

> [W]hat is reasonable doubt? It is a term often used, probably pretty well understood, but not easily defined. It is not mere possible doubt; because every thing relating to human affairs, and depending on moral evidence, is open to some possible or imaginary doubt. It is that state of the case, which, after the entire comparison and consideration of all the evidence, leaves the minds of jurors in that condition that they cannot say they feel an abiding conviction, to a moral certainty, of the truth of the charge.

The concept of reasonable doubt refers then to a state of mental certainty, not to a probability judgment (*Victor* v. *Nebraska* 1994).

The concept of *conviction intime*, which governs how judges report their decisions in French and German courts, presents similar issues, albeit with a somewhat different resolution. The principle requires that judges state they are 100% convinced of their reasoning in a particular decision, even if the evidence suggests a more probabilistic or uncertain conclusion. Judges are not allowed to make any quantitative probabilistic statements that quantify their uncertainty about their judgment (e.g., I am 95% certain that the defendant did it). Essentially, *conviction intime* asks judges to rely on their expert intuition to persuade themselves fully about the correct story. Especially in uncertain cases, this process calls on a judge to make a variety of inferences on the basis of contradictory or uncertain evidence, so as to facilitate a kind of overconfident certainty in the decision maker. As with the reasonable doubt standard, *conviction intime* may be best understood as inducing the decision maker to reach a particular mental state. Judges must all share the same sense of what constitutes this mental state or else the principle cannot produce reliable judgments. *Conviction intime* appears to demand a somewhat more rigorous, almost deductive certainty, thereby distinguishing it from the reasonable doubt standard. However, like the reasonable doubt standard, it takes advantage of a shared understanding of how mental states interact with judgment.

These three examples of how procedural rules interact with intuition suggest several important puzzles about legal systems. First, why do legal systems sometimes attempt to suppress intuition and at other times they rely on it? The answer might be mundane: some intuitions are thought to be impediments to the system's goals whereas others are seen to further its goals. Second (and relatedly), do legal systems purport to suppress unconscious processes in an effort to maintain the appearance of deliberative processing? *Conviction intime* seems to have that character, given its insistence on an expression of utmost certainty. Social order might depend on the perception that the legal system inflicts harsh punishment only in the right cases, and only for acceptable reasons. We certainly cannot rule out the alternative hypothesis; namely, that rules such as *conviction intime* do what a cursory inspection might suggest—they increase deliberative processing. If this is true, then either deliberative processing produces better judge and jury decisions, or there is an intriguing trade-off between maintaining the legitimacy of the political system and making correct legal decisions.

Third, why does the legal system seem to divide cognitive processes into conscious and unconscious, instead of sorting them at the level of psychological processes? This distinction certainly has its costs, as it impedes efforts to assess reforms that might otherwise take advantage of the subtle way that fact finders approach their decisions. The notion that some jurors process some evidence consciously and other evidence unconsciously fails to describe what it is that jurors are doing accurately. In reality, conscious and unconscious or semiconscious processes all interact to facilitate the production of an account of the facts that judges or juries can map onto various legal categories. The legal system's folk theorizing about human cognition might be a bit too wooden.

Finally, an assessment of the cognitive processes that influence judgment raises important puzzles as to the sources of difference in legal doctrines between countries. For example, the legal system in the U.S. does not have the *conviction intime* principle. Although the reasonable doubt standard is somewhat similar, as described, it tolerates doubt explicitly. Furthermore, the U.S. legal system relies heavily on juries. How these variations developed can be traced historically in each country. The observable differences seem to have come about because (a) the goals of the systems were different; (b) the nature of the decision process varies cross-culturally; or (c) one of the two systems is more effective.

To summarize, we view legal systems as relying on a distinction between conscious and unconscious processes in crafting procedural rules that govern trials. Legal systems sometimes suppress unconscious inferences, while relying on them in other contexts. As Hastie's research has shown, however, this distinction is both artificial and somewhat detrimental, as it emphasizes a particular set of questions that do not address how decision makers actually assess the facts.

Trust and Social Cooperation

Cooperation When Contracts Are Incomplete

In many social situations, individual self-interest impedes a mutually beneficial outcome that requires cooperative effort among individuals. In such situations, individuals face incentives to free ride; that is, they make no contribution to the costs for preservation while benefitting from the efforts of others. If each member acts as a free-rider, social benefits will not be realized. Game theorists formalize this situation as a public goods game, the multiplayer version of the popular Prisoner's Dilemma.

In the Prisoner's Dilemma, a row and a column player simultaneously choose to cooperate or to defect (see Figure 19.2). If both cooperate, both achieve their second best outcome. If one of them cooperates while the other defects, the defector attains her best outcome, while the cooperator gets her worst outcome. Thus, both players have an incentive to defect, producing their second-worst outcomes. A combination of greed and fear leads to the socially detrimental result (Macy and Flache 2002). Greedy individuals attempt to obtain their individual best outcome: the free lunch. Fearful individuals anticipate this and defect because they do not want to be the loser. This distribution of payoffs and the underlying preference structure are specific to the Prisoner's Dilemma. However, there are many more positive sum games that are not games of harmony (Rapoport et al. 1976).

The dilemma would not exist, if the parties involved could write a complete contract prior to playing. This would mean that each player would commit to a strategy (preferably cooperate), all subsequent actions in the game are verifiable (i.e., whether a player cooperated or defected can be confirmed beyond doubt), and the actions are enforceable by a third party. Writing such a complete contract is frequently not possible under real-life conditions. Anticipating all of the possible means of defection is rarely possible, and attempting to do so can be expensive.

Rather than draft a complete contract demanding cooperation in all circumstances, parties can rely instead on trust. In a trust relationship, a trustor deliberately takes the risk of being exploited by the trustee (Hardin 2001). How these trust relationships develop in everyday life have been experimentally analyzed in two classes of games: the trust game (Berg et al. 1995) and the gift exchange game (Fehr et al. 1993).

	Contribution	Defection
Contribution	2, 2	0, $\underline{3}$
Defection	$\underline{3}$, 0	$\underline{1}$, $\underline{1}$

Figure 19.2 Prisoner's Dilemma: the left-hand payoff is for the row player while the right-hand payoff is for the column player. Best results are underlined.

The basic setup of the trust game involves a sender, who is endowed with some amount of money (e.g., ten tokens) and a receiver. The sender may send any fraction of their endowment to the receiver, which is augmented en route, say tripled. The receiver then has the option of returning any amount of the received money back to the sender. Obviously, the joint profit of both players will be maximized if the sender transfers the entire amount to the receiver. There have been literally hundreds of experiments on the trust game conducted under very different conditions which, roughly summarized, show that the more senders give, the more is returned. A recent study has shown that this phenomenon occurs as well in market-like situations (Brown et al. 2004).

Although the evidence of widespread trust is impressive, these experiments also reveal that trust represents a fragile solution for solving the cooperation problem. Some senders do not send and some receivers do not return. In the absence of knowing whether one is facing someone who is apt to be trustworthy, one is well advised to spend the extra cost to enter into enforceable contractual protections. Any institutional intervention that increases levels of trust would therefore reduce the need to undertake such costs. By identifying the mechanisms that inspire trust, neurobiological research suggests interventions that might induce greater levels of trust and increase the probability of obtaining cooperative solutions to public goods problems.

Research in neurobiology has revealed a widespread set of mechanisms that operate in an unconscious fashion to improve trust. For example, a recent study (Kosfeld et al. 2005) has shown that the level of trust increases in subjects if oxytocin[1] has been sprayed into their nose. In the trust game subjects exposed to oxytocin sent more money. Preliminary results from imaging studies (fMRI) suggest that this effect is mediated through the amygdala, a brain structure crucial to fast emotional processing, fear conditioning, and reward learning. Oxytocin reduces activation in the amygdala, thereby muting an alarm signal that would otherwise induce avoidance tendencies. This study demonstrates a deeply embedded neurological pathway that induces trust.

In addition, preliminary studies from Tania Singer's lab suggest that subjects exhibiting mistrust do not differ with respect to their empathic brain responses elicited when others suffer pain (ACC, insula), but rather with respect to their amygdala activation elicited when they anticipate receiving painful stimulation themselves. Such subjects seem to have enhanced amygala-mediated fear responses to aversive events (Singer et al., in preparation). Going back to the Prisoner's Dilemma, these results would suggest that cooperation fails not because of greed, but rather fear. Hence, institutional mechanisms that

---

[1]   Oxytocin is a peptide produced primarily in the hypothalamus; it works both as a hormone and a neuromodulator. In nonhuman mammals, oxytocin has a central role in behavioral regulation, particularly in positive social interactions ranging from social attachment such as pair bonding, to maternal care and sexual bonding (Carter 1998; Carter et al. 2001; Insel and Young 2001; Insel and Shapiro 1992; Pedersen 1997; Uvnas-Moberg 1998). Generally it is thought to facilitate approach behavior and to overcome natural avoidance tendencies.

reduce the perceived risk of victimization would be the key to increasing trust, and hence cooperation.

Evidence from experimental economics invites a further hypothesis at the border between psychology and the neurosciences. If true, the effect would not modulate trust, but trustworthiness. In oligopoly experiments, a number of experimental subjects compete. The experimenter is interested in exploring deviations from the Walrasian equilibrium (i.e., price equal marginal cost). In principle, demand is not part of the research question. To economize on the subject pool, many oligopoly experiments have replaced demand by a computer that is programmed to buy according to a predetermined demand function. Some experimenters wondered whether this manipulation is as innocent as it seems. This turns out not to be true. Collusion plummets if the computer is replaced by human buyers (Engel 2006). One plausible interpretation is that experimental subjects are hesitant to inflict harm on their peers.

To the best of our knowledge, this hypothesis has not yet been tested experimentally. It has, however, been shown that experimental subjects exhibit empathy when they see pain inflicted on others (Jackson et al. 2005; Singer et al. 2004, 2006). This is also the case if, in a coordination game, those who have behaved fairly nonetheless get punished (Singer et al. 2006). What happens if subjects have a chance to inflict harm on their peers? This remains to be tested. Arguably, empathy results in sympathy and should make them shy away from this. If true, the definition of peers and the perception of whether a subject feels treated fairly by them becomes important.

Therefore, being vulnerable in a positive sum game appears to be beneficial for all players. If this interpretation holds, then a person might be motivated to exploit the neurological mechanism that brings about trust by projecting an image of oneself as being vulnerable. One way to do this would be to expose oneself to a serious (but not vital) risk.

Although trust may help parties secure gains from cooperation, it remains a risky choice. A solid body of experimental evidence demonstrates that actors are heterogeneous. A rough estimate has it that Western societies typically are composed of about 60% of conditional cooperators, 30% of utility maximizers, and 10% of altruists. In such populations, blind trust is not sustainable, as can be shown by modeling the situation in terms of evolutionary game theory (Boyd et al. 2003; Gintis et al. 2003). In the spirit of rational choice, in such a setting actors will watch out for information that signals the type of their interaction partners.

This insight might help explain a curious feature of both common and continental law. In both traditions, a contract represents a promise that is enforceable through the power of the courts. To be legally enforceable under the common law system, however, a contract requires an offer and acceptance of a valuable consideration; a mere promise is not enough. For example, if someone promises to give you their laptop computer tomorrow and asks for nothing in return, when this person fails to deliver the laptop, you would not be able to enforce the promise through the courts. By contrast, if a person promises to sell you their laptop for \$1 and you agree, both of you have exchanged consideration, and the promise becomes enforceable. An exchange does not need to be made up of goods of equal value; they must simply have some value. Furthermore, consideration is said sometimes to have "failed" when the consideration is too vaguely described. Hence, if I promise to give you my laptop and ask that you will "consider it as a favor," the arrangement still lacks valuable consideration. Why should the law insist on a concrete exchange? Perhaps because the exchange of concrete consideration triggers the neurological mechanisms described above: it induces people into mutual exchange, and thereby encourages the kind of cooperative thinking that will reduce the chances that the parties will exploit each other later as the conditions of the contract unfold.

Interestingly, not all legal systems require a consideration. Under many continental legal orders, a mere promise is binding, but only if it is affixed in writing (for a discussion on the actual degree of convergence, see Rothoeft 1968). The act of writing, however, might serve the same psychological function as the mutual exchange in the common law system, as the construction of a written agreement requires the type of cooperative thinking that also underlies the exchange of consideration.

Although such interventions reduce the risk that a trust relationship breaks down, or is not initiated, they are not, in and of themselves, sufficient to sustain trust. A sustainable strategy combines three elements: signal your willingness to cooperate at the outset; commit to punish defectors; in punishment, signal that you want to continue the relationship (Selten et al. 1997).

Having addressed the first element, let us now turn to the second. There is good evidence that, in a social dilemma, the chance to pay for inflicting harm on defectors improves cooperation (Fehr and Gächter 2002). From a rational actor perspective, this is surprising. Why should an individual be willing to give up some of their own utility for doing harm to cheaters? The original Prisoner's Dilemma repeats: each member of the community is best off if all others punish while the individual member does not (and keeps all her money). This is anticipated. No one ever punishes (Heckathorn 1989).

Actually, experimental subjects have a preference for punishment as an institution. If given a choice, despite a strong initial reluctance, subjects migrate rapidly to a sanctioning institution which "produces" almost full contributions and thus no punishment (Gürerk et al. 2006). This even holds if they could alternatively choose reputation to back up cooperation (Milinski and Rockenbach 2007).

Recent studies in neuroscience have started to investigate the neural foundation of such punishment sentiments. De Quervain et al. (2004) scanned subjects while they were deciding whether and how much punishment points they wanted to distribute to people who had behaved unfairly in a previous game. Activation in the dorsal striatum, a brain structure involved in processing stimulus-reward-response contingencies, was activated when subjects decided to punish, and these activations were positively correlated with the amount of punishment delivered. A recent study by Singer et al. (2006) suggests that punishment is not only rewarding when given the opportunity to execute the act, but also when subjects merely watch other defectors being punished (i.e., without executing the punishment themselves). In this experiment, subjects were scanned (and their empathic brain responses measured) as they observed people, who had either behaved fairly or unfairly in a sequential trust game, receiving painful stimulation to their hand. Both women and men showed empathic brain responses toward the suffering of fair players. Men, however, showed an absence of empathic brain responses when the unfair player got "punished," revealing instead an increased activation in the ventral striatum, an area involved in primary reward processing. The higher these men expressed subjective desires for revenge in later questionnaires, the higher their response in these reward areas. These results suggest that seeing defectors punished is rewarding and may help explain the motivation for altruistic, that is, costly punishment.

Thus prepared, we return to the greed versus fear explanation of mistrust. If indeed fear is key, society might be better off insuring trustors for the (arguably small) risk of being exploited by their counterparts. In an experimental trust game, this could be implemented the following way: at the outset, the experimenter imposes a tax. Out of her endowment, each subject has to pay a fraction into a pool. The pool compensates trusting subjects who have been exploited. Of course, punishment and insurance could also be combined. In such a scheme, not only would the defector's utility be reduced by (costly) punishment; the money thus collected by the bank would be used to (partly) compensate victims for their losses.

In the literature on punishment, this is usually seen as unilateral. The victim inflicts harm on the perpetrator. Institutional practice exhibits an alternative that engages the perpetrator. U.S. legislation, for example, propagates apologies. It does so mainly by prohibiting the apology to be introduced as evidence in a civil trial, thereby protecting the defendant from liability and reducing the cost of apology (Robbenolt 2006). Anecdotally, people injured through the negligence of others often tell their lawyers that all they really want is an apology. Furthermore, some defendants seem to want to apologize (O'Hara and Yarn 2002). One interpretation of this is that despite the defection, which led to litigation, an apology signals that one is planning to maintain a cooperative relationship. Apologies are probably effective because of the emotional content they often convey, which may be subject to automatic processing. The neuroscientific foundation of the effect of apologies has not yet been investigated. It may be hypothesized that apologies reduce reward-related signals motivating punishment behavior and, through this, reconstituting empathy. Alternatively, apologies may also have a similar effect to oxytocin in that they reduce fear signals of the amygdala and recover trust.

We now turn to the third element in the Selten et al. (1997) argument. Punishment is foolproof only in very simple settings. Whenever there is noise, the risk exists that the person on which punishment is inflicted sees this as unfair and counter-punishes (Konow 2005; Nikiforakis 2008). From this, a war of revenge can easily result, which brings cooperation to an abrupt end.

We hypothesize that "pedagogical" punishment (as found to perform best in Selten et al. 1997) and "anger" punishment are different neurologically. If institutions are able to make anger punishment unlikely (e.g. by imposing social norms), the risk of the first punishment resulting in a war of revenge is substantially reduced. Neuroscientific studies may shed some light on this suggestion. However, clever experiments will need to be designed to contrast brain signals underlying punishment motivated by retributive motives and punishment motivated purely by consequentialist motives to see whether reward-related processing is found only in the former decision. Another interesting study would be to train people in empathy-enhancing techniques and to see whether, using a similar paradigm to that used by Singer et al. (2006), subjects are able to overcome retributive motivation toward defectors after empathic induction.

Thus far, the only complications we have introduced are actor heterogeneity and noise. We have suggested minimal institutional interventions to stabilize trust. However, in many real-world interactions, a higher degree of formality is hard to avoid. Division of labor must be organized in greater detail. Some risks are so characteristic to the types of interaction that a responsible partner will specify future outcomes, should these risks materialize. In short: formal contract is advisable.

In such contexts, the contracting parties face a serious challenge, provided making the contract complete still remains impossible or inappropriate. Fehr and Rockenbach (2003) have shown that subjects who deliberately dispense the possibility of punishing undesired behavior, although it is contractually possible, reach higher efficiency than those who incorporate a punishment clause in the contract. Along similar lines, Falk and Kosfeld (2006) show that it is not beneficial for the proposer to reduce the reaction space of the opponent by withdrawing the actions that are "unfair" with respect to the proposer, because this signals distrust. Asking for a certain clause may be a strong signal of distrust. More importantly even, the parties must manage to negotiate in a way that leaves room for building trust.

Default contracts stipulated in a statute provide an alternative to this dilemma, as do standard form contracts, which are widely applied. Either way, the parties are not forced to make unlikely risks explicit. Further research is needed on the conditions under which negotiations do build, instead of erode, trust. Anecdotal evidence seems to point to the possibility that trustworthiness is signalled by the way in which negotiations are conducted.

Therefore, legal institutions governing contracts seem to take limited advantage of the kinds of mechanisms that neuroscientists studying the biological basis of trust have uncovered. Considering that common law and continental legal systems have evolved over centuries, it would perhaps be surprising if these systems took no account of the role of the human brain, as well as its strengths and weaknesses. However, once again, the law as an institution emphasizes primarily the first-level analysis of conscious versus unconscious. We suspect that the examples we have presented, in which the law incorporates some insights from neuroscience, are the exception rather than the rule. Most contract law, like procedure, treats people as rational, conscious agents who are held responsible for their actions, unless these actions can be shown to be the product of significant unconscious influences, akin to duress and deception. Hence, we anticipate that the law has much to gain from the insights of neuroscience, in particular from the light it sheds on how trust is inspired.

Standards of Criminal Responsibility

Our last case study builds on an analysis of the idea of "criminal intent" conducted by Paul Glimcher (this volume). Glimcher discusses a U.S. Supreme Court case from the early 1990s concerning a murder suspect named Solomon Hotema. In this case, the Court established the standards of criminal intent as a voluntary action and stated that subjects who are absolutely controlled by the delusions of a "diseased" brain are entitled to an acquittal. Glimcher's main argument is that this notion of voluntary action is inconsistent with the materialist view of neurobiology. Thus, in this section, we will utilize a somewhat reverse logic from that of the previous two, and begin by examining this institution with an eye toward assessing the implications of neurobiology. We discuss how the institution might change if neurobiological evidence were taken seriously.

Perhaps more so than in our previous discussions, criminal law categorizes human actions into conscious and unconscious. The law holds people responsible for their actions that it deems to be the product of conscious thought—equating conscious thought with volition. It exempts from liability people who commit a wrongful act, but who can be shown to lack the same conscious mental state as most wrongdoers. For example, courts would not treat a person who throws a knife into another as a result of an epileptic fit as they would an assassin who commits the same act as part of a contract murder. Courts approach cases of severe mental illness that lead to claims of insanity in much the same way; they try to identify whether a wrongdoer's mental state most closely approximates the cool deliberation of the assassin or the uncontrollable gyrations of the epileptic. Sufficient evidence of irrational thought leads courts to treat the mentally ill offender as the law would treat the epileptic. In cases of severe mental illness, the courts conclude that the crime is attributable to the person's (irrational, unconscious) brain, not their (rational, conscious) mind.

Neurobiology challenges this dichotomy. For example, serotonin levels in the brain have a close relationship with the likelihood of violent crime. Decreases in serotonin level are known to increase the rate of violent acts and depression in many individuals. (Rossby 2003). Imagine that the relationship was perfectly linear: more serotonin, more violent crime. It would be hard to maintain the dichotomy of criminal law in the face of such evidence. How could one say that a person is responsible for their serotonin level? Still, serotonin bears only indirectly on the distinction between conscious and unconscious processes that the courts rely on in cases of claimed insanity. Although neat linear relationships between neurological activity and behavior have yet to be identified, neurologists believe that neuroscience will uncover findings that will undermine the basic dichotomy of criminal law.

With this background, one can make a distinction between a retributive model of a criminal punishment and a consequentialist model. Most modern legal systems are built strongly on a retributive model, which asserts that punishment should be meted out to exact retribution on the criminal, punishing him for his defection from society. The retributive model is supported by experimental social dilemmas with punishment institutions, where subjects often express anger at defectors and exhibit a desire for vengeance. Retribution is critical to the justification of criminal law. A moral society must have a reason to inflict hardship on one of its members. The attribution of deliberate, intentional misconduct provides the basis for retribution against offenders. Punishing those whose conduct was the product of something other than rational, volitional thought would be no different than punishing an innocent.

The retributive model, however, rests on the assumption of voluntary action: punishing a criminal who did not voluntarily commit the crime is a morally bankrupt undertaking if done solely for retributive ends. Criminals with "diseased minds" that impair voluntary action do not deserve punishment.

Retributivism, however, is not the only motive for a criminal justice system. Punishment also serves to decrease the incidence of crime in society, either by removing violent individuals or deterring other potential criminals. This deterrent motive is a form of consequentialist justification for inflicting hardship on those who commit crime. The consequentialist model is concerned solely with improving the overall welfare of society by discouraging defection. Because retribution is irrelevant to the consequentialist view, it does not require any notion of voluntary action or freewill; its desired effect is achieved by changing the expected costs of being caught. A materialistic view of neurobiology rejects the notion of voluntary action and thus implies logically that only a consequentialist model of criminal justice is morally defensible. A consequentialist view of criminal justice would have a punishment severity function to track directly the likelihood of violent crime.

Although both retributivist and consequentialist goals animate the existence and function of most systems of criminal law, retributivism predominates today. In many instances, retributivism and consequentialism do not produce different policies. For example, neither would advocate punishing the epileptic in our earlier example, and both would assign harsh punishment to the contract killer. When the policies diverge, however, people reject consequentialism and embrace retributivism (Robinson and Darley 2003). For example, consequentialism demands that people administer punishment in ways that are sensitive to the probability that a wrongful act is detected, and yet people do not behave this way (Sunstein et al. 2000). Similarly, even though roughly two-thirds of the citizens in the U.S. support the use of the death penalty, less than one-third believe that it provides a useful deterrent[2]—retributive ends provide the support for this punishment.

Consider the implications of the relationship between serotonin and crime control. Retributivism and consequentialism implicate different policies in response to the relationship between serotonin levels and the propensity to commit crime. A retributivist would see the role of serotonin as an involuntary cause of crime that is not properly attributed to the perpetrator. Hence, for a retributivist, increased serotonin levels would justify less harsh punishment. A consequentialist, however, would view the increased propensity to commit murder as justifying an increase in the penalty for crimes committed by those with high serotonin levels. To deter crime effectively, society has to send a stronger signal to those with high serotonin levels. Although we have not done a survey, we suspect that most people would see a high serotonin level as justifying less punishment. As neuroscientists identify the precursors of crime ever more clearly, more factors like serotonin may come to affect the criminal law. Neuroscience is thus on a collision course with the intuition behind criminal law (Greene and Cohen 2004).

It is not clear whether abandoning the notion of voluntary action (favored by a retributive system) and adopting a consequentialist institution would have positive benefits for society. Research on social dilemmas suggests that the opportunity for retributive punishment is an important basis for maintaining cooperation. Thus, if the opportunity for punishment were to be removed, other people in society may be less likely to cooperate. In many ways, the legal system is designed to make punishment more efficient by providing economies of scale and by removing the need for individuals to mete out their own vengeance. Most importantly, legalizing punishment is a technology for containing the risk of counter-punishment, which we have analyzed in the previous section. This, however, is not likely to work if acts of the criminal justice system are perceived as patently unfair. This is precisely what happens if the courts punish defendants with "a broken brain." Thus adopting a consequentialist system might result in reducing a citizen's belief in the justice of the legal system, thereby diminishing cooperation on the part of an individual citizen and increasing the frequency of vigilante style justice. This potential for overall decay in social order is one reason for maintaining a retributive model of criminal justice, favored by many legal scholars. In effect, the dichotomy between conscious, rational thought and unconscious, irrational thought provides the illusion of freewill, which might be an essential intuition to a stable society.

---

[2]   ABC News/Washington Post Poll, June 22–25, 2006.

Conclusions

This report offers an analytical framework for understanding how integrating notions of deliberative and automatic processing as well as other neurobiological processes can change how we analyze institutions. Several plausible signatures of how institutions have adapted to automatic processing were presented. Most of these institutional adaptations increase the performance of decision making either by capitalizing on or contolling automatic processes in some way. The trial process relies on the intuition of its decision makers in assessing mental states of actors and in using intuitive senses of certainty of the decision makers. The contract system seems also to prod unconscious processes that produce greater degrees of trust. The criminal justice system depends on a classification of behavior as the product of conscious, rational thought or unconscious, irrational thought.

The three examples that we discussed underscore the premise that social institutions (most notably legal systems) seem to need to categorize cognitive processes into conscious and unconscious. This ignores the psychological approach of identifying many types of cognitive processes and certainly ignores the neurological level. This failure leads to difficulties as well as opportunities. In the trial process, it leads the system to underrate the value of reforms that would produce more accurate judgment. The contract system has only begun to appreciate the depth of neurological triggers to trust. The criminal justice system seems on a collision course with neurological understanding.

Still, the distinction between conscious and unconscious seems pervasive at the institutional level. Even though we can readily identify the shortcomings of this distinction, it has proven to be a valuable, workable way of categorizing human thought and action and thus is not discarded easily. Indeed, the criminal justice system's deep embrace of the dichotomy might itself motivate an enormous amount of law-abiding behavior, which otherwise might be lost were the illusion it produces to be shattered. Given the great utility of the distinction between conscious and unconscious thought at the institutional level, reformers who would rely instead on different levels of analysis bear the burden of proof that their way is better. In view of the advances in psychology and neuroscience that we might expect in the future, this burden might, on occasion, be met.

References

Berg, J., J. Dickhaut, and K. McCabe. 1995. Trust, reciprocity and social history. *Games Econ. Behav.* **10**:122–142.

Boyd, R., H. Gintis, S. Bowles, and P. J. Richerson. 2003. The Evolution of Altruistic Punishment. *Proc. Natl. Acad. Sci.* **100**:3531–3535.

Bright, D. A., and J. Goodman-Delahunty. 2006. Gruesome evidence and emotion: Anger, blame and jury decision-making. *Law Hum. Behav.* **30**:183–202.

Brown, M., A. Falk, and E. Fehr. 2004. Relational contracts and the nature of market interactions, *Econometrica* **72(3)**:747–780.

Carter, C. S. 1998. Neuroendocrine perspectives on social attachment and love. Psychoneuroend. **23(8)**:779–818

Carter, C. S., M. Altemus, and G. P. Chrousos. 2001. Neuroendocrine and emotional changes in the post-partum period. *Prog. Brain Res.* **133**:241–249.

Commonwealth v. *Webster.* 1850. 59 Mass. 295, 320.

De Quervain, D. J. F., U. Fischbacher, V. Treyer, M. Schellhammer, U. Schnyder et al. 2004. The neural basis of altruistic punishment. *Science* **305**:1254–1258.

de Vignemont, F., and T. Singer. 2006. The empathic brain: How, when and why? *Trends Cogn. Sci.* **10(10)**:435–441.

Engel, C. 2006. How Much Collusion? A Meta-Analysis on Oligopoly Experiments. MPI Collective Goods Preprint No. 2006/27. http://ssrn.com/abstract=951160.

Falk, A., and M. Kosfeld. 2006. Distrust: The hidden costs of control. *Am. Econ. Rev.* **96**:1611–1630.

Falk, A., E. Fehr, and U. Fischbacher. 2000. Testing Theories of Fairness – Intentions Matter, Institute for Empirical Research in Economics, Working Paper No. 63. University of Zurich.

Fehr, E., and B. Rockenbach. 2003. Detrimental effects of sanctions on human altruism. *Nature* **422(6928)**: 137–140.

Fehr, E., and S. Gächter. 2002. Altruistic Punishment in Humans. *Nature* **415**: 137–140.

Fehr, E., G. Kirchsteiger, and A. Riedl. 1993. Does Fairness prevent Market Clearing? An Experimental Investigation. *Qtly. J. Econ.* **108**:437–460.

Gintis, H., S. Bowles, R. Boyd, and E. Fehr. 2003. Explaining altruistic behavior in humans. *Evol. Hum. Behav.* **24**:153–172.

Greene, J. D., and J. D. Cohen. 2004. For the law, neuroscience changes nothing and everything. *Philos. Trans. R. Soc. Lond. B* **359**:1775–1785.

Gürerk, O., B. Irlenbusch, and B. Rockenbach 2006. The competitive advantage of sanctioning institutions. *Science* **312(5770)**:108–111.

Hardin, R. 2001. Conceptions and explanations of trust. In: Trust in Society, ed. Karen S. Cook, pp. 3–39. New York: Russell Sage Foundation.

Hastie, R. 1999. The role of "stories" in civil jury judgments. *Michigan J. Law Ref.* **32(2)**:1–13.

Hastie, R. 2001. Emotions in jurors' decisions. *Brooklyn Law Rev.* **66**:991–1009.

Hastie, R., and N. Pennington. 2000. Explanation-based decision making. In: Judgment and Decision Making: An Interdisciplinary Reader, ed. T. Connolly, H.R. Arkes, and K.R. Hammond, 2nd ed., pp. 212–228. New York: Cambridge Univ. Press.

Heckathorn, D. D. 1989. Collective action and the second-order free-rider problem. *Ration. Soc.* **1**:78–100.

Insel, T. R., and Shapiro, L. E. 1992. Oxytocin receptor distribution reflects social organization in monogamous and polygamous voles. *Proc. Natl. Acad. Sci.* **89**:5981–5985.

Insel, T. R., and L. J. Young. 2001. The neurobiology of attachment. *Nature Neurosci.* **2**:129–136.

Jackson P. L., A. N. Meltzoff, and J. Decety. 2005. How do we perceive the pain of others? A window into the neural processes involved in empathy. *NeuroImage* **24**:771–779.

Kahneman, D. 2003. A perspective on judgment and choice: Mapping bounded rationality. *Am. Psychol.* **58**:697–720.

Kahneman, D., and Frederick, S. 2005. A model of heuristic judgment. In: The Cambridge Handbook of Thinking and Reasoning, ed. K.J. Holyoak, and R.G. Morrison, pp. 267–293. Cambridge Univ. Press.

Konow, J. 2005. Blind spots: The effects of information and stakes on fairness bias and dispersion. *Social Justice Res.* **18**:349–390.

Kosfeld M., M. Heinrichs, P. J. Zak, U. Fischbacher, and E. Fehr. 2005. *Nature* **435**:673–676.

Macy, M. M., and A. Flache. 2002. Learning dynamics in social dilemmas. *Proc. Natl. Acad. Sci.* **99**:7229–7236.

Milinski, M., and B. Rockenbach. 2007. Spying on others evolves. *Science* **317(5837)**:108–111, 464–465.

Nikiforakis, N. S. 2008 . Punishment and Counter-Punishment in Public Good Games. Can We Really Govern Ourselves? *J. Public Econ.*, in press.

North, D. C. 1990. Institutions, Institutional Change, and Economic Performance. New York: Cambridge Univ. Press.

O'Hara, E., and D. Yarn. 2002. On apology and consilience. *Washington Law Rev.* **77**:1121–1192.

Pedersen, C. A. 1997. Oxytocin control of maternal behavior. Regulation by sex steroids and offspring stimuli. *Ann. NY Acad. Sci.* **807**:126–145.

Preston, S. D., and F.B.M. de Waal. 2002. Empathy: Its ultimate and proximate bases. *Behav. Brain Sci.* **25**:1–72.

Rapoport, A., M. J. Guyer, and D. Gordon. 1976. The 2 x 2 Game. Ann Arbor: Univ. of Michigan Press.

Robbennolt, J. K. Apologies and Settlement Levers. 2006. *J. Emp. Legal Stud.* **3**:333–373.

Robinson, P. H., and J. M. Darley. 2003. The role of deterrence in the formulation of criminal law rules: at its worst when doing its best. *Georgetown Law J.* **91**:949–1002.

Rossby, P. 2003. Serotonin Deficit and Impulsive Violence: Does Your Case Fit?, National Legal Aid & Defender Assoc. *Cornerstone:* www.nlada.org/DMS/Documents/1066920620.52/ serotonin.pdf

Rothoeft, D. 1968. System der Irrtumslehre als Methodenfrage der Rechtsvergleichung. Dargestellt am deutschen und englischen Vertragsrecht. Tübingen: Mohr.

Selten, R., M. Mitzkewitz and G. R. Uhlich. 1997. Duopoly strategies programmed by experienced players. *Econometrica* **65**: 517–555.

Singer, T. 2006. The neuronal basis and ontogeny of empathy and mind reading: Review of literature and implications for future research. *Neurosci. Biobehav. Rev.* **30**:855–863

Singer, T., B. Seymour, J. O'Doherty, H. Kaube, R. J. Dolan, and C. D. Frith. 2004. Empathy for pain involves the affective but not sensory components of pain. *Science* **303(5661)**:1157–1162.

Singer, T., B. Seymour, J. P. O'Doherty, K. E. Stephan, R. J. Dolan, and C. D. Frith. 2006. Empathic neural responses are modulated by the perceived fairness of others. *Nature* **439(7075)**:466–469.

Sunstein, C. R., D. Schkade, and D. Kahneman. 2000. Do people want optimal deterrence? *J. Legal Stud.* **29**:237–253.

Uvnas-Moberg, K. 1998. Oxytocin may mediate the benefits of positive social interaction and emotions. *Psychoneuroend.* **23(8)**:819–835.

Victor v. Nebraska, 1994. 511 U.S. 1.

Name Index

Abelson, R. P. 377
Ahn, W. -K. 372
Ainslie, G. 57, 66
Aktipis, C. A. 168, 232
Alexander, D. E. 331
Alexander, R. M. 213
Allen, W. 371
Allport, D. A. 247
Ammerman, A. J. 339
Amorapanth, P. 137
Amsterdam, A. G. 371, 376
Andersen, R. A. 73
Anderson, J. R. 174, 178, 208, 209, 213, 214, 217, 261, 273, 300, 381, 402
Anderson, T. J. 372
Aoki, K. 334
Aristotle 354
Asch, S. E. 338
Assad, J. A. 77
Axelrod, R. 167, 298, 373
Aziz-Zadeh, L. 229

Baars, B. J. 22, 41
Baddeley, A. 247
Baird, D. G. 394
Baker, C. I. 249
Bakker, C. M. 272
Balda, R. P. 327
Balleine, B. W. 52, 55, 58, 59, 61, 62
Bandler, R. 62
Bandura, A. 166, 403
Banks, M. S. 85
Bargh, J. A. 261
Barkow, J. H. 286
Barlow, H. B. 82
Baron, J. 278
Barraclough, D. J. 83
Barrett, H. C. 168
Bartlett, F. C. 13, 402
Barto, A. G. 52, 62, 65
Bartolone, J. 372
Baumol, W. J. 6
Bechara, A. 137
Ben-Haim, Y. 297
Bendiksby, M. S. 135

Bennett, W. L. 372
Berg, J. 116, 421
Bergert, F. B. 270, 329
Bering, J. M. 107
Bernheim, B. D. 149
Berns, G. S. 80
Berntson, G. G. 299
Berridge, K. C. 57, 59, 62, 133
Betsch, T. 260–262, 271–273, 278
Bettinger, R. L. 339
Bettman, J. R. 218, 331
Bischof, N. 273
Block, N. 381
Bloom, P. 160, 165, 227
Blout, S. 348
Bogacz, R. 87, 90
Bolger, D. J. 249
Bolstad, W. M. 403
Bolton, P. 6
Bostrom, A. 373
Botvinick, M. 228, 247
Bowles, S. 305, 306, 309
Boyd, D. 340
Boyd, R. 166, 225–253, 298, 305–322, 325–340, 423
Boyer, P. 310, 337
Boysen, S. T. 299, 300
Brainard, D. H. 85
Brandimonte, M. A. 243
Brandstätter, E. 260, 266
Bransford, J. D. 175
Braver, T. S. 228, 237, 247
Breland, K. 62, 66
Breland, M. 62, 66
Brendel, D. 27, 32
Bright, D. A. 417
Brighton, H. 212
Bröder, A. 267, 268, 273, 329
Brosnan, S. F. 349
Brown, J. S. 373
Brown, M. 422
Bruce, V. 351
Bruner, J. S. 371, 376
Brunswik, E. 211
Buchanan, J. M. 392

Buehler, R. 372
Bullbrook, M. E. 14
Bulthoff, H. H. 85
Buneo, C. A. 73
Burnham, T. 252
Burrel, Q. L. 216
Burstein, M. H. 380
Busemeyer, J. R. 146, 261, 279
Byrne, R. M. J. 380

Cacioppo, J. T. 261
Camerer, C. F. 112, 246
Carmel, Y. 297
Carter, C. S. 422
Caspi, A. 150
Cavada, C. 73, 76
Cavalli-Sforza, L. L. 339
Chammah, A. M. 405
Chang, F. R. 176
Changeux, J. P. 37, 42, 43
Charniak, E. 375
Charnov, E. L. 287
Chartrand, T. L. 261
Chater, N. 159, 208–212, 291, 402, 403
Chen, M. K. 251
Cheney, D. L. 226
Cherian, A. 185
Chomsky, N. 10
Chun, M. M. 43
Churchland, A. K. 71–96
Churchland, P. S. 72
Cisek, P. 72
Clark, A. 72
Clark, R. E. 35
Cleeremans, A. 166
Clements, K. C. 299
Cohen, D. 322
Cohen, J. D. 135, 225–253, 381, 429
Cohn, T. E. 82
Colby, C. L. 73
Cole, B. J. 297
Coleman, J. E. 363
Collins, A. 380
Condry, K. F. 2
Conlisk, J. 394
Cooksey, R. W. 382
Corbett, A. T. 175, 176
Corrado, G. S. 83

Cosmides, L. 135, 167, 291, 328, 329, 404
Cowan, R. 399
Coward, L. A. 395, 403
Cowey, A. 142
Critchley, M. 73
Cummins, T. D. R. 271
Cushman, F. A. 298, 299

Dallas, M. 219
Damasio, A. R. 58, 137, 261
Darley, J. M. 429
Darwin, C. 336
Davies, M. 403
Daw, M. I. 240
Daw, N. D. 55, 57, 59, 60, 64, 65, 133
Dawkins, R. 292
Dayan, P. 51–69, 125–151, 184
Deaner, R. O. 80
Decety, J. 109
de Groot, A. D. 12
Dehaene, S. 4, 9, 21–46, 125–151, 157, 226, 231, 249, 251, 279, 344
DeKleer, J. 373
Del Cul, A. 23, 27, 28, 36, 43, 140, 141
De Martino, B. 66
DeMiguel, V. 212
Denant-Boèment, L. 406
Dennett, D. C. 36, 167
De Quervain, D. J. F. 424
Descartes, R. 355, 357, 362, 367
DeScioli, P. 167
Deutsch, R. 400
Deutscher, G. 308
de Vignemont, F. 109–111, 418
Devine, P. G. 261
Devlin, J. T. 27
de Waal, F. B. M. 109, 110, 349
Dewatripont, M. 6
Diamond, J. 340
Dickinson, A. 52, 58, 59, 148
Dienes, Z. 155, 163
Dijksterhuis, A. 382, 383, 385
Ding, L. 128
Ditterich, J. 88, 185
Donald, M. 191–205, 225–253
Dorris, M. C. 83, 359
Dosher, B. A. 175
Dougherty, M. R. P. 261

Dudley, R. 331
Dugatkin, L. A. 298
Dukas, R. 286
Dux, P. E. 44

Ebbinghaus, H. 214
Eimer, M. 30
Einhorn, H. J. 379
Ellickson, R. C. 308
Elman, J. L. 228
Elston, G. N. 41
Elwork, A. 377
Engel, C. 1–18, 170, 213, 278, 391–407,
    413–430
Engstler-Schooler, T. Y. 242, 243
Ericsson, K. A. 381
Ernst, M. O. 85
Evans, J. 159

Falk, A. 414, 426
Farahany, N. A. 363
Farroni, T. 226
Fehr, E. 404, 421, 424, 426
Feigenson, L. 226
Feldman, M. S. 372
Fessler, D. M. T. 337
Fiebach, C. J. 229
Fiedler, K. 288, 405
Fischer, G. H. 322
Fischhoff, B. 11, 395
Flache, A. 393, 421
Fodor, J. A. 170, 333
Forster, M. 329
Fragaszy, D. M. 334
Frank, M. J. 228, 237
Frederick, S. 261, 397, 413
Freeman, W. T. 85
Friedman, M. 11, 393
Fries, P. 141, 142
Frings, C. 215
Frith, C. D. 107, 108, 145
Frith, U. 107, 108
Fudenberg, D. 360, 394
Fujita, K. 300

Gächter, S. 404, 424
Gaillard, R. 27, 37, 43
Gailliot, M. T. 331
Gallagher, H. L. 107, 112, 145
Gallese, V. 110

Garcia, J. 327
Garey, M. R. 401
Garland, B. 349
Garlappi, L. 212
Gauthier, I. 352
Gazzaniga, M. S. 158
Gazzola, V. 227
Gelman, S. 165
Gibson, J. J. 72
Gigerenzer, G. 13, 212, 215, 216, 218,
    260, 262, 266, 269, 270, 278, 288, 290,
    291, 296, 297, 325–340, 393–395, 402
Gil-White, F. J. 315
Gilboa, I. 403
Gillund, G. 177, 178
Gintis, H. 423
Giurfa, M. 148
Gladwell, M. 161
Glenn, C. G. 375
Glimcher, P. W. 12, 83, 128, 131, 132,
    134, 236, 272, 295, 343–368, 395,
    413–430
Glöckner, A. 6, 12, 13, 259–281, 295,
    325–340, 395, 403
Gobini, M. I. 351
Gold, J. I. 75, 76, 80, 87, 95, 126, 128,
    131, 134, 185, 279
Goldberg, M. E. 73
Goldman, S. R. 385
Goldman-Rakic, P. 73, 76
Goldstein, D. G. 215, 216, 218, 270
Good, I. J. 87
Goodman-Delahunty, J. 417
Gopher, D. 247
Gordon, P. 230, 251
Graesser, A. C. 177, 385
Granovetter, M. 392
Green, D. M. 82
Greene, J. 238
Greene, J. D. 429
Greenwald, A. G. 34, 168, 232, 405
Griffen, D. 372
Groen, G. J. 373
Gross, J. 36, 44
Gross, J. J. 149
Guglielmino, C. R. 308
Gürerk, O. 424
Güth, W. 225–253, 348

Guthrie, R. D. 321

Hagen, E. H. 286
Haidt, J. 234, 238, 401
Hallinan, E. V. 300
Hamilton, W. D. 298
Hammerstein, P. 286, 298, 299, 325–340
Hammond, K. R. 14, 291, 295, 382
Hanes, D. P. 185
Hanks, T. D. 71–96
Hansen, C. 396
Hardin, G. 394
Hardin, R. 421
Hare, B. 226
Harris, P. L. 108
Harsanyi, J. 13
Harvey, W. C. 354
Hasegawa, Y. T. 186
Hasher, L. 261
Hastie, R. 5, 170, 268, 269, 273,
    371–386, 413–430
Hauser, M. D. 2, 3, 226, 227, 298, 299
Haxby, J. V. 351, 352
Haynes, J. D. 25, 28, 36
He, S. 72
Hecht, S. 82
Heckathorn, D. D. 404, 424
Hedden, T. 298
Heekeren, H. R. 128, 129, 185, 279
Heider, F. 265
Heller, M. A. 404
Hellwig, M. 405
Henrich, J. 250, 315, 338
Herrnstein, R. J. 82
Hertwig, R. 216, 218–220
Hikosaka, K. 80
Hikosaka, O. 128
Hintzman, D. 177
Hirschfeld, L. 165, 406
Hirstein, W. 158
Hochreiter, S. 228
Hodgson, G. M. 274, 392
Hoffman, E. 113, 114, 406
Hoffrage, G. 278
Hofstader, D. 168
Hogarth, R. M. 373, 379
Holden, C. 308
Holmes, P. 87, 90
Holyoak, K. J. 262, 265, 266, 372

Horwitz, J. D. 128
Houser, D. 112, 114
Houston, A. I. 288, 294
Huettel, S. A. 144
Hug, K. 291
Huk, A. C. 88, 128, 185
Hunt, G. R. 226
Hutchinson, J. M. C. 296

Insel, T. R. 422
Ivanoff, J. 44

Jabbi, M. 109, 239
Jablonka, E. 321
Jackson, J. D. 276
Jackson, P. L. 109, 110, 423
Jacoby, L. L. 219
James, W. 157
Janetos, A. C. 297
Jaynes, E. T. 87, 96
Jiang, Y. 72
Joel, D. 53, 55, 57, 61, 66
Johnson, D. S. 401
Johnson, E. J. 218, 225–253, 331
Johnson, P. 316
Johnson-Laird, P. N. 380, 403
Jones, O. 348
Joordens, S. 141
Jorgenson, J. G. 308
Jou, J. 372
Juslin, P. 13, 288

Kacelnik, A. 286
Kagel, J. H. 6
Kahan, D. 406
Kahneman, D. 6, 53, 54, 57, 58, 82, 260,
    261, 278, 328, 381, 392, 397, 413
Kanner, L. 95
Kanwisher, N. 351, 352
Kaplan, J. 377
Karlin, S. 87
Kawagoe, R. 80
Keay, K. A. 62
Keil, F. C. 372
Kelly, R. C. 340
Keltner, D. 138
Kentridge, R. W. 32
Kersten, D. 85
Kersting, W. 393

Keysers, C. 109, 155, 156, 169, 170, 225–253, 414
Khuri, F. I. 337
Kiani, R. 71–96, 142
Kiefer, M. 27, 32
Kihlstrom, J. F. 157
Killcross, S. 59
Kim, J. -N. 128
King-Casas, B. 118
Kintsch, W. 177, 372, 385
Kirzner, I. 13, 393
Klein, G. A. 382
Knauft, B. 309
Knight, F. H. 393
Knight, J. 392
Knill, D. C. 85
Knoch, D. 115
Koch, C. 82
Koechlin, E. 34
Koelling, R. A. 327
Koffka, K. 262
Koivisto, M. 36
Konorski, J. 52
Konow, J. 406, 426
Kopp, B. 28, 30
Kording, K. P. 85, 86
Kosfeld, M. 118, 422, 426
Kouider, S. 25, 36, 44, 139
Kranczioch, C. 36, 44
Krebs, J. R. 287, 288, 296, 297
Krueger, F. 118
Kunda, Z. 262
Kunde, W. 31, 32, 35, 141
Künzler, R. 272
Kurzban, R. 155–171, 225, 325–340

Lachter, J. 32
Laland, K. N. 330, 338
Lamb, M. J. 321
Laming, D. R. J. 25
Lamm, C. 109–111
Lamme, V. A. 37
Landau, B. 226
Landauer, T. K. 215
Landy, M. S. 85
Lau, B. 83
Lau, H. C. 33, 35, 140
Leamer, E. E. 401
Lebiere, C. 174, 217, 261, 273

LeDoux, J. E. 135, 158
Lee, D. 83
Lee, M. D. 271
Lemer, C. 232
Lengyel, M. 62
Lepper, M. R. 262
Lerner, J. S. 138
Leuthold, H. 28, 30
Levi, E. 385
Levy, I. 73
Lewis, C. H. 372
Lewis, J. W. 73
Li, G. 249
Libet, B. 158, 160
Lienard, P. 337
Lindauer, M. 147
Link, S. W. 25, 82, 87
Lipton, J. S. 2
Lo, C. C. 80
Loewenstein, G. 58
Logothetis, N. K. 142
Lorberbaum, J. P. 298
Lowenstein, G. A. 138
Lubell, M. 148, 367, 413–430
Luce, R. D. 54, 82, 130, 131, 182
Luck, S. J. 28, 37
Luppino, G. 229

Ma, W. J. 87
Mace, R. 308
Machens, C. K. 129
Mackintosh, N. J. 62, 63
Macy, M. M. 393, 421
Magen, S. 325–340
Maier, S. F. 67
Mamassian, P. 85
Mandler, J. M. 375
Manski, C. 82, 131
Marois, R. 44
Marr, D. 208, 209
Marsh, B. 296
Martin, A. W. 372
Marzouki, Y. 32
Matsuzawa, T. 3, 166, 227
Mattler, U. 33, 35, 43
Maynard Smith, J. 131
Mazur, J. E. 300
Mazurek, M. E. 128, 131, 185, 186

McCabe, K. 103–120, 125–151, 298, 348, 418
McCandliss, B. D. 249
McClelland, J. L. 25, 186, 234, 247, 262, 264
McClure, S. M. 66, 68
McCoy, A. N. 80
McCrink, K. 226
McElreath, R. 148, 149, 166, 287, 317, 325–340
McKenzie, C. R. M. 379
McKoon, G. 173–186, 247
McMillen, T. 87, 90
McNamara, J. M. 288
McNamara, T. P. 177, 178
McNaughton, B. L. 247
McNeill, W. 339
Meadow, W. 399
Medin, D. L. 372
Melcher, J. M. 243
Melloni, L. 36, 141
Meltzoff, A. N. 227
Menzel, R. 125–151
Merikle, P. M. 35, 141
Merleau-Ponty, M. 72
Michalski, R. 380
Milinski, M. 424
Miller, G. F. 297
Miller, L. C. 262
Millgram, E. 262
Milson, R. 213
Mintz, E. U. 82
Mitchell, J. P. 108
Mithen, S. J. 162, 226
Miyake, A. 247
Montague, P. R. 55, 59, 62, 80, 237
Moore, A. J. 371
Morrison, I. 110
Morton, J. 179, 180
Movshon, M. E. 73
Murdock, B. B. 177, 178
Murphy, G. L. 372
Murray, E. A. 300
Myowa-Yamakoshi, M. 166

Naccache, L. 22, 23, 27, 32, 35–37, 37, 42, 72, 140
Nagel, T. 162
Nakamura, K. 27, 249

Nash, J. 6
Navarrete, C. D. 337
Navon, D. 247
Naya, Y. 236
Nelson, K. 249
Newcombe, N. 226
Newsome, W. T. 82, 128, 130, 131
Nieuwenhuis, S. 37
Nikiforakis, N. S. 426
Nimchinsky, E. A. 41
Nisbett, R. E. 158, 322, 406
Niv, Y. 53, 55, 57, 59–61, 66, 133
Noë, A. 72
Noë, R. 299
Nonacs, P. 287
North, D. C. 148, 415
Nosofsky, R. M. 270, 329

O'Doherty, J. P. 59, 62, 106
O'Hara, E. 425
O'Hear, M. M. 398
O'Regan, J. K. 72
O'Reilly, R. C. 106, 247
Oaksford, M. 159, 208, 210–212, 291, 402, 403
Ochsner, K. N. 149
Oden, N. L. 339
Olson, C. R. 128
Otto, P. E. 273, 293, 402

Packard, M. G. 62, 65
Packer, C. 299
Padoa-Schioppa, C. 77
Pandya, D. N. 73
Park, B. 268
Parker, A. J. 82, 131
Pashler, H. 43, 44
Passingham, R. E. 33, 35, 140
Patel, V. L. 373
Paton, J. J. 80
Paulesu, E. 249
Payne, J. W. 64, 218, 269, 290, 331, 381–383
Pedersen, C. A. 422
Pegna, A. J. 161
Pennington, N. 269, 372, 373, 380, 416
Pepperberg, I. M. 227
Perfect, T. J. 243
Perner, J. 155, 163

Perrett, D. I. 227
Perry, S. 334
Pessiglione, M. 33, 140
Petersson, K. M. 249
Petrides, M. 73
Petty, R. E. 261
Phelan, J. 252
Phelps, E. 125–151
Philiastides, M. G. 185
Pica, P. 230, 251
Pinker, S. 156, 165
Plassmann, H. 125–151
Platt, M. 80, 125–151, 162, 414
Plaut, D. C. 228, 247
Plessner, H. 261
Poldrack, R. A. 62, 65
Pople, H. E., Jr. 373
Poremba, A. 73, 74
Posner, M. I. 176, 247
Posner, R. A. 400
Potter, M. C. 43
Povinelli, D. J. 107
Preston, S. D. 109, 110
Prinz, W. 227
Pusey, A. E. 299
Pylyshyn, Z. W. 3

Quillian, M. R. 177

Raby, C. R. 327
Rachlin, H. 290
Rachlinski, J. J. 400, 413–430
Rangel, A. 149
Rapoport, A. 405, 421
Ratcliff, R. 25, 87, 125–151, 173–186,
    247, 261, 280
Read, S. J. 262, 265, 273
Reader, S. M. 330
Real, L. A. 328
Rehder, B. 372
Rescorla, R. A. 157
Reuter, F. 23
Reynvoet, B. 27
Richerson, P. J. 166, 253, 305–322,
    325–340
Rieskamp, J. 273, 293, 402
Rilling, J. K. 112, 115
Rips, L. J. 380
Rizzolatti, G. 72, 229

Robbenolt, J. K. 425
Robinson, P. H. 429
Robinson, T. E. 57, 59, 62, 133
Robson, A. 325–340
Rockenbach, B. 413–430
Roesch, M. R. 128
Roitman, J. D. 128, 185
Romo, R. 128, 129
Rosas, P. 85
Rosati, A. G. 300
Rossby, P. 428
Roth, A. E. 6
Rothoeft, D. 424
Rouder, J. N. 87, 180, 182
Rubinstein, A. 6, 7, 12
Rumelhart, D. E. 262, 264, 375

Salamon, S. 308
Salinas, E. 128, 129
Sanfey, A. G. 60, 61, 114, 239
Sauerland, M. 5
Saunders, J. A. 85
Saussure, F. de 194
Savage, L. J. 13, 393
Schacter, D. L. 169, 179
Schall, J. D. 142, 185
Schank, R. C. 372, 375, 377
Schelling, T. 168
Scherberger, H. 73
Scherer, K. R. 135
Schiffer, S. 329
Schlaghecken, F. 30
Schmeidler, D. 403
Schmidhuber, J. 228
Schneider, W. 247, 261
Schoenemann, P. T. 41
Scholl, B. J. 226
Schooler, J. W. 14, 225–253, 382, 396
Schooler, L. J. 179, 180, 207–221,
    225–253, 291, 300, 328, 330
Schoreit, A. 276, 277
Schubotz, R. I. 229
Schultz, W. 55, 62, 80, 106, 148
Schulz, J. 5
Schum, D. A. 372
Segraves, M. 185
Selten, R. 290, 298, 402, 413–430
Sergent, C. 23, 36, 44, 141
Serwe, S. 215

Sevón, G. 373
Seyfarth, R. M. 226
Shadlen, M. N. 71–96, 125–151, 185, 279
Shafir, E. 383
Shah, P. 247
Shallice, T. 249
Shapiro, L. E. 422
Shiffrin, R. M. 177–179, 247, 261
Shultz, T. R. 262
Siegler, R. 129
Sigman, M. 34, 44, 45, 129
Silberberg, A. 300
Simon, D. 5, 262, 265–267, 277, 372, 400, 405
Simon, H. A. 211, 212, 260, 281, 290, 297, 381, 394
Singer, M. 177
Singer, T. 103–120, 298, 413–430
Singer, W. 1–18, 125–151, 279, 280
Skinner, B. F. 291, 293
Sloman, S. A. 372, 381
Slovic, P. 261, 382
Smith, E. A. 288, 297
Smith, E. E. 380
Smith, E. R. 13
Smith, P. L. 25, 87, 128, 180
Smith, V. L. 144, 298, 377
Snyder, C. R. 247
Sober, E. 329
Softky, W. R. 82
Sokal, R. R. 339
Sol, D. 330
Soltis, J. 340
Sosis, R. 314, 315
Spaniol, J. 184
Spelke, E. S. 2, 3, 225–253
Sperber, D. 165, 406
Sperry, L. L. 377
Spitzer, M. L. 406
Spivey, M. J. 75
Sporer, S. L. 4, 5, 401, 405
Squire, L. R. 179, 238
Stanescu, R. 231
Stanovich, K. E. 159, 292, 381
Stark, R. 316
Stein, N. L. 375

Stephens, D. W. 287, 288, 296, 297, 299, 300
Stevens, J. R. 163, 207, 285–301, 325–340
Stewart, L. 249
Steyvers, M. 179
Stoerig, P. 142
Stone, M. 182
Stone, T. 403
Strack, F. 400
Straffin, P. D. 6
Sugrue, L. P. 82, 128, 134
Summerfield, C. 279
Sunstein, C. R. 399, 404, 429
Suppes, P. 130
Sutton, R. S. 52, 62, 65
Swensson, R. G. 182
Swets, J. A. 82

Tanner, W. P., Jr. 82
Taylor, H. M. 87
Tetlock, P. E. 396, 398, 402
Teubner, G. 392
Thagard, P. 262, 279
Thapar, A. 184
Thomson, D. M. 175
Thurstone, L. L. 82
Tinbergen, N. 286
Tirole, J. 360, 394
Todd, P. M. 260, 262, 278, 288, 297
Tolman, E. C. 61
Tomasello, M. 195, 249
Tomb, I. 137
Tononi, G. 141
Tooby, J. 135, 167, 291, 328, 329
Townsend, J. T. 146, 261, 279
Trabasso, T. 372, 375, 377
Tremblay, L. 80
Trick, L. M. 3
Trivers, R. L. 298, 299
Trommershäuser, J. 85, 225–253
Tuerlinckx, F. 183
Tullock, G. 392
Tulving, E. 164, 174–176, 179
Tversky, A. 6, 260, 328, 392
Twining, W. 372

Uppal, R. 212
Usher, M. 25, 186

Uvnas-Moberg, K. 422

Valenza, E. 226
van Aalderen-Smeets, S. I. 36
van Alphen, J. J. M. 296
van den Broek, P. 375
van Ee, R. 85
Van Essen, D. C. 73
van Gaal, S. 34, 35, 43
van Olden, Z. 382
Van Wallendael, L. R. 379
Vaughan, W. 82
Vesalius, A. 354
Vinckier, F. 249
Vohs, K. D. 249
von Neumann, J. 44, 45
Vorberg, D. 25, 30, 140

Wagar, B. M. 279
Wagenaar, W. A. 372
Wajnberg, E. 296
Wakano, J. Y. 334
Wald, A. 87
Wallis, J. D. 76
Wang, X. J. 42, 80, 129
Ward, D. 297
Wason, P. C. 207, 208, 210–212
Wasserstrom, R. 385
Watanabe, K. 80
Watanabe, M. 80
Watkins, C. J. C. H. 56, 58
Watkins, M. J. 207
Weber, E. U. 11, 396, 413–430
Wechsler, D. 11
Wegner, D. 261

Wegner, G. 392, 398
Weick, K. E. 403
Weinreb, L. L. 385
Weiskrantz, L. 36, 161
West, R. F. 159, 381
Wicker, B. 109, 239
Wigmore, J. H. 372
Wilensky, R. 372
Wilson, C. 339
Wilson, D. 165
Wilson, R. A. 372
Wilson, T. D. 158, 159, 169, 244, 382, 383, 396
Winterhalder, B. 288, 297
Wittenbrink, B. 269, 273, 382, 384
Wixted, J. T. 299
Wolfowitz, J. 87
Wolpe, P. R. 349
Wolpert, D. M. 85, 86
Wong, K. F. 42, 129
Wynn, K. 2, 226, 227

Xiao, E. 114
Xu, F. 226

Yang, T. 92, 93
Yarn, D. 425
Young, L. J. 422
Young, P. 309
Yovel, G. 351
Yuille, A. 85

Zacks, R. T. 261
Zárate, M. A. 13
Zhang, J. 298
Zwaan, R. W. 177

Subject Index

ACT-R 217–220, 240–241
actor-critic learning rule 62
adaptive toolbox 260, 266–271, 273
agriculture 306, 335–336, 339
amygdala 59, 80, 84, 111, 422, 425
anterior cingulate cortex (ACC) 37, 41,
  80, 110, 111, 114, 422
anterior insula (AI) 110, 111, 239
anterior intraparietal region (AIP) 73
anterior paracingulate 107, 118, 145
aphasia 143
apologies, role in civil trials 425
attention 37, 141, 194, 203, 233
  executive 31–32
  joint 248–249
  role in subliminal processing 30–33
  shared 107, 112
  top-down 40, 44, 141
attentional blink 28, 36–37, 43–44, 139
  masking in 44
attentional load 241–242
attitudes 136, 138, 267, 322
autism 95, 107, 195
automatic processes 94, 173–176, 193,
  203–204, 231–237, 242, 247, 260–262,
  265, 269, 328
  implications for the legal system 418,
    430

Bayesian reasoning 71, 84–93, 119, 214,
  291, 395, 403
Bechara gambling task 137
behavior
  involuntary-irrational 344, 349–350,
    355–356, 361, 363
  legal classes of 344–346, 357
  voluntary-rational 344–346, 349, 351,
    354–357, 359, 361, 366
behaviorism 157, 193
beliefs 108–109, 126, 136, 267, 306,
  340, 393, 418
  false beliefs task 107, 112
  transmission of 310, 312, 316

benzodiazepines 133
bidirectional reasoning 266
binocular rivalry 95, 141–142, 235
blindsight 22, 32, 36, 139, 142
bounded rationality 211, 260, 271,
  280–281, 289–290, 296–297, 329
brain-mind-culture coevolution 197–201
brainstem 57, 110, 133–134
brightness discrimination 129, 143

cached values 55–59, 61, 63–64, 133
Callithrix jacchus 300
capital punishment 347
causal agent 353–355, 358
cerebellum 110
cheater detection 291, 299, 391,
  404–406
chess 12, 64, 191, 204, 212, 401
chimpanzees 226, 286
  foraging in 285, 288, 296
  numerical reasoning in 3
  social learning in 165
choice 82, 94, 126, 204, 266, 291, 293
  See also rational choice, Wason selec-
    tion task
  defining uncertainty 401–402
  delayed outcomes 56–57
  deliberation-without-attention 383
  forced recognition test 175, 242
  inter-temporal 230, 238
  Luce rule 54, 131
  selection 126–129
  set 373, 377, 383, 396
  strategies 382–384
  two-choice tasks 180, 184
city-size task 216, 267–268
cognitive-cultural networks
  (CCNs) 195–199, 203, 248–249
coherence 291–294, 378
  -based reasoning 400, 405
  shifts 265–267
commitment 126–129
  threshold for 146

Commonwealth of Massachusetts v. Johnson 373–377
Commonwealth of Massachusetts v. Webster 419
competition 6, 13, 15, 54, 63, 134
  institutional 314–315, 340
  instrumental 64–65
  Pavlovian 65–67
  top-down attentional 44
compound cue models 177–178
computational level of information processing 208–211, 213–215
condition–action rule 380
conformity in social learning 312–314, 338
consciousness
  defined 9, 23–25, 139–140, 346, 395, 414
  measuring 236
  neural bases of 22, 141–142
conscious processing 40, 44
  defined 24, 139
  explanation-based framework 380–384
consequentialism 346–350, 428–429
contract system 394, 404, 421–430
control
  goal-directed 52, 60–61, 64–65, 106
  value-based systems 60–63, 133–135
conviction intime 5, 419–420
cooperation 195, 298–300, 421–429
  in-group 319
  role of apologies 425
criminal justice system 344–347, 356, 362–363, 427–430
  standards of responsibility 427–429
cue-dependent retrieval 174–177
culpability 149, 343, 347, 350, 355–356, 367, 368, 418 *See also* guilt determination
  legal categories of 345–346
cultural evolution 252–254, 334–336
culture
  -gene coevolution 305–322
  role in decision making 191–204, 248–253
Cyanocitta cristata 300

decision
  components of 82, 84, 288–292
  defined 9, 126–128
  evidence-based 77, 80–83, 94
  evolution of individual 327–333
  rules in multiple-judge courts 277
  times 268–269
  variable (DV) 77–83, 86–92, 127–128, 131, 134
decision making
  agents of 8–9
  evolution of 155–169, 295–297, 333–334
  explicit 155–171
  impact of natural selection on 286–297
  implementation costs 331–332
  individual differences in 143–146
  legal 149–150, 262, 371–385, 415–420
  moral 245–246, 248–250, 354
  neurobiology of 71–96, 125–151, 343–368, 355
  numerical comparison task 26
  origins of variability in 130–132
  perceptual 82, 94, 125–126, 143–144
  randomness in 82–83, 130–131
  social 103–119
declarative memory system 217, 240
deliberative reasoning 230, 273, 321, 333–334
depression 362, 428
determinism 355–358
dictator game 113–114, 250
discounting 56–57, 66
domain specificity 235, 247, 270
dopamine 59, 62, 118, 133, 134
  -gating hypothesis 106
dorsal lateral prefrontal cortex (DLPFC) 76, 114–115, 133, 141
drift diffusion model 128–130, 143
dual diffusion models 183, 186
dualism 136–137, 159, 343–368
dynamic programming 53–57
dyslexia 193, 249

economic decision making 144–146

emotions 138–139, 149, 239, 318, 361, 418
  defined 135
  face perception 111
  physiological response 137–138
  role in decisions 126, 135–139
  Scherer's model 135–136
empathy 103–104, 108–111, 118, 418, 423
  defined 109
encoding 26, 73, 108, 173–176
  verbal 333
episodic cognition 199–201
episodic control 62, 65, 68, 134
equal weight heuristic 268, 270
event representation 201–202
evidence 71–74, 86, 94, 127, 130
  accumulation 34, 42–46, 76–80, 112, 140, 142, 186, 279
    influence of age on 143
    model 21, 25, 30–31
  based decisions 77, 80–83, 94
evidentiary rules 416–417
exculpatory behavior 346, 349, 351, 355–359
  influence of emotions on 361
expected utility 53, 55, 77
  theory 291
expert intuition 399, 419
explanation-based judgment 372–373, 384, 416–418
  certainty principles 373, 378–379
explicit system 155–159, 165, 169, 232
  defined 159
  evolution of 162–164
  properties of 159–160

face perception 111, 204, 244, 351–352
fairness 348–349, 367, 391, 406, 418
false beliefs task 107, 112
Faroe Islands 325
fast and frugal heuristics 215, 260, 262, 267–271, 273, 296, 402
fear conditioning 422, 425
fitness payoffs 287–288, 294, 297, 310
fluency heuristic 219
footbridge scenario 238, 245

foraging 94, 294, 296
  patch model 285, 287
Fore 340
forgetting 216, 218–220, 299
  computational level analysis of 213
forward model 54–55, 58, 60–61, 67–68
  system 133, 139
free will 94, 150, 158, 249, 250, 351, 353–354, 357, 359, 361–362
Freudianism 157, 391
functional evaluation 291–295
fusiform cortex 27, 352

gambling task 144, 145, 260
  Bechara 137
game theory 6–7, 13, 104–106, 298, 402, 421, 423
  evolutionary 310
Gebusi (Papua New Guinea) 309
gene-culture coevolution 305–322
gift exchange game 421–422
global memory models 177–178
global workspace 37–41, 43
  defined 21
  model 37–42, 279
  role of 45
goal-directed control 52, 60–61, 64–65, 106, 133
Google 216–217
grammar 166, 193, 228–229, 320
Gratton effect 31
grindadráp 325–326
group
  identification 251, 308, 310, 319, 339
  selection 312–316
  stability 309, 338
guilt 318 *See also* culpability
  determination 4–6, 15, 17, 149–150, 347, 416
    reasonable doubt 419–420

habitual control 52, 61–62, 68, 133, 134
  in artificial systems 64
hardware implementation level 209
heritable variation 314–318

heuristics 12, 212, 307, 379
  equal weight 268, 270
  fast and frugal 215, 260, 262,
      267–271, 273, 296, 402
  fluency 219
  recognition 215–220
  simple 212, 290, 296, 329, 394–395
  Take the Best 270, 274
Hill v. Ozmint 363
hominid evolution 198–201
honeybee 147–148, 330
Hotema v. the U.S. 355–357, 363, 427
human cognition
  evolution of 199–200
  uniqueness of 226–231
human migration 308, 313, 339
human soul 353–355
hypothalamus 57, 133

if-then logic 76, 83
imitation 227, 230–231, 307, 308, 310,
    314–315, 318
implicit
  association task 168, 232
  decision making 162–163
    evolution of 155–171
  memory 173, 179–180
  system, properties of 159–160
incentive story 393–400
individual decision making, impact on
  institutions 335–337
inference 290–291, 418
  defined 288
  in jury decisions 377–380
information processing 288–289, 296
  elementary 218
  goal of 96
  Google 216–217
  multilevel analysis of 208–209
information retrieval, cue-depen-
    dent 173–177
insight 14, 126, 143
institutional design 17, 274–276, 308,
    336, 349, 368, 392, 396–401, 413–430
institutions
  defined 148, 305–306, 326
  evolution of 149, 305–322, 325–340

heritability of 307–308
  influence of individual decisions
      on 335
  marriage rules 336
  religious communes 314–315
  symbolic marking in 309, 316–319
instrumental control 62–63, 66, 68
intentional architecture 74–79, 90, 96
inter-temporal choice 230, 238
intraparietal sulcus 72–74
intuition 5, 8, 136–137, 204, 210, 244,
    261, 272, 319, 322, 381–382, 391,
    395–397, 402–404, 420
  expert 399, 419
  misled 405–406
involuntary-irrational-exculpatory
    behavior 344–345, 349–350, 355–356,
    361, 363
involuntary trust game 146
Irakia Awa (Papua New Guinea) 340

judgment 191, 204
  explanation-based 372–373, 378–379,
      384, 416–419
  legal 150, 397, 400
  moral 354
  strategy 382
jury system 414
  decision making in 371–385, 415–420
  presentation of evidence 416–417
  selection 418
justice, notion of 367

language 164–166, 194, 199, 201,
    227–229, 308, 330
  evolution of 230–231, 320
lateral intraparietal area (LIP) 73–76,
    128, 135
legal accountability 343–368
legal decision making 149–150, 262,
    371–385, 415–420
liability 349, 398, 418, 425
  exemption 427
liking 57, 62, 67, 133
literacy 192–193, 248–249, 249

neuropsychology of 193
log likelihood ratio (logLR) 25–26, 81, 88
long-run average utility 59–60, 66
long-run expected value 133–134
Luce choice rule 54, 131

Markov decision process 228–229
masking 22–24, 28, 36, 39, 139–140
  paradigm example 24
materialism 357–359
medial prefrontal cortex (mPFC) 107–108, 112, 115
memory 173, 202, 209, 243, 300
  cue-dependent retrieval 174–177
  decay 218, 220, 299
  declarative 217, 240
  episodic 62, 164, 167
  external 216–217
  global models 177–178
  implicit 173, 179–180
  procedural 238, 240
  recognition 143, 174, 180, 182
  TODAM model 178
  working 160, 233–234, 247
mentalizing 104, 107–112, 418
migration, human 308, 313, 339
mimetic cognition 199–200
moral decision making 245–246, 249–250, 354
motives 149–150, 267, 339, 418
motor learning 156, 234, 238
music skill 156, 193, 203, 234, 237, 333
mythic cognition 199–200

narrative *See also* story model
  defined 376
  verdicts 377–378
Nash equilibrium (NE) 6, 104, 106, 335
native values 57–58
  system 133, 139
natural selection 286–297, 306, 327, 330, 332
  influence of conformity on 312–314
negative automaintenance 63, 65

negligence 398, 400
neurobiology of decision making 71–96, 125, 129, 343–368, 355
  evolution of 147–148
  implications for institutes 148–150
nonconscious processing 8–9, 139–142
  See also preconscious processing
  brain imaging evidence for 28
  defined 24
norms 14–17, 316, 393
  fairness 367, 391, 406, 418
numerical reasoning 10, 25–26, 143, 191, 226–227, 230, 241–242
  cultural variability in 251
  in chimpanzees 3

optimal outcomes 294–297
optimization 11, 212–214, 287, 294–296
orbitofrontal cortex (OFC) 59, 77, 80, 84
oxytocin 118, 422, 425

parallel constraint satisfaction (PCS) 260–271, 328
  defined 395
  network structure 264
  PCS rule 278–281
    implications for institutions 274
  predictions 265–266
  primary network 271
  secondary network 272
parietal reach region (PRR) 73
Parkinson's disease 236
Pavlovian control 62–66, 68, 134, 139
perception 72–73, 196, 261
  face 111
  impacts of culture on 193–194
  of pain 108–109, 119
perceptual decision making 82, 94, 125–126, 143
  drift-diffusion models 128–130
pilot whale hunts 325–326
policy 54–55, 94, 127
posterior probability 84–86, 90, 128, 214
preconscious processing 40–45
predestination 353–354

predictability 397–398, 400–401
predicted utility 54, 58, 63–64
preferences 290–291
  defined 288
  heterogenity in 144
primary network 271–278
priming 140, 142, 177–179
  numerical masked 32
  numerical repetition 27, 29
  orthographic 28
Prisoner's Dilemma 111, 167, 298–300,
  393–394, 403–405, 421–424
probabilistic behavior, models 130–131
professional training, institutional arrangements for 396, 399–400
public goods game 250
punishment 298, 346–347, 364–367,
  425–428
  mitigation 363
  moralistic 312–313
  third-party 250–251

quantum theory 358
Q values 53–56, 58–60

Ratcliff diffusion model 180–184
rational behavior 344, 346, 349, 352,
  356
  defined 207–208, 345–346
rational choice 346, 365, 394, 404, 423
  See also Prisoner's Dilemma
  theory (RCT) 260, 266, 391–393, 395,
  398
reasonable doubt 419–420
reciprocal altruism 117–118, 298–300
recognition heuristic 215–220
recognition memory 143, 174, 180, 182
red/green motion task 76, 228, 360
reductionism 366–367
reflective processes 234–237, 240–242,
  247
reflexive processes 234–237, 240, 242,
  247
reinforcement learning 52–57, 65, 119,
  240, 289–293, 295, 327, 330

religious communes 314–315
representation and algorithm level 208–
  209, 211–213, 216–217
Rescorla-Wagner learning rule 54–55
retributivism 346–350, 354, 428–429
retrieval, information
  cue-dependent 173–177
risk 393, 397
  aversion 138, 145
rituals 310, 316, 319, 340

Saguinus oedipus 295
Sarbanes-Oxley Act 397
semantic processing 25–27, 30, 164,
  175, 196
sequential probability ratio test (SPRT)
  87–90
sequential sampling 71, 86, 88, 91
serotonin 59, 134, 362–365, 427, 429
shared attention 107, 112
signal-detection theory 4, 23, 71
simple heuristics 212, 290, 296, 329,
  394–395
social cognitive interface 168
social decision making 103–121,
  144–146
social evolution 310, 319
  through differential extinction 339–
  340
social instincts 318–320
social institutions *See* institutions
social learning 334–335
  conformity in 312–314, 338
  role of environmental change 334,
  339–340
somatic marker 58, 137
split brain patients 158
stimulus onset asynchrony 24, 30
stopping rule 34–35, 83, 86–89, 91–94,
  126–127, 296
story model 269, 371–373, 384–385,
  416–418
  structure of 375–377
striatum 54, 58–62, 80, 133, 424–425
Stroop effect 32, 35, 332
subjective expected utility (SEU) 270

subjective reporting 23–24, 139–142, 232, 236, 381, 386
subliminal processing 22, 25, 40–45, 279
  accumulation of evidence 28–30
  limits to 34–36
  modulated by attention 31–32
  semantic 27–29
substantia nigra pars reticulata 84
superior colliculus 185
superior temporal sulcus (STS) 107–108, 115
symbolic marking in institutions 309, 316–319
system 1 233, 241, 346, 381–382, 413–414
system 2 233, 241, 346, 381–382, 385, 413–416

Take the Best 260, 268, 270, 274
technology 196, 306, 335, 338
termination rule *See* stopping rule
termite fishing 165, 285, 287, 296
text processing 175–177
thalamus 84
theory-of-mind (ToM) 103, 112, 114, 118–119, 145, 228, 248, 298, 333
  See also mentalizing
  defined 107
third-party punishment games 250–251
Tit-for-Tat (TFT) 167, 298–300
tool use 165, 226–227, 230, 285
tort law 397, 400
trial process 371–385, 415–420, 430
trust 118, 402, 421–429
  investment/trust game 103, 116–118
  involuntary trust game 146
  voluntary trust game 144–145

ultimatum game 103, 114–115, 239, 250–251, 348
unbounded rationality 289–290, 295

uncertainty 13, 16, 393
  defined 401–402
unconscious processing 32, 68, 143, 157, 203, 220, 237
  defined 139
utility 53–55, 58, 127, 131
  long-run average 59–60, 66
  role of time in 89–90
  subjective expected 270

value 71, 80, 94, 127
  -based decisions 77, 80–83, 94, 132–135
    choice in 81
  cached 55–59, 61, 63–64, 133
  culturally transmitted 310
  of a state defined 132
  role of time in 89–90
  systems 51–69, 132–134
ventral medial prefrontal cortex 137
ventral tegmentum 84
verbal overshadowing 243–245
verdicts, role of narrative in 377–378
Victor v. Nebraska 419
voluntary-rational behavior 345–346, 349, 351, 354–357, 359–361, 366
voluntary trust game 144–145

Walrasian equilibrium 423
Wason selection task 207–211, 291–292, 328
weighted compensatory models 266, 270
Western Scrub Jay 327–328
word recognition 179, 193, 262
working memory 160, 233–234, 247
workspace neurons 39–42
writing 192, 248–249